MW01252935

CHALLENGES FOR QUALITY OF LIFE
IN THE CONTEMPORARY WORLD

Social Indicators Research Series

Volume 24

General Editor:

ALEX C. MICHALOS
University of Northern British Columbia,
Prince George, Canada

Editors:

ED DIENER
University of Illinois, Champaign, U.S.A.

WOLFGANG GLATZER
J.W. Goethe University, Frankfurt am Main, Germany

TORBJORN MOUM
University of Oslo, Norway

MIRJAM A.G. SPRANGERS
University of Amsterdam, The Netherlands

JOACHIM VOGEL
Central Bureau of Statistics, Stockholm, Sweden

RUUT VEENHOVEN
Erasmus University, Rotterdam, The Netherlands

This new series aims to provide a public forum for single treatises and collections of papers on social indicators research that are too long to be published in our journal *Social Indicators Research*. Like the journal, the book series deals with statistical assessments of the quality of life from a broad perspective. It welcomes the research on a wide variety of substantive areas, including health, crime, housing, education, family life, leisure activities, transportation, mobility, economics, work, religion and environmental issues. These areas of research will focus on the impact of key issues such as health on the overall quality of life and vice versa. An international review board, consisting of Ruut Veenhoven, Joachim Vogel, Ed Diener, Torbjorn Moum, Mirjam A.G. Sprangers and Wolfgang Glatzer, will ensure the high quality of the series as a whole.

The titles published in this series are listed at the end of this volume.

CHALLENGES FOR QUALITY OF LIFE IN THE CONTEMPORARY WORLD

Advances in quality-of-life studies, theory and research

Edited by

WOLFGANG GLATZER

Johan Wolfgang Goethe Universität,
Frankfurt am Main, Germany

SUSANNE VON BELOW

Johan Wolfgang Goethe Universität,
Frankfurt am Main, Germany

and

MATTHIAS STOFFREGEN

Johan Wolfgang Goethe Universität,
Frankfurt am Main, Germany

KLUWER ACADEMIC PUBLISHERS
DORDRECHT / BOSTON / LONDON

A C.I.P. Catalogue record for this book is available from the Library of Congress.

ISBN 1-4020-2890-3 (HB)
ISBN 1-4020-2903-9 (e-book)

Published by Kluwer Academic Publishers,
P.O. Box 17, 3300 AA Dordrecht, The Netherlands.

Sold and distributed in North, Central and South America
by Kluwer Academic Publishers,
101 Philip Drive, Norwell, MA 02061, U.S.A.

In all other countries, sold and distributed
by Kluwer Academic Publishers,
P.O. Box 322, 3300 AH Dordrecht, The Netherlands.

Printed on acid-free paper

Printed in the Netherlands.

CONTENTS

ACKNOWLEDGMENTS

This book evolved from an international conference, which was organized by the International Society for Quality of Life Studies and carried through at the Johann Wolfgang Goethe-University in Frankfurt am Main in July 2003. This conference offered an interdisciplinary forum for presentations and discussions concerning the challenges for quality of life in the contemporary world.

Such a conference is not possible without sponsors and supporters to whom we extend our gratitude. We want to thank our university and its president Prof. Rudolf Steinberg for considerable financial and practical support, as well as the city of Frankfurt, especially its mayor Petra Roth. We gratefully obtained financial support from the association of the "Freunde und Förderer der Johann Wolfgang Goethe Universität" with its president Hilmar Kopper. We also want to thank the Deutsche Bundesbank and its former president Ernst Welteke for hosting a session in the representative rooms of the German national bank, where the relationship between money, wealth, and satisfaction was discussed. Furthermore, we extend our thanks to the Hans Böckler Stiftung, represented by Erika Mezger, whose support allowed participants from Eastern European and developing countries to participate in the conference.

There was additional support by the Springer/Kluwer Academic Publishers and the Institut für Glücksforschung. Also, university institutions like the Social Science Department at the Center for North American Studies and the Center for Work, Social Security and Quality of Life gave us their assistance. Last but not least, we want to thank the many helpers who worked with us in preparing and managing the conference.

Some contributions from the conference have already been published in Social Indicators Network News, including the statements of the opening and the award sessions by the sponsors Ursula Fechter, Rudolf Steinberg and Ernst Welteke as well as by the social scientists Abbott L. Ferris, Kenneth C. Land, Don Rahtz, M. Joseph Sirgy, and Wolfgang Zapf (SINET Nr. 74 & 75). Some papers have been submitted for publication in Social Indicators Research, the Journal of Happiness Studies as well as others.

An important task for this volume was the production of the typoscript, for which Matthias Stoffregen held the main responsibility. The three of us formed the editorial group which was responsible for selecting and improving the manuscripts for the conference volume. We thank our colleagues who were engaged in assisting the editorial team, and we are especially grateful for the support given to us by Maya Becker, Juliane Reitzig, Joachim Ritter and Usch Büchner.

The book is serving its purpose if it gives many readers a substantial insight into the quality of life research in recent times.

Wolfgang Glatzer, Susanne von Below, Matthias Stoffregen

1

1. CHALLENGES FOR QUALITY OF LIFE

Introduction

Wolfgang Glatzer

Johann Wolfgang Goethe-Universität Frankfurt am Main, Germany

ABSTRACT

Challenges for the quality of life in the contemporary world were the focus of the Fifth International Quality of Life-Conference in Frankfurt am Main in the year 2003, hosted and organized by the International Society for Quality of Life Studies. The first part of this introductory article is concerned with a general assessment of contemporary quality of life research. At present, the concept of quality of life is a kind of umbrella which keeps together a reasonable number of international social scientists who have similar research interests. The second part of the introduction describes the topics of this book: The five chapters are concerned with the societal goal discussion on quality of life, the scientific monitoring of quality of life, the economic challenges for quality of life, its cultural challenges, and finally the options and restrictions for improving quality of life. Altogether, the contributions are related to present international investigations and discussions of basic questions of quality of life.

ATTENTION FOR QUALITY OF LIFE

Challenges for the quality of life in the contemporary world were the focus at the Fifth International Quality of Life-Conference in Frankfurt am Main in the year 2003, hosted and organized by the International Society for Quality of Life Studies. There are new threats and new prospects for the quality of life in each generation, and securing and improving quality of life is a never-ending task. Sometimes the challenges for quality of life are worldwide and dramatic, sometimes they remain nearly unnoticed and its effects are restricted to one or just a few individual life courses.

The dream of a decent quality of life seems difficult to preserve in the shadow of terrorism and natural disasters. Rather than weakening the striving for improved quality of life these events are challenging and strengthening the idea of quality of life. Social processes are always characterized by counter reactions and ambivalences. Thinking about quality of life seems to have gotten stronger world wide in the past years and many research activities, which are documented in this volume, are related to this process. They are concerned with various social processes that are significant and precarious for shaping the quality of life.

Wolfgang Glatzer, Susanne von Below, Matthias Stoffregen (eds.), Challenges for Quality of Life in the Contemporary World, 3-9.
© *2004 Kluwer Academic Publishers. Printed in the Netherlands.*

The concept of challenge is related to threats, dangers and risks in various life domains, which – if they are taken into account by individuals or governments – could be reduced or avoided. Challenges for quality of life in the contemporary world are manifold and always changing. Among them there are, on the one hand, unexpected events, which easily catch the public's attention, while on the other, there are structural challenges, which are often forgotten and remain hidden in the back – and underground.

ASSESSMENTS OF CONTEMPORARY QUALITY OF LIFE RESEARCH

Surely, each individual is thinking about her or his quality of life – be it with respect to one's everyday life, the quality of life in the nation as a whole or the quality of the world's life. Due to its complexity, no individual can claim to evaluate its quality of life with full validity depending alone on the individual experience; however, the social sciences – in the broadest sense – are necessary to engage in the definition, measurement, exploration, and explanation of quality of life and its troubles. My remarks are based upon a number of theses on the term and the concept of quality of life. In fact, quality of life research is at present not a strictly defined discipline, rather it functions as an umbrella, which attracts people sharing similar research interests worldwide.

1. Quality of life is a term which doesn't exclusively belong to the International Society for Quality of Life Studies (ISQOLS) or another quality of life-researcher group; it is not only the preferred term within ISQOLS, but rather it is used in many fields. This means that we have only partial influence on the meaning and the use of this term. Even in the same scientific field, there are many actors beside our association, for example we have a sister society, the "International Society for Quality of Life Research" (ISOQOL), which is rather strictly related to the health sector and the significance of quality of life in reducing illness and disease. But far from being a purely scientific term, quality of life is used in everyday language, presumably in all our languages and societies. There are multiple organizations and associations that define their tasks within the field of quality of life. Applications can be seen in politics and the economy; the German chancellor Gerhard Schröder, for instance, mentioned quality of life and sustainability in Germany in a recent government declaration. Hardly a day goes by without being confronted with advertisements that declare a certain product to be contributing to your quality of life – if you buy it. The positive connotation of quality of life is employed in many fields to attract people. With "quality of life", we have a term which is used in different contexts and especially its popular meaning is influenced by different sources. So it is inevitably a shifting concept.

2. Nevertheless, the term quality of life is also a scientific term and the quality of life network is not far from constituting a scientific discipline. Let me give you the reasons why I think that quality of life research shapes a new scientific discipline: There are networks of social scientists working on quality of life issues using a similar recognizable perspective with respect to theoretical, methodological, and empirical questions. There is now a large number of books defining itself as belonging to the qol-discipline and using its main term (see the selected book-list at the end of the article). A scientific discipline needs a journal for communication and several journals are available which carry quality of life in their title. We also find bibliographi-

cal publications, interim assessments, and quality of life has found entrance into reference books and dictionaries. The weak point is surely that the textbooks of the field have gotten already somewhat old and we lack an up to date introductory text-book which illustrates the actual basic knowledge of the field to newcomers. It is interesting to see that an editorial team of ISQOLS is planning a special encyclope-dia about quality of life.

3. Quality of life in social sciences is a concept related to different dimensions of a society, it is on the one hand related to the goal and value discussion of societies, and on the other hand to the quality of societies, of its social conditions and social trends. With respect to the goal dimension and the goal discussion, the research questions are concerned with goals, values and norms as they are defined by indi-viduals, associations, governments and international authorities. Prevalent is the analytical use of the quality of life concept. It is used to guide the analyses of living conditions and the perceived quality of life. The new trend in quality of life research is often a strong emphasis on the subjective perception of life by the people.

4. Quality of life implies a positive view of the world, but it does not neglect the negative features of society, like alienation and exclusion, anxieties and fears, as well as worries and loneliness. The concept of quality of life is aware of the multi-plicity and ambivalence of human life. Besides positive and negative dimensions of life there is also the future dimension which has to be taken into account addition-ally. The future perspective constitutes another independent dimension of individual and societal well-being: What people hope and fear for their future is an essential part of their quality of life.

5. Quality of life is a multi-level term and this is essential for the questions con-nected with the concept. With respect to the contrasting cases, quality of life can be defined on the one hand for the individual and on the other for the global world. It is conceived and measured differently in the individual case, in local areas, in commu-nities, regions, nations, continents or in global terms. Consistency in theoretical and practical respect is a serious problem.

Most challenging is the aggregation problem in quality of life studies; if each in-dividual could realize its preferred life style it is questionable, whether the result would be tolerable. If a few individuals behave in a certain way it may have positive consequences for their quality of life, if many do the same, the positive consequence will often be destroyed. The total outcome of a social process is usually not the sum of its parts. One central question for quality of life research is therefore how the dif-ferent concepts of quality of life fit together on different levels.

6. Quality of life is a term used internationally in many languages. Speaking of quality of life seems to be universal. The participants of the conference came from 43 countries and they were all conducting quality of life research in one way or an-other. Not only the term quality of life is international, moreover, the task of creat-ing quality of life is multinational, respectively global. It is problematic if one coun-try defines its quality of life exclusively for its own. Others can set restrictions and exert severe influence. To produce and to secure quality of life is, in the last in-stance, a world wide task. Many international and supranational organizations have dedicated resources to this task. Worldwide communication about quality of life research is therefore indispensable.

7. Quality of life, in the full sense of the term, is interdisciplinary: different ap-proaches use it in varying ways. I do not know of another area of research, where so

many scientific fields are involved: sociology, political science, economics, (social) psychology, medicine, philosophy, marketing, environmental sciences and others. Thus, in quality of life research, a new discipline is emerging under the influence of very different traditional disciplines. We should cultivate this network and hope for synergetic effects.

8. As it seems the first generation of quality of life researchers is on the way to retreat and to retire. To mention a few names which have exerted significant influence, one has to refer to early founders in the United States such as Frank Andrews, Angus Campbell, Philip E. Converse, and Stephen B. Withey. The first generation in Europe ranges from Erik Allardt to Wolfgang Zapf. Others like the social psychologist Michael Argyle have already passed away. The most prominent contributor to the quality of life concept is surely the Nobel prize winner Amartya Sen.

The second and the third generation of quality of life researchers is now facing the challenge to routinize and to improve quality of life investigations. Their advantage is that they are standing on the shoulders of the first generation but nevertheless the tasks for quality of life research are endless. Theory, methods, empirical studies and social reporting are waiting for improvements and continual application.

THE TOPICS OF QUALITY OF LIFE RESEARCH IN THIS BOOK

The contributions on quality of life in this book are related to five main fields of discussion and research. The first one takes account of the fact that we still have an ongoing goal discussion in our societies, in modernized countries as well as in developing ones. Quality of life and complementary respectively competing concepts are in question. The second section focuses on a selection of scientific institutions and procedures, which are necessary for monitoring quality of life in a valid and reliable manner. Here, the task of establishing quality of life research as a societal resource is put into the foreground. The third part deals with various (socio-) economic challenges for quality of life in the economy and the working life. Direct and indirect influences from economic developments are influencing the quality of life. Then follows, as the fourth section, a set of contributions on (socio-) cultural challenges for quality of life. Here, for example, goals related to freedom and complementary values, but also to the family and child well-being are under consideration. The fifth section of the book is devoted to fundamental options and restrictions for improving quality of life, starting with the question of quality of life in a divided society and ending with the question, whether life satisfaction can be produced at all. In total, the contributions investigate the challenges for quality of life on the different levels of the individual, the local and the regional communities up to the quality of a nation's life and the quality of life in the global world.

1. Goal discussions in society are going on permanently, but they are on the agenda especially when new states or state unions are founded. No wonder that for the emerging European Union goal discussions have a special significance. In this context, the concept of social quality has been developed in critical contrast to the concept of quality of life (Alan Walker/Laurent van der Maesen). This scientific dispute will go on and it will also penetrate into the public discussion. From a more worldwide perspective, the concept of sustainable development, which is partly similar and partly different to quality of life, has a high rank (Martina Schäfer/Benjamin Nölting/Lydia Illge). In both concepts, the natural environment

receives significant attention; but in contrast to quality of life, the concept of sustainability places more emphasis on the living conditions of future generations. Quality of life and well-being were in the past mainly introduced as goals for modernized societies; now efforts are made to transfer them to developing countries as well. Given the precarious socio-economic situation in the poorer areas of the world, it is a difficult task to define subjective measures of well-being in developing countries (Laura Camfield). In contrast to this subjective approach for developing countries, a more traditional approach refers to social indicators which are relatively close to living standard and level of living. The argument is here that the task of securing the basics for a decent quality of life will in the long run remain the highest priority in Africa (Patrick E. Edewor). Altogether this first chapter gives an impression of the societal discourse about the concept of quality of life and related concepts in advanced industrialized and developing countries.

2. Given acceptable concepts of quality of life in our societies, the analyzing and monitoring of quality of life over time gets a new task: methods of measurement among them quality of life surveys and their assembling in data archives have been successfully institutionalized. Surely, the most prominent example is the World Database on Happiness (Ruut Veenhoven). Its approach is new insofar as it goes beyond a simple data archive and contains a bibliography, a catalogue of valid indicators and of findings and investigators in the field. Another example for the development of a quality of life related infrastructure is the "Dynamic Information Centre" (Michaela Hudler-Seitzberger). It offers information about comparative national and cross-national survey questions and survey programs, which are of relevance to welfare and quality of life measurement.

The reduction of an overload of information is a normal challenge and the final goal of extensive approaches often aim at one comprehensive index which represents a complex situation. The development of comprehensive indices for measuring quality of life is demonstrated with respect to child well-being in the long run (Kenneth Land). But one or just a few indicators are often insufficient for a complex situation and therefore the question is rather the right selection of indicators. There are a lot of difficulties connected to monitoring the social state, which is shown for the Netherlands, and a systematic overview of quality of life and living conditions needs a clear theoretical guidance (Jeroen Belhoewer/Theo Roes).

Without any doubt, the quantitative methods, which have almost a qualitative-theoretical background, were clearly preferred in the beginning of quality of life research. The prevailing idea was to get representative data, where each person was included with one vote. But the qualitative methods have also detected the field of quality of life and one example are biographical analyses of quality of life processes in migration (Maria Kontos). Theoretically, this approach is built on the concept of capabilities, introduced in the books of Amartya Sen.

Each of the five contributions in this chapter offer a view of some of the big methodological problems of quality of life research and how they are solved today.

3. Economic challenges are structural and occasional concomitants for quality of life. For example, inflation, which is at first glance independent from quality life, shows a lot of connections if one looks more closely (Heinz Herrmann). Monetary stability is a positive value seen from the standard of living and from quality of life. Another economic challenge lies in the quality of working life, which is conceived as a substantial segment of quality of life. In the context of growing global competi-

tion, new division lines on the labor market are emerging, which are especially significant for non-regular workers (Byoung-Hoon Lee/Yoo-Sun Kim).

One of the most frequently investigated problems in quality of life research is the question if income and wealth generate happiness. Just the opposite view is taken if one asks "Does happiness pay?". This question is answered positively insofar as the hypothesis is proven by panel data that economic success is based on certain psychological factors (Carol Graham/Andrew Eggers/Sandip Sukhtankar). It is shown, that happy people are economically more successful than unhappy people. Altogether, there seems to be a circle between happiness and economic success which means that one enforces the other. But the relationships are not so strong that they could create a divided society of the rich and happy on the one side and the poor and unhappy on the other.

4. Cultural challenges for quality of life often arise when societal values are threatened. The relationship between satisfaction with life and freedom in decisions is a constellation of this kind. The value of freedom is one of the most prominent goals of western societies and related analyses have found that it is rather significant for the perceived quality of life (Max Haller/Markus Hadler). With a similar background, the relationship of life satisfaction with salient values for the future is the problem of a cross-cultural study (Ferrran Casas/Cristina Figuer/Mònica Gonzáles/Germà Coenders). Gender and age are very influential variables in this context.

The changing family structure of modern societies with increasing divorce rates and fewer complete families could be a source of impairments for individuals' quality of life. The differences between complete and single parent families is analyzed as astonishingly small in the course of time in the Netherlands (Anna Lont/Jaap Dronkers). Values and their realization are a very old problem which challenges societies and individuals. The question, how belief in personal values and the perceived level of realization of these values in one's community determines the subjective quality of life, is answered positively. Though this result is found in a small population in the Kibbutz, it may be of general validity (Uriel Leviatan).

5. The final set of contributions is on basic options and restrictions for quality of life with the intention to enlighten dilemma constellations for quality of life. The first essay is related to the problem of ethnically and socio-economically divided societies, where the opportunities to participate in quality of life differ considerably (Valerie Møller). In divided countries there is no average measure of quality of life which could guide national development.

Satisfaction with health and its relation to health care systems is another challenge for improving quality of life. In a broad comparison of different institutional characteristics within the European Union, the minor relevance of health expenditure is shown (Jürgen Kohl/Claus Wendt). There are a lot of restrictions for the welfare state to influence the perception of health and social security.

There are a few things in human life which concern everybody without exception, and, one of which is death. But the process of dying has developed socially very differently and there is a rising demand to regard the process of dying as a component of quality of life (Maria Angeles Durán). The concept of quality of life is of relevance also for the dark sides of life and the last phase of life will increasingly become part of the discussion for a good quality of life.

At the end of the final book chapter, one fundamental question is raised: Can we produce life satisfaction? (Richard Easterlin). Exactly at this point, it becomes clear what the meaning of options and restrictions is. If the setpoint model for individual satisfaction would be correct, struggling for satisfaction would be no convincing option. If mainly pecuniary success ("more is better") would make us happier in the long run, there would be an option without serious restrictions or alternatives. But of course, we are in an uncertain field of options and restrictions, where our own decisions influence the outcome. According to the experience of Easterlin "most people could increase their life satisfaction by devoting more time to family life and health".

As this book is conceived it should offer innovative information from quality of life research, stimulate interdisciplinary research on quality of life, and encourage international cooperation and it could play the role of a social change agent. According to the constitution of the International Society for Quality of Life Studies, it should be a contribution to the international communication, discussion and exchange about quality of life questions.

RECOMMENDED READING LIST OF RECENT QUALITY OF LIFE-BOOKS

Cummins, R. & E. Gullone (2002): The Universality of Subjective Wellbeing Indicators. Social Indicators Series, Vol. 16, Dordrecht, Boston, London: Kluwer Academic Publishers.

Diener, E. & E. M. Suh (eds.) (2000): Culture and Subjective Well-Being. Cambridge, London: MIT Press.

Easterlin, R. (1997): Growth Triumphant: The 21st Century in Historical Perspective. Ann Arbor: University of Michigan Press.

Frey, B. & A. Stutzer (2002): Happiness and Economics. How the Economy and Institutions Affect Human Well-Being. Princeton/Oxford: Princeton University Press.

Hagerty, M., J. Vogel & V. Møller (eds.) (2002): Assessing Quality of Life and Living Conditions to Guide National Policy – The State of the Art. Social Indicators Research Series vol. 11, Dordrecht, Boston, London: Kluwer Academic Publishers.

Nussbaum, M. & A. K. Sen (1993): The Quality of Life. Oxford et al.: Oxford University Press.

Offer, A. (1996): In Pursuit of the Quality of Life. Oxford: Oxford University Press.

Prescott-Allen, R. (2001): The Well-Being of Nations. A Country-by-Country Index of Quality of Life and the Environment. Washington/DC: Island Press.

Rapley, M. (2003): Quality of Life Research. A Critical Introduction. London, Thousand Oaks, New Delhi: Sage Publications.

Sirgy, M.J., D. Rahtz & D.-J. Lee (2004): Community Quality of Life Indicators – Best Cases. Social Indicators Research Series, Vol. 22, Dordrecht, Boston, London: Kluwer Academic Publishers.

Veenhoven, R. (1993): Happiness in Nations. Subjective Appreciation of Life in 56 Nations, 1946-1992. Erasmus University of Rotterdam (2004 update available at www.eur.nl/fsw/research/happiness).

Vogel, J. (1997): Living conditions and Inequality in the European Union. Eurostat: Population and Social Conditions E/97-3, Luxembourg.

PART I:
GOAL DISCUSSIONS
ON QUALITY OF LIFE

2. SOCIAL QUALITY AND QUALITY OF LIFE

Alan Walker and Laurent van der Maesen

University of Sheffield, United Kingdom,
and European Foundation for Social Quality, Amsterdam, The Netherlands

ABSTRACT

The two purposes of this paper are to introduce the concept of social quality and to discuss the main differences between it and the idea of quality of life. The concept of social quality was introduced in 1977 as an alternative to economic growth as a yardstick for social and economic progress. Subsequently it has been extensively theorized and, on a practical policy level, became a core part of the EU's social agenda. In this paper we explain the concept of social quality and its development, and then go on to outline the theory of social relations underlying it. Finally, discussion of the differences between social quality and quality of life leads to the conclusion that the latter is too ill-defined and amorphous to provide a useful guide for policy making even if its scientific heritage is substantial.

INTRODUCTION

The main purpose of this paper is to examine the differences between the concepts of social quality and quality of life. This assessment is necessary for both theoretical and practical reasons. On the one hand it is important to explore any differences in their theoretical underpinnings while, on the other, it is essential to understand their respective strengths and weaknesses as potential adjuncts to policy making. At the same time it is important to acknowledge the tentative nature of this comparison which is caused by the recent origins and relative under-development of social quality, which contrasts with the long history of quality of life studies. To start with the background to the concept of social quality is explained and its theoretical underpinning is discussed. Then the current phase of work on social quality, its operationalization, is described. Finally the main elements of social quality are contrasted with those of quality of life.

BACKGROUND TO SOCIAL QUALITY

The concept of social quality originated in a series of expert meetings in Amsterdam on European Social Policy. The first meeting in 1991 was convened to examine processes of transformation in both western and central-eastern Europe and their consequences for senior citizens. A follow-up meeting in 1993 discussed the causes of social inequalities among older people in the EU. Both meetings were specifically intended to build on the work of two of the European Commission's Observatories –

13

Wolfgang Glatzer, Susanne von Below, Matthias Stoffregen (eds.), Challenges for Quality of Life in the Contemporary World, 13-31.
© 2004 Kluwer Academic Publishers. Printed in the Netherlands.

on Social Exclusion and Ageing – and both reached similar conclusions. Most importantly, it was the unequal relationship between economic policy and social policy, and the increasing tendency for the former to define the content and scope of the latter, that was identified as the main source of the recent crises in European social policy. In short the social dimension appeared to be viewed increasingly as being in conflict with the economic or monetary one and, as a consequence, risked serious downgrading. It seemed to us that this process was taking on an air of inevitability and that, therefore, the European model of development itself was in jeopardy. That was the problem that stimulated the thinking which led to the concept of social quality.

The conflict between the economic/monetary and social dimensions of the EU was most visible in the reductions in social spending and unemployment resulting from the convergence criteria for EMU (Meulders & Plasman, 1998). Less obvious is the implied residualization and individualization of social policy in the emerging US style "third way" politics in Europe – the transatlantic consensus – and the attempt to re-cast the EU's social protection systems into a narrow production-orientated US model (Walker & Deacon, 2003). It was the risk posed by these developments which led to the conclusion that a new approach to social policy was required. Of course we are not claiming originality for the insight that the European social policy model is in danger, it has been articulated many times, including by the European Commission and the Comité des Sages (1996).

What was required to address the unequal relationship between economic and social policy was a new conceptualization, one which would help to establish a balance between economic and social development in Europe by re-examining the foundations and goals of social policy. Our search for a concept that both represented what the European model had sought to embody and that focused attention on the goals of social policy – re-cast from its narrow administrative form to a broader societal one (Walker, 1984) - led rapidly to the term "social quality". This appealed to us because it conveyed, on the one hand, the achievement of the EU Member States in creating a unique blend of economic success and social development not found in either the US or East-Asia. While, on the other, it suggests a mission that is unfinished: a reminder of what the EU should be striving for and a guiding star for plotting the required direction of change. In other words, the European model is characterized by elements of social quality but it has not been articulated in this way before.

CONCEPTUALISATION OF SOCIAL QUALITY

What do we mean by the term "social quality"? Social quality was originally proposed as a standard by which to measure the extent to which the quality of the daily lives of citizens have attained an acceptable European level (Beck, van der Maesen & Walker, 1998). Social quality, therefore, is a reflection of European citizenship. To measure this social quality requires a broad multi-dimensional standard, broader than more familiar social indicators like poverty and social exclusion. Moreover, social quality is a feature of societies and their institutions even though it is assessed with reference to its impact on citizens. Therefore the concept of human needs did not capture what we were looking for (Doyal & Gough, 1991). Also, given the highly developed nature of the EU, it would have been inappropriate to employ a concept such as basic needs. It also had to incorporate a mixture of structural factors and individual-level ones. We were mindful of the need to properly represent the delicate balance in Europe between collective and individual responsibility. Standard quality of life scales were not adequate for the purposes outlined above for the reasons set out below.

In the light of all these considerations we defined social quality as: "the extent to which citizens are able to participate in the social and economic life of their communities under conditions which enhance their well-being and individual potential" (Beck et al., 1998, p. 3). That is the extent to which the quality of social relations promotes both participation and personal development (The term "citizen" is meant to denote any resident rather than a legal status.). In order to achieve an acceptable level of social quality it is hypothesized that four conditions have to be fulfilled.

First, people have to have access to *socio-economic security* – from whatever source, including employment and social security – in order to protect them from poverty and other forms of material deprivation. Socio-economic security in the EU requires good quality paid employment and social protection to guarantee living standards and access to resources: income, education, health care, social services, environment, public health, personal safety and so on.

Second, people have to experience *social inclusion* in, or minimum levels of social exclusion from, key social and economic institutions such as the labor market. Social inclusion concerns citizenship. This may be a wide and all embracing national or European citizenship or "exclusive" with large numbers of outcasts and quasi-citizens (denied citizenship completely or partially by means of discrimination). Room (1999) for example, has argued that exclusion is the denial or non-realization of social rights.

Third, people should be able to live in communities and societies characterized by *social cohesion*. Social cohesion refers to the glue which holds together communities and societies. It is vital for both social development and individual self-realization. The contemporary discussion of cohesion often centers on the narrow concept of social capital but its legacy stretches back, via Durkheim, to solidarity, shared norms and values. Reference to social cohesion does not mean that traditional forms of solidarity must be preserved at all costs but, rather, it requires a recognition of the changing social structure (e.g. family formation) and the need to renew those that continue to underpin social cohesion, such as intergenerational solidarity, and to find new forms to take the place of those that are weakening.

Fourth, people must be to some extent autonomous and *empowered* in order to be able to fully participate in the face of rapid socio-economic change. Empowerment means enabling citizens to control their own lives and to take advantage of opportunities. It means increasing the range of human choice. Therefore it goes far beyond participation in the political system to focus on the individual's potential capacity (knowledge, skills, experience and so on) and how far these can be realized.

Diagram 1: Conditional Factors of Social Quality

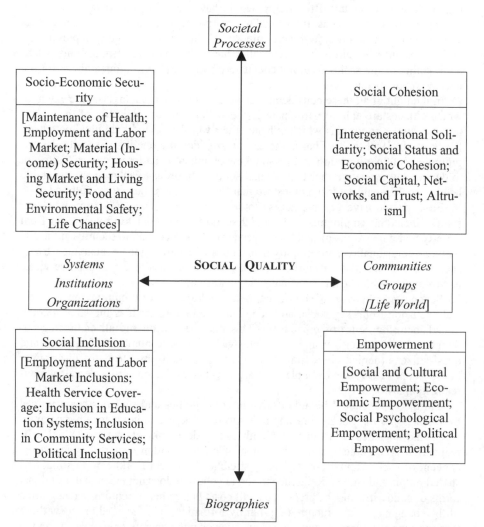

These four components may be represented diagrammatically in a two-dimensional quadrangle (diagram 1). On the one hand there is the distinction between the macro and micro levels – between structure and agency in sociological terms, while, on the other, there is the horizontal relationship between the formal and the informal, between institutions and organizations and communities, groups and individuals. Thus the vertical axis represents the tension between societal development and biographical development; while the horizontal axis represents the tension between institutional processes and individual actions (between, in Lockwood's (1999) terms, system integration and social integration or, in Habermas' (1968) terms, between the system and the life world). Of course each cell in the quadrangle is itself represented by a continuum: socio-economic security/ insecurity; social cohesion/ fragmentation; social inclusion/ exclusion; and autonomy/ dependency. Obviously the underlying assumption is that each of these components may be operationalized and, thereby, the model, or a more refined version of it, could become a practical tool for policy makers and policy analysts. It has recently come to our notice that parallel work by Keyes (1998) has led to a very similar conceptualization of 'social well-being' which encompasses social integration, social contribution, social coherence, social actualization and social acceptance.

SOCIAL QUALITY AS POLICY

Remarkably, before the ink was dry on the first formulation of social quality in 1997, the idea of social quality had been translated into policy when the Netherlands Ministry of Welfare and Sport employed it as a guiding principle in evaluating the impact of its policies. Gradually, over the last few years, European policy-makers have been seeing potential in the term – as an embodiment of European ideals and a touchstone for the European model. Thus the *Social Policy Agenda* of the European Commission includes references to social quality and 'quality' has been adopted as one of the key themes of European social policy (European Commission, 2000, p. 13; even if the location of the term in the EU policy triangle is wrong conceptually; cf. diagram 2).

Diagram 2: The EU Policy Triangle

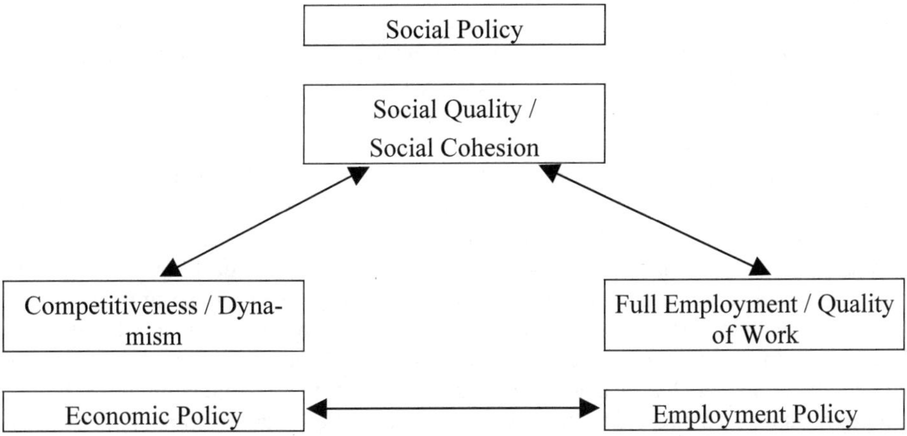

Source: European Commission, 2000, p. 13: The policy mixes to be established to create a virtuous circle of economic and social progress should reflect the inter-dependence of these policies and aim to maximize their mutual positive reinforcement.

The following statement, from the Commission's Social Policy Agenda, could have been extracted from the first book on social quality: "A key message is that growth is not an end in itself but essentially a means to achieving a better standard of living for all" (European Commission, 2000, p. 13). The Commissioner for Employment and Social Affairs Anna Diamantopoulou (2001) has acknowledged the influential role of the first book on social quality in the development of the new European Social Policy Agenda, and both she and President Romano Prodi (2001), have endorsed the idea of social quality and welcomed the publication of the Foundation's second book (Beck, van der Maesen, Thomèse & Walker, 2001).

THEORIZING SOCIAL QUALITY

One of the early criticisms of the concept of social quality is that it lacked a theoretical foundation and, therefore, could be mistaken for a purely instrumental idea, like other terms in the quality domain such as TQM, or one of the very many quality of life scales. Our own theoretical journey into the philosophical foundations of social quality made us realize that the search for a rationale for social policy was too restricting and, instead, what was required was a scientific framework which establishes whether the *social* component of social quality is an authentic entity in its own right and, if it is, that would enable us to develop conclusions about its quality. It is the failure to pursue this endeavor that has left social policy trapped in a limited domain defined by economists as non-economic (Donzelot, 1979; Walker, 1984). Classical economists defined society's problems as "social" rather than "economic" and social policy has been working within that straightjacket ever since.

The heart of what is social, we argue, is the self-realization of individuals, as social beings, in the context of the formation of collective identities. Thus the "social" is the outcome of constantly changing processes through which individuals realize themselves as interacting social beings. Rather than being atomized economic agents we argue, from Honneth (1994), that a person's self-realization depends on social recognition. The processes whereby we all achieve self-realization, to a greater or lesser extent, are partly historically and, therefore, structurally determined and partly determined by the agents themselves (structure and praxis).

According to our theory, first of all as previously stated, the social world is realized in the interaction (and interdependence) between the self-realization of individual people as social beings and the formation of collective identities. We call this the *constitution* of "the social". Secondly, four basic conditions determine the opportunities open for social relations to develop (diagram 1). People must have the capability to interact (empowerment); the institutional and structural context must be accessible to them (inclusion); they must have access to the necessary material and other resources that facilitate interaction (socio-economic security); and the necessary collectively accepted values and norms, such as trust, that enable community building (cohesion). This refers to the *opportunities* for "the social". Of course there may be substantial variations between individuals on one or all of these conditions. Thirdly, therefore, the actual nature, content and structure of what is the social component of human relations is a function of the relationship between two axes. Each axis represents a set of tensions: on the horizontal axis it is between systems, institutions and organizations, on the one hand, and communities and groups on the other; while on the vertical axis the tension is between social processes and biographical ones. These twin tensions create the dynamic which influences both self-realization and the formation of collective identities and which determines the specific quality of the social (diagram 3). This refers to the *concretization* or production of "the social". In other words it is the process whereby human subjects become social actors, who are then confronted with variable opportunities for social action.

Diagram 3: Constitution, Opportunities, and Concretization of "the Social"

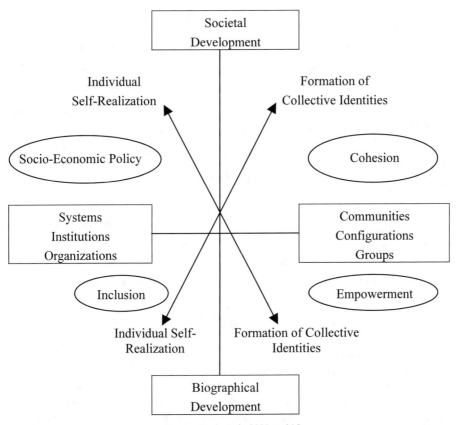

Source: Beck et al., 2001, p. 315.

This process whereby the social world is realized by the dynamic relationship between the two axes in the context of the interaction between the formation of collective identifies and self-realization is illustrated in diagram 4. On the horizontal axis we see the contrast between rationality and subjectivity, between demos on the left and ethnos on the right. So, on the left side we are concerned with the relationship between the individual and the world of systems and institutions, in short with *participation*. On the right side there are relations between individuals and social groups and communities in the negotiation of everyday life. Access and belonging in these relationships concern *social recognition and appreciation*. The vertical axis represents the worlds of societal and biographical processes and, within them, are embedded values, norms, principles, rights, conventions and so on. The top half of the axis concerns the *social justice* while the bottom half indicates *compassion or social responsiveness* (the manner in which people interact).

Diagram 4: Quadrangle: The Constitution of Social Actors

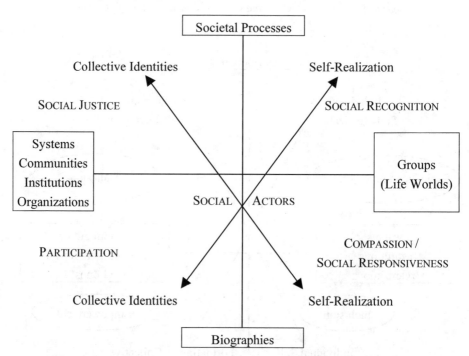

It is obvious that the outcome of this set of processes which produce the social world may be positive and negative. Self-realization may mean autonomy or egocentrism while collective identities may be open and liberating or closed and authoritarian. Therefore ethical guidelines are required to distinguish between acceptable and unacceptable outcomes. This means that social quality must have an ideological dimension. As previously noted, from the beginning there were dual – scientific and political – engines behind the social quality initiative and the two are brought together in the campaign for human dignity in Europe. This is centered on the Amsterdam Declaration on Social Quality (1997) which, above all, calls for respect for fundamental human dignity. The four components of the social quality quadrant (four ontological conditions of "the social") also reflect this perspective: Socio-economic security points to social justice; inclusion refers to the social rights of citizens; cohesion implies an interdependent moral contract and solidarity; and empowerment means equity in life chances. Social quality concerns the dignity of individuals as social beings.

Having conceptualized the idea of what is unique about the description "social" in such a way that we will be able to develop conclusions about its quality, the final unresolved issue was what do we mean by "quality"? The answer comes in six parts.

First, because the heart of the social world concerns the self-realization of individuals as social beings, the main point of reference for quality must be the circumstances of daily life. Second, therefore, quality is a function of permanently changing interactions among actors in everyday life and cannot be reduced to processes between systems and communities and groups. Thirdly, quality does not have a one-dimensional nature. There are no quality standards independent of the dynamic historical and situational circumstances in which the social world is manufactured. Fourth, the interpretation of European quality in terms of minimum standards for everybody is not an option. In Therborn's (2001) terms social quality implies an "open horizon" rather than a "social floor". Fifth, quality depends on capacity. In other words, quality will be realized if people are enabled to develop communicative capacities in the ever more complex circumstances that confront us all. Sixth, quality is not only a question of outcomes but of processes as well. The nature of interventions, the choice of strategies for action, and the type of organization have an important bearing on the quality of the process.

INDICATORS OF SOCIAL QUALITY

Having created a theoretical platform for the understanding and development of social quality – by seeking an independent rationale for the term "social" – the next and current chapter in the story is to operationally the concept. As noted already, any index of social quality must be multi-dimensional and, in particular, it is necessary to derive indicators for the four components of the social quality quadrangle. Then these have to be combined to produce an aggregate indicator of social quality. These aims raise substantial methodological problems, not the least of which are how to operationally each component and how to aggregate them. But there is already a lot of existing material on two of the four – socio-economic security and inclusion – and a substantial body of work on social indicators and, therefore, we are not starting from scratch. A further crucial question is who decides what quality is? Of course with a concept that reflects European citizenship the perspective of citizens must be uppermost but, in addition, there has to be a role for experts and policy makers.

These are just some of the questions that we aim to resolve in the current 14 country European Thematic Network on Indicators of Social Quality that is being funded under the Fifth Framework Programme. The Network is in the process of constructing an index of social quality that is intended eventually to be used as both a policy tool and as a basis for citizen empowerment in the policy process.

QUALITY OF LIFE

Having outlined the background to, current work and aspirations of the social quality project we turn, now, to its relationship with the idea of quality of life. First, a few words about the latter concept. In contrast to the very recently arrived concept of social quality the study of quality of life has a long tradition in the social and related sciences. Pigou (1929) was the first social scientist to mention the term "quality of life" in the context of discussion of economics and welfare. He was writing about government welfare provision for the lower classes and the way it is affected by work: "First, non-economic welfare is liable to be modified by the manner in which income is earned. For the surroundings of work react upon the quality of life" (Pigou, 1929, p. 14). The term then disappeared for nearly two decades. It resurfaced in the US at the latter part of the Second World War when it was used to imply the good life or material wealth as indicated by ownership of houses, consumer goods and cars (Fallowfield, 1990). In the 1950s the Eisenhower Commission on National Goals began the task of trying to measure life quality and the results revealed different environmental and social influences (Oliver, Huxley, Bridges & Mohamad, 1996). The term "quality of life" was used in the report by the President's Commission published in the mid-1960s (Wood-Dauphine, 1999). This was the beginning of the social indicators movement in the US which was intended to provide regular reports on social progress in order to inform the planning and evaluation of social policy. An important international impetus to quality of life research was the expansion by the WHO of its definition of health to include physical, emotional and social well-being, which also broadened the discussion about the measurement of this new approach to health.

In the US, where most of the early social research into quality of life was conducted, quality of life researchers tried to pin down its meaning by identifying and investigating various proxy states such as life satisfaction, happiness, morale and subjective well-being (Campbell, Converse & Rogers, 1976; Diener, 1999). The dominance of positivism in US social science meant that those approaches amenable to quantification were favored even when the scientific constructions being used were remote from the life worlds in which people live their lives (Bradburn & Caplowitz, 1965; Bradburn, 1969; George & Bearon, 1980; Bowling, 1991). A theoretical model of quality of life as "the good life" was first proposed by Lawton (1983) who defined it as behavioral competence, the objective environment and perceived quality of life. Unfortunately there was a false objectivity about the subjective aspects of this and other approaches to quality of life, such as Bradburn's (1969) negative affect. The summation of scores on such scales and their subsequent imposition on individuals or groups involves glossing over subtle variations and nuances in the way that people construct quality in their lives. These psychological well-being and morale scales are often quite negative too (Bradburn, 1969; Neugarten, 1961). In the UK research was dominated, until recently, by health and health-related issues and, within that field, economic assessments of quality of life have been particularly influential (Bowling, 1995a). The best known example is the Quality Adjusted Life Years (QALY) measure which uses health professionals' definitions of the constituents of quality of life in order to assess the value of clinical interventions.

It is only in the last decade or so that the perspectives of the people – especially patients and service users – have been brought more fully into research on quality of life by the development of open-ended subjective inquiries which put individuals at the center of judgments about the quality of their own lives. A leading example is the Schedule for the Evaluation of Individual Quality of Life (SEIQoL) which operates by eliciting from respondents those aspects of life which are considered to be crucial to the overall quality of life (O'Boyle et al., 1993). Thus, in contrast to normative measures of health-related quality of life, which reflect the judgments of researchers and, usually, a disease-oriented model of quality of life, it is the individual concerned that rates the importance of different elements. Nonetheless there is plenty of room for distortion in the operation of scales such as SEIQoL, caused for example by the location of the interview, the expectations generated by the study and the cumulative effects of the previous questions (Bond, 1999).

The simple direct method of asking members of the public themselves what is most important in their lives has been used surprisingly little in this field. Bowling (1995b) was one of the first in the UK and she asked a random sample of 2000 adults what they regarded as important in their lives (good and bad). People taking part in the research were asked open ended questions about the most important things in their lives. They could mention as many as they wanted but only five responses were coded. Respondents then chose show cards to represent the five most important things and these items were recorded. Free responses and coded selections were found to be quite consistent. People were then asked to organize the mentioned items 'in rank order of importance' (Bowling 1995b, p. 1451). The results were, in priority order, relationships with family and relatives, the person's health, the health of another (close) person and finances/standard of living/housing. When all the various priority areas were combined the most frequently mentioned aspect was the material one (finances etc.) followed by relationships with family and friends. This research demonstrated that several of those items regarded by the general pubic as important to their quality of life do not feature in the most commonly used assessments of health status.

Thus there is a wide variety of attempts to operationally the assessment of quality of life and the literature is periodically dominated by methodological disputes concerning objective versus subjective assessments. At one end of the spectrum is the Scandinavian approach which has focused on objective living conditions (Erikson, 1993), whilst at the other end, the American Quality of Life approach has emphasized the subjective evaluation of psychological well-being and individual need satisfaction (Argyle, 1996). The approach developed by Fahey, Nolan and Whelan (2002) for the Dublin Foundation encompasses both objective and subjective dimensions, as do those of Zapf and colleagues and the ZUMA model developed by Berger-Schmitt and Noll. The ZUMA quality of life model is a highly sophisticated attempt to both conceptualize and measure quality of life. Its conceptual framework is based on three concepts: quality of life, social cohesion, and sustainability. Berger-Schmitt and Noll are at the forefront of attempts to theories as well as operationally quality of life and their ultimate aim is "to measure and analyze changes in the welfare of European citizens using theoretically and methodologically well-grounded indicators derived from an overarching conceptual framework". The ZUMA model, therefore, is closer to that of social quality than most of the others within the quality of life school although, as we will show, the theoretical framework which has been developed by Berger-Schmitt and Noll, is not as far-reaching as that of social quality.

In attempting to classify the various different approaches to aspects of quality of life Noll (2000) helpfully distinguishes between concepts which focus on individual quality of life and those that emphasize the distribution of welfare and social relations or the quality of societies (diagram 5). He further delineates specific approaches to the quality of societies (such as social capital) from comprehensive ones (such as human development).

Diagram 5: Welfare Concepts

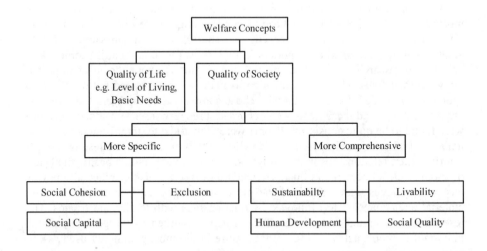

Source: Noll, 2000.

The conceptual framework of quality of life developed by Berger-Schmitt and Noll (2000) combines objective living conditions and the enhancement of subjective well-being, with quality of life as the "overarching perspective of observation and measurement" (p. 64). This ZUMA approach is embedded in the EuReporting project, initiated by Habich, Zapf, and Noll, which is at the forefront of the endeavor to create robust social indicators for the systematic monitoring of living conditions and quality of life. This European Framework Five research project also led to the creation of Euromodule, a core set of survey questions to provide comparative data on living standards and quality of life in European countries (Delhey, Böhnke, Habich, and Zapf, 2001). In constructing the European System of Social Indicators the EuReporting project followed the ZUMA approach, which in turn reflects the tradition of the quality of life school, and focused on life domains. Thus a comprehensive system of indicators was constructed covering 13 life domains – such as housing, transport, health, environment and public safety and crime – with an additional one for total life situation (Berger-Schmitt & Noll, 2000). Two of the goals of the ZUMA approach to quality of life measurement are a reduction in disparities and inequalities (including social exclusion) and the strengthening of connections and social ties to include an enhancement of social capital. The ZUMA approach therefore acts as an overarching model of quality of life which includes social capital, social inclusion and social cohesion.

CONTRASTING SOCIAL QUALITY AND QUALITY OF LIFE

In this final section we turn to the similarities and differences between the two concepts under examination. Our aim is not to portray them as competing concepts but, rather, to understand their respective strengths and weaknesses and, therefore, to draw conclusions about their appropriate usage. This contrast focuses on three dimensions: theory, methods and policy application. Before proceeding let us be clear about the nature of the two concepts under consideration. The diagrammatic classification of social quality by Berger-Schmitt and Noll (2000) as a "quality of society" concept which attempts to integrate social cohesion, social exclusion and human development under a common policy perspective, is misleading (diagram 5). In fact social quality comprises aspects of *both* quality of life and quality of society (where this is interpreted as quality of social relations). In social quality it is the dynamic interaction of the individual with society that determines the quality of the social. Thus a more appropriate representation is shown in diagram 6.

Diagram 6: Quality Constructs for Research and Policy Making

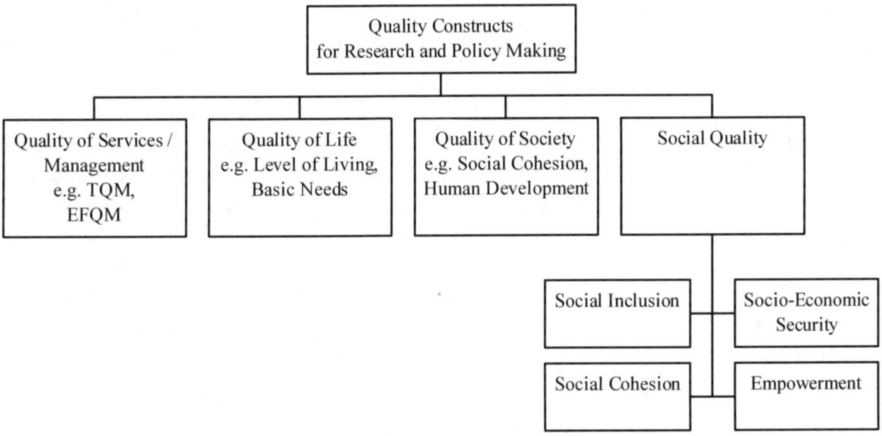

Theoretical Foundations

A key difference between the concepts of social quality and quality of life is the extent to which each is theoretically grounded. In this respect social quality lies at one end of the spectrum, while the majority of the quality of life literature lies at the other.

As we have explained, a concerted effort has been made to construct a firm theoretical foundation for social quality in terms of the constitution of social relations. The relationship between "the formation of collective identities" and "self-realization" within and between each of the four components – socio-economic security; cohesion; inclusion; and empowerment – forms the unified theoretical basis of the components. Because the theory of social quality is focused on social relationships it is able to examine them critically, indeed operationalization *by definition* must emphasize the varying quality of human relationships and social arrangements. As previously indicated ENIQ is attempting to link this theory of the "social" to empirical reality through the use of domains, sub-domains and indicators that are specifically constructed to reflect the theory underlying social quality. At this stage therefore, while the theory is robust, the theoretically-determined construction of indicators is an aspiration.

In the quality of life school things are quite different: for decades it has been preoccupied with the development of indicators which are designed to act as measuring tools. Many experts in the field of quality of life studies have themselves noted the lack of theoretical foundations underlying the concept (Hörnquist, 1982; Gill & Feinstein, 1994; Bowling, 1997; Hunt, 1997). As a result, in practice there are many definitions and formulations of quality of life (as in the case of social capital) which contrast with the single unified social quality approach. According to Farquar (1995, p. 1440): "definitions of quality of life are as numerous and inconsistent as the methods of assessing it (since) different people value different things". In the absence of the vital source of coherence provided by a theoretical framework quality of life can easily become a reflection of the researcher's preferences. This means assembling the required number of life domains and, although there are usually common dimensions, such as health, financial resources and social networks, the list may vary considerably from project to project. Of course this "fit for purpose" aspect of quality of life can be an advantageous source of flexibility but it results in a lack of consistency and comparability in quality of life studies. There is a danger too, in contrast to the social quality approach, that existing social relations and structures are taken-for-granted aspects of the assessment of quality of life rather than being analyzed critically. There is also a tendency in research to treat quality of life as a fixed concept that is made up of different domains. An alternative approach might see it as being more fluid and reflecting the dynamic strategies and actions that people evolve to promote the quality of their lives or a "life of quality" (Peace et al., 2003). As an action theory social quality has the potential to reflect the phenomenological meanings and identities that people invest in such strategies but this aspect of the social quality methodology is not yet developed (Beck et al., 2001, p. 367).

The theoretical framework which underpins the quality of life approach is often weak and individualistic. Indeed, some of the quality of life advocates seem to be actively avoiding any in-depth theoretical discussion. For example, in their justification of utilizing an analytical as well as descriptive approach Fahey, Nolan and Whelan (2002, p. 1) argue that "an analytical approach to social and economic processes can generate knowledge that contributes to the policy making process without the need to become bogged down in philosophical discussions of causality". The ZUMA model of the quality of life, however, is more theoretically based than most of the others in the quality of life movement. As noted previously, Berger-Schmitt and Noll (2002) have developed a framework based around three concepts: sustainability (within which social capital is incorporated); social cohesion; and quality of life. This brings the model very close to the social quality approach but, as yet, there is no theory which links these three concepts. Moreover, while the list of life domains is comprehensive there is no theoretical justification for the selection process.

Methods

The scope of quality of life is potentially vast, comprising a potentially endless list of domains and indicators and covering the whole world, whereas social quality is defined tightly around its four core components and was intended, initially, as a European concept. Also, in contrast to quality of life, social quality has an openly political or ideological dimension – being linked to a vision of participative social relations. However this does not mean that quality of life is an apolitical concept: It entails value judgments regardless of the attempts to portray it as neutral.

For the quality of life school indicators are used to *measure* changes over time and to compare the quality of life between different countries and between individuals within each of the countries. There is an attempt to utilize indicators which can help in the evaluation of policy interventions through both descriptive and analytical monitoring, and through the use of objective and subjective data sources. While some attempt is made to make judgments on what the resulting data sources mean for the quality of life of citizens, the subjective nature of many of the variables mean that there is room for political debate and negotiation. Some may believe, for example, that an increase in the proportion of children under the age of five being cared for in a nursery setting is beneficial, while others will see it as detrimental. The same variable, in a social quality setting will have a normative judgment attached to it, although (as previously stated) at the present time some of these normative judgments are yet to be confirmed finally.

In terms of measurement the quality of life approach attempts to move beyond a simple description and comparison of a set of indicators across time and countries, to include an understanding of the processes that influence the distribution of these quality of life indicators within and between countries. Social quality is also concerned with *why* such differences occur and the processes involved. The quality of life movement has developed a methodologically sound approach to its empirical work, while the new-comer social quality school has only just embarked on its methods journey. Both the social quality and quality of life perspectives have attempted to provide a set of indicators as a measuring tool. The quality of life indicators are commonly individual subjective ones.

The quality of life movement, in its various guises, focuses on a series of domains which attempt to cover all aspects of life and reflect what is important to citizens. The ZUMA based quality of life model consists of a large series of indicators and domains which cover all aspects of life (Berger-Schmitt & Noll, 2000). The Dublin-based quality of life approach developed by Fahey, Nolan and Whelan, has identified 12 domains and the intention is to utilize the indicators with varying degrees of detail, some indicators will be examined at a descriptive level and some in more depth at an analytical level depending upon the importance which is attached to them at any one time. This reflects a close link to the policy arena.

The domains and indicators for social quality are based specifically on the four components outlined previously and, within these, a very small sample of indicators are being drawn up by the ENIQ. The tri-partite uniqueness of this selection process is based on the boundary set by each component (i.e. its concise definition), its essential focus or essence and the nature of the "social" embedded in each domain, sub-domain and indicator. This is what makes them social quality domains, sub-domains and indicators as opposed to quality of life domains. Of course this does not preclude them being used as quality of life domains, sub-domains or indicators.

Policy Application

Both quality of life and social quality are promoted as positive concepts that have the potential to benefit society. While social quality provides a vision for the future, a normative statement about how the social quality of the people of Europe can and should be improved, the quality of life approach aims to measure changes in objective living standards and subjective well-being through a series of social indicators. However the absence of a theoretical rationale for quality of life tends to undermine its usefulness in the policy world. Thus the inclusion or exclusion of particular domains may be a matter of common sense or up to the individual researcher or policy maker. In other words the content of any index constructed on the basis of quality of life is always likely to be open to question and, therefore, its role in the policy process may be, at best, contested and, at worst, manipulated to suit particular interests (a deficiency that the ZUMA group has tried to address in its comprehensive framework).

The architects of social quality were motivated by a perceived imbalance in policy priorities at EU and national levels and, notwithstanding the necessity of scientific legitimation, it is to the policy making process and, by implication, the everyday circumstances of people, that the concept is directed. Thus the social quality indicators network is intended to deliver practical yardsticks to both policy makers and citizens. But the proponents are not content to stop there: the bold claim being made for social quality is that it provides a guideline for policy makers in the development and implementation of policies. It claims the ability to do so because it provides the essential connection between needs, actors and policies. Thus it can transform the abstract relationship between economic policy, social policy and employment policy in the EU policy triangle (diagram 2) into a concrete and practical one by providing the connections between them.

This integrative role of social quality requires some explanation (diagram 7). It means, first, that it encompasses all policies (economic, social, cultural, and so on). Second, it covers all phases of policy making (from design to evaluation). Third, success in the interrelationships between needs, actors and policies depends on the existence of basic conditions for social relations to develop (public fora, public ethics, systems for communication and understanding). Fourth, the appropriate method to develop policies promoting social quality is an iterative one (which depends on communication and dialogue). Fifth, policies have to be integrative in order to produce social quality (which implies, at the very least, mechanisms for coordination). Finally, the definition of problems has to be adequate – legal, legitimate and functional (which depends on consensus with regard to the notion of justice).

Diagram 7: Connecting Needs, Actors, and Policies

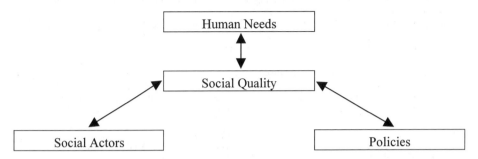

Operationalized in this way it is argued that social quality has the potential to make policies more effective and policy processes more democratic. It is not only that policy makers need more evidence about policy outcomes but also that these outcomes must be anticipated. Anticipating policy impact with regard to social quality assumes strongly and clearly formulated goals, which have to be the outcomes of a dialogue with the actors involved. However many of the actors are not represented in the policy making process. This implies a radical change in policy making processes towards democratization and the introduction of formally accepted guidelines for the promotion of dialogues between citizens and policy makers.

CONCLUSION

While quality of life has had a global reach, over the last decade in Europe its development has been striving towards comprehensiveness and, therefore, its path has mirrored the development of social quality. Indeed it is possible to see some convergence in the ZUMA formulation of quality of life and social quality. However there are still important differences between them in their theoretical foundations, in their focus (individuals versus social beings) and their potential in the policy domain. Moreover there are multiple quality of life models and, in practice, it is difficult to distinguish their respective claims for superiority. Like quality of life, social quality aims at comprehensiveness, but does so from a theoretical starting point concerned with the constitution of social relations. Providing the theory is accepted (and of course, like all theories, it may be contested) then the creation of indices should follow from the theory. This is the process that ENIQ is engaged on at present. Depending on the outcome of this work social quality could offer the prospect of consistent policy guidelines.

REFERENCES

Amsterdam Declaration on Social Quality (1997): Amsterdam, European Foundation on Social Quality.
Argyle, M. (1996): Subjective Well-Being. A. Offer (ed.): In Pursuit of the Quality of Life, Oxford: Oxford university Press, 18-45.
Beck, W., L. van der Maesen, F. Thomèse & A. Walker, A. (eds.) (2001): Social Quality: A Vision for Europe, The Hague: Kluwer International.
Beck, W., L. van der Maesen & A. Walker (eds.) (1998): The Social Quality of Europe, Bristol: Policy Press.

Berger-Schmitt, R. & H.-H. Noll (2000): Conceptual Framework and Structures of a European System of Social Indicators, EuReporting Working Paper 9, Mannheim: Centre for Survey Research and Methodology (ZUMA).

Bond, J. (1999): Quality of Life for People with Dementia: Approaches to the Challenge of Measurement. Ageing and Society 19, 561-79.

Bowling, A. (1991): Measuring Health: A Review of Quality of Life Measurement Scales, Buckingham: Open University Press.

Bowling, A. (1995a): Measuring Disease, Buckingham: Open University Press.

Bowling, A. (1995b): What Things are Important in People's Lives? A Survey of the Public's Judgements to Inform Scales of Health Related Quality of Life. Social Science and Medicine 41 (10), 1447-62.

Bowling, A. (1997): Measuring Health: A Review of Quality of Life Measurement Scales, Second Edition, Philadelphia: Open University Press.

Bradburn, N.M. (1969): The Structure of Psychological Well-Being, Chicago, Ill.: Aldine.

Bradburn, N.M. & D. Caplovitz (1965): Reports on Happiness: a Pilot Study of Behavior Related to Mental Health, Chicago, Ill.: Aldine.

Campbell, A., P. Converse & W. Rogers (1976): The Quality of American Life: Perceptions, Evaluations and Satisfactions, New York: Russell Sage Foundation.

Comité des Sages (1996): For A Europe of Civic and Social Rights, Brussels: European Commission.

Daimantopoulou, A. (2001): Foreword. Beck et al. : xv.

Böhnke, P., R. Habich & W. Zapf (2001): The Euromudule, Berlin: Social Science Research Centre.

Diener, E. (1999): Subjective Well-being: Three Decades of Progress. Psychological Bulletin 125, 276-301.

Donzelot, J. (1979): The Policy of Families, London: Hutchinson.

Doyal, L. & I. Gough (1999): A Theory of Human Need, Basingstoke: Macmilllan.

Erikson, R. (1993): Descriptions of Inequality: The Swedish Approach to Welfare Research. M. Nussbaum & A. Sen (eds.): The Quality of Life, Oxford: Oxford University Press, 67-83.

European Commission (2000): Social Policy Agenda, Brussels: DG Employment and Social Affairs.

Fallowfield, L. (1990): The Quality of Life: The Missing Measurement in Health Care, London: Souvenir Press.

Farquar, M. (1995): Elderly People's Definitions of Quality of Life. Social Science and Medicine 41 (10), 1439-46.

George, L. K. & L. B. Bearon (1980): Quality of Life in Older Persons: Meaning and Measurement, New York: Human Sciences Press.

Gill, T. M. & A. R. Feinstein (1994): A Critical Appraisal of Quality of Life Measurements. Journal of the American Medical Association 272, 619-26.

Habermas, J. (1968): Legitimation Crisis, London: Macmillan.

Honneth, A. (1994): Die soziale Dynamik von Mißachtung. Zur Ortsbestimmung einer kritischen Gesellschaftstheorie. Leviathan 22, 78-93.

Hörnquist, J. O. (1982): The Concept of Quality of Life. Scandinavian Journal of Social Medicine 10, 57-61.

Hunt, S. M. (1997): The Problem of Quality of Life. Quality of Life Research 6, 205-12.

Keyes, C. (1998): Social Well-Being. Social Psychology Quarterly 61 (2), 121-40.

Lawton, M. P. (1983): Environment and Other Determinants of Well-being in Older People. The Gerontologist 23, 349-57.

Lockwood, D. (1999): Civic Integration and Social Cohesion. I. Gough & G. Olofsson (eds.): Capitalism and Social Cohesion: Essays in Exclusion and Integration, Basingstoke: Macmillan.

Meulders, D. & R. Plasman (1998): European Economic Policies and Social Quality. Beck et al., op. cit., 19-40.

Neugarten, B. L., R. J. Havighurst & S. S. Tobin (1961): The Measurement of Life Satisfaction. Journal of Gerontology 16, 134-43.

O'Boyle, C., H. McGee, A. Hickey, C. Joyce and K. O'Malley (1993): The Schedule for the Evaluation of Individual Quality of Life, Dublin: Department of Psychology, Royal College of Surgeons in Ireland.

Oliver, J., P. Huxley, K. Bridges, and H. Mohamad (1996): Quality of Life and Mental Health Services, London: Routledge.

Peace, S., C. Holland and L. Kellaher (2003): Environment and Identity in Later Life: A Cross-setting Study, GO Findings 18, Growing Older Programme: University of Sheffield, Sheffield.

Pigou, A. C. (1929): The Economics of Welfare, London, Macmillan.

Prodi, R. (2001): Foreword. Beck et al., o. cit., xiii.
Therborn, G. (2001): On the Politics and Policy of Social Quality. Beck et al., op. cit., 19-30.
Walker, A. & B. Deacon (2003): Economic Globalisation and Policies on Ageing. Journal of Societal and
    Social Policy 2 (2), 1-18.
Walker, A. (1984): Social Planning, Oxford: Blackwell.
Wood-Dauphine, S. (1999): Assessing Quality of Life in Clinical Research. From Where Have We Come
    and Where Are We Going?. Journal of Clinical Epidemiology 52, 355-63.

3. BRINGING TOGETHER THE CONCEPTS OF QUALITY OF LIFE AND SUSTAINABILITY

Martina Schäfer, Benjamin Nölting, Lydia Illge
Center of Technology and Society, Technical University Berlin and German Institute for Economic Research Berlin, Germany

ABSTRACT

The two subjects – quality of life and sustainable development – have so far mostly been treated separately from each other, although they have a lot in common. Those engaged in either one of these fields typically ask questions like: What is a "good" life characterized by? What dimensions and qualities does it have? What is the importance of material and immaterial aspects for achieving a "good" life, and what interactions are there between them? In both debates the quality of the natural environment plays an important role.

Of course there are also differences in the debates. While the discussion about quality of life concentrates on the present well-being of groups of individuals, a large part of the discussion about sustainable development focuses on a "good" life for all people living today as well as future generations. However, this "good" life can only be maintained in the long run when natural limits – such as the carrying capacity of ecosystems and resource availability – are respected. In this way, the sustainable development concept extends the perspective from "today" to the future, from "here" to the people on the rest of the planet, and from human beings alone to their coexistence with the natural environment.

Within the following article an analytical framework "sustainable wealth" is developed which employs dimensions of the two concepts "quality of life" and "sustainability".

INTRODUCTION

The project "Reconsidering Regional Wealth. The Contribution of the Organic Agriculture and Food Sector to Quality of Life" (TU Berlin/DIW Berlin) makes an effort to bring together aspects of the concepts "quality of life" and "sustainability". The aim of the project is to uncover the contributions of the organic agriculture and food sector to quality of life, taking into consideration the requirements of sustainable development. In the first phase of the project, we have developed an analytical framework for operationalizing "sustainable wealth" by employing dimensions of both quality of life and sustainability. While the concept of sustainable development chosen for this project defines minimum criteria for global sustainable development, the concept of quality of life concentrates on criteria for objective or subjective well-being of humans.

We decided to integrate both concepts assuming that implementing the concept of sustainability at the regional level can be supported by including questions of quality of life. In this paper we first present our understandings of sustainable devel-

Wolfgang Glatzer, Susanne von Below, Matthias Stoffregen (eds.), Challenges for Quality of Life in the Contemporary World, 33-43.

opment and quality of life, the latter being an interpretation of "wealth". In a second step we lay out our approach to integrating the two concepts into a general analytical framework. Finally, we outline how we are planning to adapt this framework to the regional industrial sector namely the organic food sector in the Berlin-Brandenburg region of Germany.

THE CONCEPT OF SUSTAINABLE DEVELOPMENT

The Constitutive Elements

We refer to the approach of the German Helmholtz Association (HGF) (Kopfmüller et al., 2001) which defines the following constitutive elements: an equal treatment of intra- and intergenerative justice, a global orientation, and an anthropocentric approach.

In contrast to some other definitions of sustainable development we consider equal access (to natural, social and cultural resources) *within generations* as being a precondition for equal access *between generations*. Otherwise already existing distributive injustice would be carried over into the future (Brown-Weiss, 1989, p. 14). Given this assumption, we have to treat regional sustainability as being part of a global concept. As a consequence, it is not sufficient to look at the local or regional effects of, for instance, economic activities. Rather, the effects on the living conditions outside the region have to be considered as well. Furthermore, we assume that the main goal of sustainable development is to maintain opportunities for human development – and not preserving nature per se. However, this interpretation of human interest is not understood as a short sighted exploitative "use" of nature but refers to the conservation of the multiple functions of nature for human beings.

Thus, sustainable development within the project is defined as maintaining a minimum stock and development potentials within and between the generations, in a global perspective, and based on a broad understanding of anthropocentrism.

The Integrative Approach and the Definition of Basic Requirements

The problems sustainability research deals with are very complex and can – from our point of view – be handled best by using an integrative approach. In contrast, using an approach that treats several dimensions (e.g. social, economic, ecological) separately may exclude interactions between the dimensions. Furthermore, an integrative approach also promotes interdisciplinary work.

Unlike those integrative approaches that are based on sustainability dimensions, the HGF approach formulates *basic requirements* for sustainable development which are supposed to be valid worldwide. They are related to each other, consistent, and of equal significance. This very general approach provides the basis for our research project and will be applied to a specific societal context (e.g., a region, see below).

Modifications of the HGF Approach

We found it necessary to modify the set of objectives and rules of the HGF approach. Referring to theoretical concepts of feminist economics (Biesecker, 1997; Biesecker & Hofmeister, 2000) we find it essential to consider *reproduction processes in nature and society* (typically outside of the market economy, e. g., providing food, shelter and care at home) as being of equal importance to *production processes* (typically within the market economy).

Table 1: The General Objectives of Sustainable Development and the Basic Requirements (Rules)

General Objectives	1. Ensuring human existence	2. Preserving the potential for production and reproduction*[1]	3. Maintaining Development Potential
Rules	1.1. Protection of human health	2.1. Sustainable use of renewable resources	3.1. Equal access to education, occupation, and information
	1.2. Securing the satisfaction of basic needs	2.2. Sustainable use of non-renewable resources	3.2. Participation in societal decision making process
	1.3. Autonomous self-support	2.3. Sustainable use of the environment as a sink	3.3. Maintaining cultural heritage and cultural diversity
	1.4. Just distribution of access to the natural environment	*2.4. Preserving and supporting reproductivity of nature*	3.4. Maintaining cultural functions of nature
	1.5. Compensation of extreme differences in income and wealth	2.5. Avoiding unjustifiable technical risks	3.5. Maintaining social resources
		2.6. Sustainable development of the material conditions for production and reproduction[2]	
		2.7. Sustainable development of human potentials and knowledge for production and reproduction[2]	

Source: Kopfmüller et al., 2001, p. 172; modified and extended. Extensions of the HGF approach are printed in italics. *[1]=original: preserving the production potential; *[2]=original: Sustainable development of material, human and knowledge capital (ibid.).

We therefore extend the second general objective of the HGF approach as follows: ensuring human existence, preserving the potentials for production and reproduction of society (original: Preserving the productive potential of society) (Kopfmüller et al., 2001), maintaining the development potentials of society. Table 1 shows the set of objectives and rules that are used within our project to operationalize sustainable development.

THE CONCEPTS OF WEALTH AND QUALITY OF LIFE

In order to link sustainability to a "daily life perspective" more closely we connect sustainability research with the question of regional wealth, interpreted as quality of life. In doing so, we stress the *chances* of sustainable development in addition to the *limits* that are implied by it.

Since there is no overall set of dimensions that characterizes quality of life, we surveyed existing concepts of welfare economics, ecological economics, theoretical and empirical quality of life research, as well as local and regional grass roots initiatives. We also considered the transdisciplinary input of people from the region who are involved in the organic agriculture and food sector and who were asked to define regional wealth. – Within the project there is an ongoing cooperation with people engaged in the organic agriculture and food sector; these people are members of the project's advisory board.

From the literature survey we draw the following conclusions:
- Firstly, the monetary concept of *economic welfare* with its normative premises (individual freedom and the market as the main regulative force) is not compatible with sustainable development.
- Secondly, it is not sufficient for the empirical analysis of a "good life" (as described, e.g. by Biesecker & Hofmeister, 2000) because it concentrates on aspects to be measured in monetary terms.
- Finally, the concept of *quality of life* as a multidimensional approach seems to be compatible with the normative premises of sustainable development. Also, by considering material and immaterial, objective and subjective as well as individual and collective aspects it can be adapted well to the empirical questions of the project.

Based on a collection and categorization of the basic elements of the philosophical, empirical and participatory research on quality of life, we distinguish the following spheres:

Material sphere: The material standard of living is generally defined by the amount and the quality of goods and services offered to individuals. Besides individual consumption it is described by the public goods supply, including education, public transport, health care, child and senior care etc. We also consider the quality of the natural environment as belonging to this sphere.

Social sphere: This sphere contains interpersonal aspects and refers to the need for social affiliation which is characterized by family, friendship and care. It therefore stresses the importance of those reproductive activities for quality of life that take place outside of the market (although there is, of course, also reproduction within the market system).

Personal development and self-realization: The aspects of this sphere are very heterogeneous; they include status, professional self-realization, fun and playing, as well as societal and political participation. In a broader understanding we also include development options, meaning of life, availability of time, and aesthetics etc. in this category.

Societal sphere: In this category we consider collective values like freedom, security, participation, solidarity and justice. In table 2 we summarize the dimensions of quality of life.

The four spheres and the dimensions are – generally speaking – not contradictory to each other. However, in a specific situation they can compete with each other. In our opinion – and this is a normative predefinition – the task is to find a balance between the different values like material standard of living, freedom, justice, security, self-realization, participation and care. Quality of life is not achieved if one of the aspects is neglected or dominates. Herein, we find similarities to the concept of sustainable development aiming at integrating ecological, economic, cultural and social demands.

Table 2: Dimensions of Wealth and Quality of Life

Spheres of Quality of Life	Dimensions of Wealth and Quality of Life
Material Sphere Basic Values: Material Wealth, Well-Being	• assets (Noll, 1997) • employment, material security (Noll, 1997) • quality of food and housing (Korczak, 1995; Noll, 1997; Nussbaum, 1999; Canadian Policy Research Networks, 2001) • health (Noll, 1997; Jacksonville Community Council, 2002) • quality of the natural environment (quality of the drinking water, air quality, soil quality, diversity of animals and plants, natural landscapes) (Korczak, 1995; Independent Commission on Population and Quality of Life, 1998; Nussbaum, 1999) • supply with mobility, education, care for children and seniors, culture and leisure; regional supply (Korczak, 1995; Canadian Policy Research Network, 2001; Jacksonville Community Council, 2002)
Social Sphere Basic Value: Care	• family life (Gatersleben, 2000; Krause & Habich, 2000) • friendship (Nussbaum, 1999; Gatersleben, 2000) • love, affection, attention (Nussbaum, 1999) • sexuality (Nussbaum, 1999) • care by the social net and the community (Glatzer, 1984)

Table 2: Dimensions of Wealth and Quality of Life (continued)

Personal Development and Self-Realization Basic Values: Self-Realization, Freedom	• work (labor, caring work, community work) (quality, challenge, and development options) (Noll, 1997; Gatersleben, 2000) • learning (Independent Commission an Population and Quality of Life, 1998; Gatersleben, 2000; Jacksonville Community Council, 2002) • options for participation (Jacksonville Community Council, 2002) • esteem, reputation, status (Gatersleben, 2000) • humor, games (Nussbaum, 1999) • sense of life, aims in life (Nussbaum, 1999; Schmuck & Sheldon, 2001) • joy of life, well-being (Noll, 1997; Czikszentmihalyi, 1999) • availability of time (project's advisory board; Politische Ökologie, 1999) • aesthetics (aesthetic landscapes, cities, things, etc.) (Gatersleben, 2000; Jacksonville Community Council Inc., 2002) • regional identity (project's advisory board) • capabilities, options (Sen, 1993) • manifold socio-economic structures (project's advisory board)
Societal Sphere Basic Values: Justice, Security, Participation	• freedom (Independent Commission on Population and Quality of Life, 1998; Krause & Habich, 2000) • justice (Independent Commission on Population an Quality of Life, 1998; Krause & Habich, 2000) • equal opportunity (Krause & Habich, 1997) • solidarity (Glatzer, 1990) • security (Korczak; Krause & Habich, 2000) • participation (Independent Commission on Population and Quality of Life, 1998; Krause & Habich, 2000; Canadian Policy Research Networks, 2001)

Source: Own synopsis.

Our second normative premise is that our analysis of quality of life is gender-sensitive. This includes an acknowledgement of the differing living conditions for men and women, which are influenced by culture and society, the different subjective perspectives, interests and preferences of men and women.

INTEGRATION IN AN ANALYTICAL FRAMEWORK "SUSTAINABLE WEALTH"

The two concepts – sustainable development and quality of life – are, as has been shown above, multidimensional and normative. Furthermore, they deal with existing and desirable living conditions of human beings. In this section, we want to analyze whether it is possible to combine both concepts from an analytical and a normative perspective into a framework of "sustainable wealth".

To describe the relationship between the concepts of sustainability and wealth we bring together the rules of sustainability and the dimensions of quality of life in a cross-impact-matrix. The columns represent the rules of sustainable development. They refer to preserving basic requirements for human existence (material and im-material). They therefore define *goals*, which have to be achieved by certain meas-ures and activities. The lines of the matrix represent the dimensions of wealth and quality of life, describing the actual *status quo* at a certain point in time.

Table 3: Relationship between the Dimensions of Wealth/Quality of Life and the Rules of Sustainable Development in a Cross-impact-matrix

Rules of Sustainable Development (cf. table 1) Dimensions of Quality of Life (table 2)	Ensuring Human Existence (rules 1.1 – 1.5)	Preserving the Potentials for Production and re Production (rules 2.1 – 2.7)	Maintaining the Development Potentials (rules 3.1 – 3.5)
Material Sphere			
Social Sphere			
Personal Development and Self-realization			
Societal Sphere			

Source: Own matrix.

In the matrix, the relationship between each rule of sustainability and each dimen-sion of quality of life can be checked. We can distinguish three types of relation-ships:

a)   Relationships that apparently exist. One example is the relationship be-tween the goal "sustainable use of environment as a sink" and the qual-ity of life dimension "quality of the natural environment". Yet, only when adapting the framework to the regional level it will be possible to describe more precisely what kind of interaction exists. We expect the following cases:

Win-win-situations, which are profitable in the present and in the future. One example are measures of environmental protection which have a positive impact on the quality of life today and in the future.

Conflicting interests, which exist when development options for future generations can only be preserved by reducing the material standard of living in the present. Reducing the quantity of resource use today can for example maintain them for the future. Conflicting interests can also be expected with respect to intragenerative justice: The standard of living in some countries prevents the fulfillment of basic requirements for sustainability in other countries.

b)   In many cases it is not possible to estimate today whether there are interactions between certain rules of sustainability and quality of life dimensions; this depends very much on the *way* in which certain goals are achieved.

c)   Finally, there are cases where the realization of sustainability does not have an apparent influence on quality of life – and vice versa. Here, we refer especially to qualities that depend very much on the individual perception and way of living (like humor, friendship, sexuality etc.).

The matrix also shows which aspects of quality of life are not a constitutive part of sustainable development. Dimensions like friendship, humor or availability of time contribute to quality of life without necessarily endangering the goals of sustainable development. Systematically revealing these aspects, helps to identify options for realizing a "good life" within the limits defined by the concept of sustainable development. It is no coincidence that this category contains first of all immaterial aspects that are also mentioned in research projects about "new concepts of wealth".

Further more, the concept of quality of life draws attention to basic values like freedom, options and care, which are not a constitutive part of sustainable development at first sight. The basic requirements of sustainable development include, however, some of these basic values implicitly, for instance elements of individual freedom (equal chances, participation). Stressing values like freedom and care, and associated aspects like self-realization and options within the debate about wealth and quality of life helps to amplify the concept of sustainable development on an analytical level and increases its attractiveness for society.

The combination of the two concepts into one integrative framework seems to be possible from an analytical perspective as well as concerning the normative background. This framework may be applied to different research fields such as industrial sectors, regions, human needs, etc. Concerning conflicting interests, in our understanding the basic requirements of sustainable development have to be given priority in comparison to the dimensions of quality of life. For example individual freedom would be limited by the rules of sustainability at the point where the existence and development of human beings today or in the future are endangered.

Most conflicting interests will arise in specific situations when individual aspects of sustainability have to be balanced with certain aspects of quality of life. These questions can be dealt with systematically and transparently if – firstly, the relation to the normative premises is clear and – secondly, if those involved are included in a participatory way.

APPLICATION TO A REGIONAL INDUSTRIAL SECTOR

During the upcoming phase of our project, the integrative framework will be applied to the regional organic agriculture and food sector. To reduce the complexity of empirical research, we want to apply a sectoral analysis of problems and activities. On the one hand we want to identify the *relevant problems* for this regional industrial sector. On the other hand we want to outline which *relevant activities* of the industrial protagonists may contribute to achieving the goal of "sustainable wealth". This analysis of problems and activities will be carried out in a participatory way.

The identified fields of relevant problems can further on be described by "state" and "pressure" indicators of sustainable development, the relevant activities by "response" indicators.

The analysis of problems and activities can be structured by the rules of sustainability and the dimensions of quality of life. For each rule the following may be described:

1.   analysis of problems of the agricultural and the food sector as a whole and of the organic sector on the national and regional level.
2.   potentials for the enhancement of sustainable wealth
   a)   general structural conditions that support the fulfillment of the rules
   b)   further activities of the organic sector that contribute to the fulfillment of the rules
3.   relationship between the rules of sustainability and the dimensions of wealth in those locations that are impacted by the regional sector.

The analysis of relevant problems and activities in the region – concerning this particular sector – will be discussed with regional protagonists of this field. In addition, we will also consider the results of a "Q study" that we have carried out (a method that allows us to define different regional wealth discourses in Berlin-Brandenburg, Germany). The various "wealth discourses" in the region will provide information on the importance of certain dimensions of quality of life for certain groups of the population and allow for deriving successful ways of communicating sustainability goals.

The results will be the basis for developing a set of qualitative criteria and indicators to describe and measure sustainability and quality of life effects of a regional sector.

DEVELOPMENT OF THE EVALUATION METHOD

Within the project, we want to develop an evaluation method that analyses the contribution of the organic agriculture and food industry to regional wealth. The analytical framework and the methodological steps may also be applied to other industrial sectors, regions and fields of interest.

The evaluation has two target groups: *policy makers* of structural and regional politics (on the European, national, regional, and local level) and *protagonists of the organic agriculture and food sector*.

In direct exchange with relevant policy makers and evaluators (e.g., of LEADER + projects, the national support program for the ecological agriculture and food industry, programs for the development of regional economy etc.) the project wants to contribute to the completion and modification of evaluation methods in use with the focus on "sustainable wealth".

Another goal is to contribute to further developing companies and projects of the organic food sector and the sector as a whole. The companies and projects will receive information about their strengths and deficits. This can be the basis for improving communication about the benefits they generate for the region (and beyond). The information is also expected to reveal needs for actions – either by single companies or by the complete sector.

The evaluation method analyses multidimensional effects of the sector by using qualitative and quantitative indicators and criteria. It also combines the analysis from a macro-perspective (regional economic sector) with the analysis from a micro-perspective (single companies or projects). Some of the qualities mentioned in the concepts of wealth and quality of life can be described by objective criteria, others by subjective attitudes (for example, quality of existing cultural or educational facilities). Thus, the analysis will be carried out by collecting both objective and subjective data.

The main task for the upcoming phase of developing the evaluation method will be to find instruments and methods for presenting and evaluating the collected data.

SUMMARY AND OUTLOOK

So far, the project "Reconsidering regional wealth" has developed an analytical framework which integrates the two concepts of sustainable development and quality of life. Our motivation for combining basic requirements for sustainable development worldwide with positive qualities for a "good life" on a regional level is to achieve higher acceptance for this type of development and to find ways of a more "popular" communication. The analytical framework allows for a systematic analysis of the interactions between certain rules of sustainability and certain dimensions of wealth or quality of life and can be applied to various fields, industrial sectors and regions. In our project it will be used to analyze the contribution of the organic agriculture and food sector to "sustainable wealth".

In a next step, we will reduce the complexity of the analytical framework by analyzing the relevant problems and activities of this regional sector. This will be the basis for developing a set of indicators and criteria for the empirical analysis. This set will include quantitative and qualitative as well as objective and subjective indicators. However, questions of how to present and evaluate data appropriately still have to be dealt with.

At several stages of the project we employ participatory elements. For instance, we considered discussions with members of our advisory board (protagonists of the organic agriculture and food sector) in order to develop a broad understanding of wealth and quality of life.

In the upcoming analysis of relevant problems and activities we will first take into account the results of an empirical method that allows us to define regional discourses of wealth (Q-method). This will give us information on the weight of different quality of life dimensions. Secondly, we will discuss the relevant problems of the regional sector with regional stakeholders, including the members of our advisory board.

The evaluation method aims at supporting evaluation of European, national and regional promotion programs and of companies and projects of the organic agriculture and food sector. For this purpose, we are currently contacting evaluators in different contexts in order to find out more about their methodological needs and demands.

REFERENCES

Biesecker, A. (1997): Vom Eigennutz zur Vorsorge. Über sozial-ökologische Grundlagen einer feministischen Ökonomik. Bremer Diskussionspapiere Nr. 19, Bremen: Universität Bremen.

Biesecker, A., S. Hofmeister (2000): Vom nachhaltigen Naturkapital zur Einheit von Produktivität und Reproduktivität. Bremer Diskussionspapiere Nr. 41, Bremen: Universität Bremen.

Brown-Weiss, E. (1989): In Fairness to Future Generations. International Law, Common Patrimony and Intergenerational Equity, New York, Tokyo et al.: The United Nations University.

Canadian Policy Research Networks (ed.) (2001): Asking Citizens What Matters for Quality of Life in Canada. A Rural Lens. Quality of Life Indicators Project. Ottawa: Canadian Policy Research Networks.

Csikzentmihalyi, M. (1999): If we Are so Rich, why Aren't we Happy? American Psychologist 54 (10), S. 821-27.

Gatersleben, B. C. M. (2000): Sustainable Household Metabolism and Quality of Life. Examining the Perceived Social Sustainability of Environmentally Sustainable Household Consumption Patterns. Groningen: De Regenboog.

Glatzer, W. (1984): Haushaltsproduktion. W. Glatzer & W. Zapf (eds..): Lebensqualität in der Bundesrepublik. Objektive Lebensbedingungen und subjektives Wohlbefinden, Frankfurt/Main: Campus, 366-88.

Glatzer, W. (1990): Messung der Lebensqualität. Kruse, L., C.-F. Graumann, E.-D. Lantermann (eds.): Ökologische Psychologie. Ein Handbuch in Schlüsselbegriffen, München: Psychologie Verlags Union, 240-4.

Independent Commission on Population and Quality of Life (1998): Visionen für eine bessere Lebensqualität, Basel u.a.: Birkhäuser.

Jacksonville Community Council Inc. (2002): Quality of Life in Jacksonville. Indicators for Progress 2002: http://www.jcci.org/qol/qol.htm (30.04.2003).

Kopfmüller, J., V. Brandl, J. Jörissen, M. Paetau, G. Banse, R. Coenen & A. Grunwald (2001): Nachhaltige Entwicklung integrativ betrachtet. Konstitutive Elemente, Regeln, Indikatoren. Berlin: Edition Sigma.

Korczak, D. (1995): Lebensqualität-Atlas. Umwelt, Kultur, Wohlstand, Versorgung, Sicherheit und Gesundheit in Deutschland, Opladen: Westdeutscher Verlag.

Krause, P., R. Habich (2000): Einkommen und Lebensqualität im vereinigten Deutschland. Vierteljahreshefte für Wirtschaftsforschung 69 (2), 317-40.

Noll, H.-H. (1997): Wohlstand, Lebensqualität und Wohlbefinden in den Ländern der Europäischen Union. S. Immerfall (ed.): Die westeuropäischen Gesellschaften im Vergleich, Opladen: Leske & Budrich, S. 431-73.

Nussbaum, M. C. (1999): Gerechtigkeit oder Das gute Leben, Frankfurt/Main: Suhrkamp.

Politische Ökologie (1999): Von der Zeitnot zum Zeitwohlstand. Auf der Suche nach den rechten Zeitmaßen. Politische Ökologie 17 (57/58).

Schmuck, P., K. M. Sheldon (2001): Life Goals and Well-Being. To the Frontiers of Life Goal Research. P. Schmuck, K.M. Sheldon (eds.): Life Goals and Well-Being. Towards a Positive Psychology of Human Striving, Seattle: Hogrefe and Huber Publishers, 1-17.

Sen, A. K. (1993): Capability and Well-Being. M. C. Nussbaum & A. K. Sen (eds.): The Quality of Life. A Study Prepared for the World Institute for Development Economics Research (WIDER) of the United Nations University, Oxford: Clarendon Press, 30-53.

4. SUBJECTIVE MEASURES OF WELL-BEING IN DEVELOPING COUNTRIES

Laura Camfield

ESRC Research Group on Well-being in Developing Countries,
University of Bath, Great Britain

ABSTRACT

The paper explores the conceptual and methodological issues entailed in using subjective measures of well-being in developing countries. In the first part I define, situate, and contrast subjective quality of life (QoL), subjective well-being (SWB), and well-being. I also look at the conceptual and methodological shortcomings of subjective measures of well-being and suggest ways of overcoming these by combining different approaches. I then explore how an expanded concept of subjective quality of life fits into the theoretical framework of the UK-based Well-being in Developing Countries study (or WeD), specifically how it plans to produce a new, "development-related" profile of quality of life, drawing on the methodology of the WHOQOL group (1995; 1998).

INTRODUCTION

This paper addresses the conceptual and methodological issues entailed in using subjective measures of well-being, especially outside the Euro-American context in which they were developed. Initially I look at definitions and relationships between key terms such as subjective quality of life (QoL), subjective well-being (SWB), and well-being. I then examine the conceptual and methodological shortcomings of subjective measures of well-being and suggest ways of overcoming these by combining different approaches to investigating and measuring quality of life. The final part of the paper explores how an expanded concept of subjective quality of life fits into the theoretical framework of the UK-based Well-being in Developing Countries study (or WeD)[1]. I describe how our research will "draw insights from the psychological literature on subjective well-being and quality of life" and "explore how these approaches can add to our understanding of development processes" [WeD Research statement 2003]. I also explain how the quality of life research will "seek to reflect local understandings in constructing a new, "development-related" profile of quality of life" [2003], provisionally called the "DevQoL", using a simplified version of the definition of quality of life[2] and "spoke-wheel" methodology developed by the Quality of life group of the World Health Organization (WHOQOL 1995; 1998).

Wolfgang Glatzer, Susanne von Below, Matthias Stoffregen (eds.), Challenges for Quality of
Life in the Contemporary World, 45-59.

SUBJECTIVE QUALITY OF LIFE

I prefix quality of life with "subjective" to distinguish my understanding of it as a subjectively valued experiential state ("to have good quality of life") from its more common use as an objective composite indicator. Like health (another notoriously difficult concept to define), quality of life can be simultaneously an evaluation, a state, a goal, and an indicator, depending on context. Measuring subjective quality of life should not only involve "self-report" by the subject in response to direct questions about their quality of life, but should also enable them to indicate the importance to them of each aspect of life or more radically, specify the aspects that they consider most influential on their quality of life.

SUBJECTIVE QUALITY OF LIFE IN HEALTHCARE

Although subjective quality of life measures originated in social indicators research in the mid 1970s (e.g. Andrews and Withey's General Well-being Scale 1976), they have been used most extensively within healthcare. Quality of life measures have grown exponentially over the past decade, funded by national health services, pharmaceuticals and the US health insurance industry. Medline, the main index for medical papers, first used the phrase "quality of life" as a heading in 1975. Since then tens of thousands of papers have been published, nearly 18,000 between 2000 and 2003 alone, and there have been a proliferation of study groups, conferences and special journal issues. This remarkable growth can be linked to increasing cost consciousness in medicine, risk management by health care providers, and the need for more sensitive measures to compare treatments for chronic illness. The same pressures operate on development practitioners and their funders who need to focus their activities on demonstrably effective interventions, which have minimal negative impact on their host communities. While donors are not quite at the stage of using "Happiness-adjusted Life Years" to decide which projects to fund (Veenhoven, 2003)[3], simple tools for assessment and evaluation are needed to supplement conventional economic indicators.

There are three types of subjective quality of life measure used in healthcare:

generic (or *universal*), which can be used in sick and "healthy" populations, cover all conditions, and are brief and easier to translate (for example, the MOS Short form 36-item health survey or SF-36 [Ware, 1994]);

disease-specific (or *local*, referring to the concerns of a specific "imagined community"), which are generated from interviews with clinicians and people with particular conditions and are only appropriate to that condition; and

individualized, where individual respondents specify the areas of life that are important to them and evaluate their performance in those domains (for example, the Patient Generated Index or PGI [Ruta et al., 1994]).[4]

Although disease-specific measures are obviously relevant, generic measures are widely used as they express outcomes in a standard numerical format. This makes it possible to compare the quality of life of people with different conditions and, by combining the scores with clinical information and population preferences, to estimate the impact of different conditions and make ostensibly participatory decisions about funding priorities using metrics like the quality-adjusted life year. Individualized measures are rarely used in either healthcare or health services research, however, they offer an interesting model for our research as they are designed both to "elicit the value system of individual respondents and to quantify quality of life using this elicited system" (Browne et al., 1997, p. 742. quoted in Kavita, et al., 2003). They also enable us to investigate whether subjective quality of life is simply "the extent to which our hopes and ambitions are matched by experience" (Calnan, 1984).

MEASURING SUBJECTIVE QUALITY OF LIFE:
METHODOLOGICAL CHALLENGES

Researchers can use quality of life very loosely: One popular edited collection entitled *Quality of Life after Open-heart Surgery* focused on common medical outcomes like clinical measures and survival times. Descriptions of the measures like quality of life, health status, or well-being are used interchangeably, even though they have different histories and problems. For example, "heath-related quality of life" which is the term currently in vogue in healthcare implies that quality of life can be separated into health and non-health related components.[5]

Although quality of life is defined as a holistic concept, namely what a person feels about their life when they evaluate it as a whole, this is not necessarily what quality of life measures assess as they are biased towards "physical function" (e.g. Leplege & Hunt, 1997), despite the fact that population and patient surveys suggest it is not the most important determinant of quality of life (e.g. McDowell & Newell, 1987; Bowling, 1995). Valued aspects of life like feeling a sense of identity or belonging have been excluded for the pragmatic reason that the majority would not respond to medical interventions.[6] In the case of the WHOQOL, this would have prevented it from being used in international clinical trials, which was an important objective for the most powerful of its user groups. Another reason for exclusion is the tendency for measures to replicate themselves: Many "new" items come from reviews of existing measures which new measures are then validated against[7] (c.f. Hacking, 1995, on the tautologousness of measures of multiple personality disorder). Measures therefore need to be different enough to be perceived as new, but not so different that other measures cannot be used to "validate" them or contextualize their results.

Even studies undertaken from the individualistic perspective of biomedicine suggest the main determinants of quality of life are social and environmental. This is obscured, however, when quality of life is located solely in the "natural" body of the individual. A regression analysis of mean happiness scores from eleven quality of life surveys carried out by Michalos (2001) found that *satisfaction* with health was never the strongest predictor of happiness and in five studies failed to qualify for the final regression due to lack of statistical significance. Although self-reported health (measured with the SF-36) accounted for 4 % of explicable variance in happiness scores, this was entirely due to the scores on the mental health domain.[8]

We might also ask how the individualistic focus of the majority of quality of life measures affects their comprehensibility in societies that operate with different models of the person, for example, what is characterized as internal or external to a person. On a purely practical level, many of the normative reference points for functional scales may be irrelevant; for example, the majority of the functional items in French blindness scales (e.g., "Can you drive a car?", "Can you see street lamps?") needed to be reworked ("Do you know which way is east?" –necessary to establish orientation for prayer, "Do you fall into holes?"), so they could be used in francophone Mali (Leplege et al., 1999). Problems of translation go beyond vocabulary to the tacit models underlying the measures, which exemplify the operation of Lukes's second and third levels of power (1986). The models not only set the agenda but shape the ways in which the issues can be thought about in the first place; for example, the Cartesian dualism of separate physical and psychological domains and the way the social domain, if it has been included, is represented as external to the person. The veteran quality of life researcher Hunt observes ironically that "the ethnocentricity of assuming that a measure developed in, say, the USA, or England, will be applicable (after adaptation) in pretty much any country or language in the world (…) is highlighted if one imagines the chances of a health questionnaire developed in Bali, Nigeria, or Hong Kong, being deemed suitable for use in Newcastle, Newark, or Nice" (1999). Bearing in mind the way these methodological issues multiply when quality of life measures are used cross-culturally, we might ask what is driving the international expansion of quality of life measurement?

MEASURING SUBJECTIVE QUALITY OF LIFE CROSS-CULTURALLY: THE WHOQOL MEASURE

Internationally, the World Health Organisation or WHO has been one of the keenest advocates of quality of life, which is consonant with its definition of health as "a state of complete physical, mental and social well-being, and not merely the absence of disease or infirmity (…) whose realization requires the action of many other social and economic sectors". In 1991 the WHO formed the WHOQOL group to develop a measure that would assess quality of life, rather than merely the impact of disease and impairment, perceived health, or functional status, as existing "quality of life" measures did. This measure would combat "the increasingly mechanistic model of medicine" and use quality of life assessments to introduce a "humanistic element into healthcare", supporting the WHO's "continued promotion of an holistic approach to health and healthcare".

The WHOQOL's "spoke-wheel" development process, where a common and consensually derived methodology enabled it to be developed simultaneously in 15 countries, is now recognized as the gold standard for international projects (WHO-Quality of Life, 1998). However, it is a resource-intensive process that requires access to translation and transcription facilities, which may not be available in most developing countries.[9] The original WHOQOL process was also not fully participatory as the six domains of quality of life were defined in advance by a small group of "experts", setting the agenda for the population focus groups who generated the items. Although there was some iteration between the advisory group and the focus groups, the structure of the instrument did not change substantially (a domain with a single facet was added on spirituality, religion and personal beliefs) and continued to reflect similar measures in the field. We plan to approach the topic as openly as possible with a diverse sample of respondents from the rural and urban sites where we are working. The researchers will use a range of qualitative methods, including semi-structured interviews with individuals and groups and participatory techniques, and will already have spent some time in the site building relationships with local people. The findings of the exploratory fieldwork will be combined with data from the country workshops on quality of life[10] to create a "quality of life framework", which will be discussed with "focus-groups" of local people and development practitioners. Although focus group research has been criticized for lack of representativeness and power imbalances, these can be surmounted by choosing an appropriate activity (e.g. exploring areas of consensus rather than difference), sampling carefully, and using skilled and reflexive facilitators. Historically the qualitative contribution to measure development has been neglected, possibly due to researchers' discomfort with the less scientific aspects of the process. We plan to use the expertise of the WeD team in qualitative methods (and their field experience) to ground the DevQoL, enabling it to provide a more nuanced analysis of people's lives.

We will get people to prioritize aspects of quality of life using either the methodology of the WHOQOL-100 or the Person Generated Index[11], depending on which works best in the field. This will enable us to measure what effect a gap between people's aspirations and achievements has on their evaluations of quality of life, a theme already identified as important by researchers like Michalos (1985), Calnan (1984) and Skevington et al. (Skevington & O'Connell, 2003).

Despite the apparent comprehensiveness of the 24 WHOQOL facets, which range from self-esteem to transport, the WHOQOL-100 presents a fragmented and disembodied view of life. It clearly needs strengthening in areas like economic, political and financial relationships, security, and social inclusion; omissions confirmed by our theoretical frameworks and empirical data from the quality of life workshops. Working from the WHOQOL model in the way we have described will hopefully enable the DevQoL to fulfill the promise of the WHOQOL group's original definition by setting individual perceptions of quality of life in their cultural and social context.

The observations we have made about the WHOQOL apply with greater force to other quality of life measures in its field. But is it surprising that measures designed by western psychologists for use by doctors and economists should be individualistic, non-political, and curiously disembodied? Having discussed the slightly different use of quality of life measurement within healthcare, in the next part of the paper, I will define SWB and Well-being, examine conventional indicators of life satisfaction and happiness, and draw some methodological conclusions.

SUBJECTIVE WELL-BEING (SWB)

SWB is usually defined as a subjective measurement that combines the presence of positive emotions and absence of negative emotions with overall satisfaction with life (Diener, 1984). As with quality of life, however, measures of SWB can present a different picture. For example, Cummins includes subjective and objective measures of material well-being, health, productivity, intimacy, safety, place in community, and emotional well-being (Cummins, 1997), which may be why it has been described as a measure of "need satisfaction" rather than SWB.[12] Ryff's six factor measure of SWB is similarly expansive, though possibly more culturally specific[13], comprising self-acceptance, personal growth, purpose in life, positive relations with others, autonomy, happiness and environmental mastery (Ryff, 1995).

SWB is most commonly measured using self-report questions about happiness or life satisfaction, the results of which have become increasingly important to the social indicators movement, "economists of happiness" like Clarke and Oswald, and policy makers (e.g. the recent Cabinet Office report on the implication of "life satisfaction" for UK government policy, Strategy Unit, 2002). In the next part of the paper I explore some of the problems with standard measures of happiness and life satisfaction and link my critique back to the WHOQOL through its characterization as a measure of life satisfaction rather than quality of life.

HAPPINESS AND LIFE SATISFACTION

Standard questions about happiness and life satisfaction[14] are a routine part of data sets like the World Values Survey (http://wvs.isr.umich.edu/), the Eurobarometer (http://europa.eu.int/comm/public_opinion/), and the South African General Household survey (http://www.statssa.gov.za/) and have been collated for comparative purposes in the World Database of Happiness (http://www.eur.nl/fsw/research/ happiness/). There are, however, some problems with using this data. Firstly, the phrasing of the questions and the response scales used were not uniform across countries and time periods, which may have affected responses. Secondly, "global" questions on subjective well-being (e.g. "Taking everything as a whole, how is your quality of life?") are more prone to cognitive or mood biases than domain specific ones (Schwartz & Strack, 1999) and may also be very difficult to answer sensibly! We hope to avoid this problem by making the questions sufficiently specific to ensure that they are comprehensible, meaningful and can be answered accurately. It is more useful to know that people are unhappy with their working conditions, or that they were happier before their employer used a loan from a micro-credit scheme to install unsafe machinery, than it is to know their level of satisfaction overall, whether this is measured on a 5, 11 or 100 point scale!

Although positive and negative feelings represent only two of the 24 domains of the WHOQOL, half the items are phrased in terms of satisfaction (for example, "how satisfied are you with your sleep?"), possibly due to the fact that the English language offers a limited number of ways to ask people to evaluate aspects of their life. This prompted the quality of life researchers Williams (2000) and Hagerty (Hagerty et al., 2001) to controversially suggest it be compared with measures of life satisfaction rather than quality of life. This is not necessarily a compliment. Although life satisfaction has been widely used as a more "cognitive" (and thus scientific) measure of SWB than happiness[15], the concept has its own problems: The coordinator of a project investigating well-being in the UK stopped asking people how satisfied they were because the word sounded "dead" and provoked responses like "well, I mustn't grumble..." (Nick Marks, New Economics Foundation, personal communication). Similarly, initial research by the WeD teams in Thailand and Peru questioned the meaningfulness of the concept when it related to circumstances that people could not control or change, as their only option was satisfaction (personal communication). Life satisfaction becomes redundant in situations where people have little control or choice in the areas that matter to them and unhelpfully evokes Western discourses of voluntarism and consumer power.

While the word satisfaction is described as universally meaningful, this does not mean it has the same meaning universally: Killian's review of "patient satisfaction" studies in the UK described how being satisfied with a treatment can encompass feelings of resignation and helplessness and a belief that the treatment is useless (Kilian et al., 1999). Recent psychological research (Schimmack et al., 2002) also suggests a personality "trait-level" propensity to be satisfied with life is a more important determinant of life satisfaction scores than objective life circumstances, which may reduce its utility as a social indicator. This is an interesting addition to the studies of identical and non-identical twins carried out by Hamer (1996) and Lykken and Tellegen (1996) which measured the happiness of twins raised apart and together and concluded that up to 80 % of the stable differences in life satisfaction were heritable. Less than 3 % of variance was explained by socio-economic status, educational attainment, family income, marital status and religious commitment.

Although being happy and/or satisfied with life are intrinsically valuable states, and ones that have been neglected in development (Clark, 2000), we cannot presume that they have the same meaning or priority in every country or situation. Consequently, a measure is needed that assesses the presence of both locally valued experiential states and the fulfillment of more prosaic needs for material, relational, and cultural resources. This state of optimum experiential and need satisfaction we have provisionally called "development-related quality of life", drawing on the WeD group's stipulative definition of "development" as interventions aiming to produce a state where the needs that people value are satisfied. The prefix "development-related" functions in the same way as "health-related" quality of life to focus our attention on the aspects of quality of life that will be affected by development projects, recognizing that their effects may be multi-dimensional and unintended. Perhaps an exploration of the comparatively uncontested concept of well-being can help us move towards a better understanding of how development-related quality of life should be defined and measured?

WELL-BEING

The "constituent elements" of well-being or a good form of human life have been understood respectively as satisfaction of desires or preferences, prudential values (arguably the human desire account taken to its logical limit), positive freedoms, and human capabilities or needs. All these accounts present certain problems, for example, desires may be other-directed, ill informed, adaptive, or not reflect the person's values. While certain shared values or concepts of quality of life are necessary for mutual intelligibility, they do not comprise a comprehensive vision of good quality of life. Nor can their priority be assumed in any situation; I am reminded of an Angolan child refugee who when asked how it felt to be chased from her home by a murderous gang – yes, journalists do ask these sort of things – said that the worst part was losing her one good set of clothes because she now could not appear in public without shame. This kind of understanding (what Saltmarshe calls "seen from the corner of the eye", 2003) is highly valued by qualitative researchers. The need to avoid foreclosing on it inspired Clark's open-ended questionnaire for exploring poor South Africans' conceptions of a good life (2000)[16], which may be included within the WeD project. Although the lists it produced closely resemble lists of basic needs or core values, the process also produced some surprises. For example, the priority given to Coca-Cola™, offered a greater understanding of the rationality underlying people's choices through an exploration of the many different functionings this product could support.[17]

While Subjective Quality of life and SWB are often treated as interchangeable, I argue that Subjective Quality of life actually has more in common with well-being. Both concepts are multi-dimensional, context specific, and incorporate things people have reason to value, as well as their wants and needs. The similarity is apparent when we compare Clark's definition of well-being as "the constituent elements of a good form of human life – whatever that may be" (2000) with the WHOQOL group's definition of quality of life as "an individual's perceptions of their position in life in the context of the culture and value systems in which they live and in relation to their goals, expectations, standards and concerns" (1995). They differ only in two respects: firstly, Clark's method for measuring well-being reflects his foundational definition in a way that the WHOQOL-100 does not. For example, unlike individualized measures of quality of life like the Schedule for the Evaluation of Individual Quality of Life (SeiQoL) (O'Boyle et al., 1992) or Patient Generated Index (PGI) (Ruta et al., 1994) the WHOQOL -100 does not allow people to specify their concerns or goals although they can indicate priority among the choices offered to them.

The reasons for this are pragmatic – setting parameters for people's responses ensures the process is quick, comparable, easy to analyze, and more "scientific", especially if you believe people cannot reliably articulate what is important to them. Secondly, Clark's definition does not explicitly acknowledge the cultural and structural constraints on people's conception of the good life, or the potential tension between the individual and the collective if a good life for one individual involves exploiting or abusing another. The additional elements of the WHOQOL definition, for example, the role of social norms in shaping people's expectations, aims, perceptions of success and failure, and overall evaluations of quality of life, may be best explored qualitatively.[18]

COMBINING APPROACHES TO MEASURING SWB

I suspect that the elision of subjective Quality of life and SWB has occurred for two reasons; firstly, similarities in their language of measurement, which I describe below. Secondly, both are perceived as the domain of psychologists, which may account for their individual and ethnocentric focus. Current debates over measurement have obscured the theoretical distinctions between Quality of life and SWB, due to what Veenhoven describes as their "domination by psychometricians, who focus [...] on factor loadings, reliability issues and inter-test correlations" at the expense of a "clear answer to the question of what these measures actually measure" (Veenhoven, 2000, pp. 19-20).

Some theorists from quality of life and SWB backgrounds have also attempted to bring the two concepts into a fruitful relationship. For example, Kahneman, Diener, and Schwarz in their preface to "Hedonic Psychology" (1999). Kahneman et al. suggest that analyses of quality of life should include cultural and social context, individual values, capabilities and objective circumstances, and SWB. They claim that "any evaluation of quality of life is embedded in the cultural and social context of both the subject and the evaluator [...and] cannot be reduced to the balance of pleasure and pain, or to assessments of subjective life-satisfaction" (ibid., p. X). However, they place experiences of pleasure and SWB "at the centre of the story" (undoubtedly influenced by their disciplinary and cultural backgrounds), which may not be true of less hedonistic societies.

Veenhoven also observed little consensus over the meaning of quality of life and well-being (2000). Meanings are often confined to their own discursive communities, there is marked divergence between scientific definitions and common usage, and the inclusiveness of the terms makes them difficult to operationalize. He attempts to overcome this by restating the fundamental questions of "what is quality?" and "whose life quality are we talking about?" He divides quality of life into opportunities and outcomes and external and internal, for example, environmental "livability" and personal "life-ability" or capabilities. Veenhoven also distinguishes between the objective utility and subjective appreciation of life, basically its social meaning or significance versus the degree of felt satisfaction or happiness. He admits that the former is more difficult to measure quantitatively than the latter, especially as in the short-term individual happiness is a very poor indicator of social utility!

USING MEASURES OF SUBJECTIVE WELL-BEING IN THE WED FIELD SITES

In the remainder of the paper I argue that, especially for work in developing country contexts, we need to develop a measure that combines the most useful concepts and methods from Quality of life, SWB and well-being literatures. This would be based on a more expansive and actor-oriented conception of Quality of life and supplemented by extensive, in-depth qualitative work. This is essential not only so that the measure will be meaningful to its respondents but also so the data will be meaningful to the analysts. For example, curves plotted with WHOQOL data from different countries tend to show that responses to the items are concentrated around points 3 and 4 of the 5 point response scale, "neither satisfied nor dissatisfied" and "satisfied" (e.g. WHOQOL Group, 1998). While this could mean that the WHOQOL represents dimensions that are common to all humans, another interpretation has been offered by Bourdieu in his critique of methods of surveying opinion (1989). He suggests this represents nothing more than the human tendency to circle the middle number in a questionnaire, particularly when you are uncertain what is being asked or for what purpose the data will be used. This finding could also support the characterization of the WHOQOL as a life satisfaction measure since life satisfaction measures have a similar response pattern of means of 75+2.5 in western nations and 70+5 in non-western nations (Cummins, 2002). This may be due to the Positive Cognitive Biases described in Cummins and Nistico's homeostatic theory of SWB (2000), or less charitably, because they share the methodological shortcomings identified by Bourdieu.

In the case of the WHOQOL, this may be exacerbated by the abstract and general nature of the questions, for example, "how available to you is the information that you need in everyday life?" which were designed so they would be equally meaningful (or less) across all countries. When the questionnaire is interview-administered to respondents who cannot read or write (the majority of participants in our study) it puts the researcher in an unenviable position since the protocol forbids them from answering the obvious question "information for what?"

The question of how much support to give to respondents is an important one – on the one hand we do not want to inadvertently bias the results of the measure (producing results that would not be acceptable to our psychological peers), but on the other the interview-administration needs to be a relaxed and almost conversational interaction where respondents feel able to ask the interviewer for clarification or decide on a response category in negotiation with other household members. Sadly, the realities of field research bears little resemblance to the quasi-experimental conditions demanded by protocols for instrument administration (for example, most measures contain a check box to indicate if they have been filled in unassisted; if this has not been checked, the data is usually excluded).

This is particularly problematic for the WHOQOL's social domain as while qualitative research (e.g. Resource Profiles research in South Asia, Thailand, and Eastern Europe, cf.. McGregor, 2000) suggests it is one of the most important aspects of people's lives, the domain is psychometrically weak (O'Carroll et al., 2000; Hagerty et al., 2001). The reason for this is that it only has three facets, one of which, sexual activity, is prone to missing data even when the person is responding in the privacy of their own bedroom, rather than to an interviewer of a different gender or generation, in front of their entire household. The example highlights the fallacy of assuming that responses to the measure will be anonymous and unmediated, as would be expected in a similar study in Britain.[19]

Length is a more obvious problem when measures are interview administered and researchers coming from health-related quality of life can tend to over estimate the enthusiasm of respondents (I recall one study that sent pancreatic transplant recipients eleven different measures, Milde et al., 1992). People with limiting conditions are an unusually compliant and conscientious group (survey response rates average 85 %) and may have plenty of time to fill. They may also have grown up in a culture where surveys are a common form of democratic participation and self-exploration; I doubt many participants in our study will thank us for the opportunity to respond to a very personal questionnaire because they "learnt so much about themselves"![20] There is an obvious tension within WeD between creating a measure that will be more inclusive and locally relevant than anything that has gone before but will not take hours to administer. It also needs to be scientific (i.e. valid and replicable) but able to be administered in a relaxed and conversational way. In short, it needs to be an "appropriate technology". I do not believe these aims are irreconcilable, but it is important to be aware of the issues that have impeded similar projects in the past.

WED'S MIXED-METHOD APPROACH
TO EXPLORING SUBJECTIVE WELL-BEING

Having explored some of the problems with the existing forms of quality of life measurement, the question still remains as to how the WeD project will investigate subjective quality of life. In order to capture the different dimensions of quality of life explored in this paper, we will be triangulating our data using a mixed methodology, or, in lay terms, covering our bets. We plan to combine detailed qualitative research with the development of a quality of life measure that is recognized as sound in quality of life circles, works well with rural respondents in developing countries, is acceptable to local development practitioners, and does not contradict our commitment to bringing together "local" and "universal" perspectives on quality of life and well-being. This commitment is theoretically as well as methodologically significant since one of the roles of the quality of life input is to facilitate communication between the universal, represented by Doyal and Gough's *Theory of Human Needs* (1991), and the local, represented by the *Resource Profiles Approach* (McGregor, 2000). The *Theory of Human Needs* develops a cross-cultural concept of basic needs as universal prerequisites that enable sustained participation in a chosen form of life. Its original dimensions of participation, physical health and autonomy may be extended to include psychological well-being and competences, and affiliation and belongingness (Gough, personal communication). The *Resource Profiles Approach* works at the local level using an actor-oriented perspective. It posits that individuals, households and communities in developing countries actively "manage" a complex of resources (material, human, social, cultural, and natural) to achieve the best possible outcome. Communication between the levels is conceptually facilitated by the notion of quality of life. The quality of life research will be attempting to produce a universal measure that is grounded in local realities, and supplement it with qualitative investigations of people's understandings of good quality of life and strategies for achieving it.

Developing the measure will involve investigating the categories and components of quality of life in the WeD field sites through semi-structured 'interactions' with a diverse range of informants and validating the emergent quality of life framework with local people and other key stakeholders. This will enable us to distinguish between components of quality of life at the universal level and those of the locality and the culture-group, and explore the relationship between them. We will also assess the level at which it is possible to produce a measure of quality of life that is meaningful to respondents, analysts and development practitioners and develop methods that will best achieve this. I will not elaborate further on the proposed methodology as this information is available in papers produced by the WHOQOL group (1995; 1998). It has been expanded to include the new technique of "cognitive debriefing", which involves extensive interviews exploring how people interpret and respond to the measure. This will ensure that in every country we are measuring not only what we *should* be measuring but what we think we are measuring. We will use two "global" questions about happiness and life satisfaction (translated into the appropriate local terms) as these will enable interesting comparisons with existing data sets and may also adapt the Satisfaction with Life (SWLS) (Diener et al., 1985) and Positive and Negative Affect (PANAS) (Watson et al., 1988) scales.

Additionally, we plan to use a modified version of the SEIQoL or the "global" version of the PGI (now called the "Person Generated Index") (Ruta, 1997), where people would be asked to nominate the areas of their life that have most influence on their quality of life (or that of their household) and indicate their relative importance. This would be done using a common participatory technique like distributing a number of coins across the areas to represent their relative influence.[21] We could then ask them to assess their current status in each of these areas using the same technique. The advantage of this process is that it is quick, simple, can be carried out using participatory techniques, and, compared to a 100 item questionnaire, involves minimal translation. This means it can be repeated many times during fieldwork to explore issues of seasonality. Although the data produced will have intra rather than inter-personal comparability, it will be possible to compare the extent of the gap between expectations and achievements, which we expect to correlate significantly with SWB. It also provides a good starting point for discussions about how the respondent defines quality of life and prioritorizes the different elements within it, and why their quality of life has changed over the preceding period.

Using these approaches we hope to cover all aspects of people's subjective quality of life and communicate with people who find responding to a questionnaire or heavily structured interview an alienating experience. Objective quality of life will not be neglected, of course, and we hope to have sufficient data, combined with reflexive accounts of process, to enable a fruitful exploration of any discrepancies between the two. Perhaps by refusing to prioritize objective over subjective or qualitative over quantitative we are storing up trouble for the data analysis phase, but we hope this radical openness will enable us to learn from all the approaches used and ultimately provide methodological guidance as well as comprehensive data sets to future researchers in this field.

NOTES

1   WeD is developing a framework for studying poverty, inequality and quality of life in four developing countries (Bangladesh, Thailand, Ethiopia, and Peru).
2   "An individual's perception of their position in life, in the context of the culture in which they live" (adapted from [WHOQOL Group 1993 & 1995])
3   These combine life satisfaction scores with life expectancy and were proposed as a possible measure at the ISOQOLS conference 2003 (see also Veenhoven, 1996).
4   Individualized measures are becoming increasingly influential within medicine because they have high 'face' and 'content' validity and directly address the changes that are important to patients (see Joyce et al [1999] for a useful review). In relation to development practice they could perform an analogous role in highlighting areas of people's lives where intervention could be focused, or warning where poorly researched interventions might damage the quality of life of the people they are intended to benefit.
5   See Michalos (2001) for a critique of this concept, which he sees as both an example of biomedical expansionism (health = quality of life) and confounded (if health = quality of life, then the concept of health-related quality of life is as meaningless as "quality of life-related quality of life" would be!)
6   I observed this process during the creation of the Multiple Sclerosis Impact Scale-29 item (Hobart et al., 2001) where statements that the researchers did not think related to quality of life (e.g., reactions

to diagnosis) were excluded from the first draft of the measure. Subsequently, items related to "coping with multiple sclerosis" and the "positive impact of multiple sclerosis" were excluded as "irrelevant", although they were obviously relevant to the people who generated them.

7   Fox-Rushby attributes this to the "nature of research careers" where "any one researcher has the opportunity to influence the development of more than one instrument, either by moving between research institutions, by sitting on different steering committees, or by becoming part of the many flourishing international groups" (for example, one WHOQOL researcher has also been involved in the IHQL and EuroQOL and another in the SIP and QWB) (1995).

8   This is good news for critics like Ravallion (2000) who argue that the effects of personality and mood make subjective measures unreliable (or for global manufacturers of anti-depressants who were quick incorporate disease rankings from the Global Burden Disease study in their marketing strategy, WHO, 2000).

9   We estimated that if we followed the WHOQOL protocol exactly, each language version of the DevQoL would require 680 hours of transcription and 920 hours of translation.

10   These were conducted in all four countries during our initial visits between June and October 2003, using a protocol piloted among Country representatives at the WeD inaugural workshop in Bath (January 2003).

11   The WHOQOL asks people to rate each item using a 5 point Likert scale, for example "How important to you is your quality of life? 1: Not important […] 5: Extremely important" and the PGI invites them to distribute points or coins across their five priority areas.

12   It also contains an element of individual weighting through importance weightings and is usually administered alongside a measure of "national well-being".

13   Christopher (1999) makes a powerful critique of the cultural specificity of the model of well-being underlying Ryff's measure.

14   For example, "All things considered, how satisfied or dissatisfied are you with your life-as-a-whole now? 1 dissatisfied… 10 satisfied" (Veenhoven, 2001, 20022; www.eur.nl/fsw/research/happiness).

15   Cf. Veenhoven's "World Database of Happiness Research", which, despite its name, uses a standard life satisfaction question.

16   Clark's approach is an interesting mix of philosophy (fully formed conceptions of the good life can be accessed through philosophical enquiry) and inverted snobbery (ordinary people are the best judge of what constitutes a good life and it does not include opera!) There has been debate within the WeD group over whether people's values can be explored through abstract questioning, or, setting this question aside, how they translate to behavior (a point also made by critics of health economic methods for generating population valuations of different health states).

17   Unfortunately, due to the limitations of survey research on a small budget, these meanings could not be fully explored in subsequent qualitative work. This lack of follow-up has also been a problem in quality of life work where bizarre or intriguing results have not been investigated or contextualized (for example, why participants from a study using the Rosser Well-being Scale described "feeling a lack of ambition" as 45 % worse than "complete bowel incontinence", Rosser et al., 1992).

18   One of the WeD team members is piloting a protocol in 21 villages in Ethiopia, which explores these themes through participatory and qualitative work with groups and individuals (for example, identifying local understandings of well-being, quality of life and poverty) (Ethiopia WeD Research Programme 2003).

19   Of course, even this cannot be assumed. During my Ph.D. I interviewed six people who had responded to a pilot questionnaire measuring quality of life in Dystonia (Camfield, 2002). Their accounts illustrated the ways questionnaires can be "destabilized" by respondents not behaving in the expected manner or engaging in "anti-programs" (Latour, 1992) like using a proxy respondent, missing out questions, answering "sarcastically", or responding on the basis of age or other conditions.

20   This interaction was described to me by a researcher on a project designing a measure of the health-related quality of life of older adults.

21   See Bevan et al, 2003 for an account of a 'very informal pilot' of this technique, which took place in Ethiopia during our grounding and piloting phase.

REFERENCES

Andrews, F., Withey, S. (1976): Social Indicators of Well-being: American Perceptions of Quality of Life, New York: Plenum Press.

Bevan P., K. Kebede & A. Pankhurst A. (2003): A Report on a very Informal Pilot of the Person Generated Index© of Quality of Life in Ethiopia (unpublished).

Bowling, A. (1995): A Survey of the Public's Judgements to Inform Scales of Quality of Life Social Science and Medicine 41, 1411-17.

Calnan, K. C. (1984): Quality of Life in Cancer Patients – A Hypothesis. Journal of Medicinal Ethics 10, 124.

Camfield, L. (2002): Measuring Quality of Life in Dystonia: An Ethnography of Contested Representations, London: PhD thesis, University of London.

Christopher, J. C. (1999): Situating Psychological Well-being: Exploring the Cultural Roots of its Theory and Research. Journal of Counseling and Development 77, 141-52.

Clark, D. (2000): Visions of Development: A Study of Human Values, Cheltenham: Edward Elgar.

Cummins, R. A. (1997): Comprehensive Quality of Life Scale – Adult. Manual, 5th edition, Melbourne: School of Psychology, Deakin University.

Cummins, R. A. (2002): Normative Life Satisfaction: Measurement Issues and a Homeostatic Model. Social Indicators Research 64, 225-56.

Cummins, R. A & H. Nistico (2002): Maintaining Life Satisfaction: The Role of Positive Cognitive Bias. Journal of Happiness Studies 3 (1), 37-69.

Diener, E. (1984): Subjective Well-being. Psychological Bulletin 95 (3), 542-75.

Doyal, L. & I. Gough (1991): A Theory of Human Need, London: Macmillan.

Ethiopia WeD Research Programme (2003): Well-being and Ill-being Dynamics in Ethiopia. A Study in 20 Rural Sites (unpublished).

Fox-Rushby, J. & M. Parker (1995): Culture and the Measurement of Health-related Quality of Life, European Review of Applied Psychology 45 (4), 257-63.

Hacking, I. (1995): Rewriting the Soul. Multiple Personality and the Sciences of Memory, New York: Princeton.

Hagerty, M. R., R. A. Cummins, A. L. Ferriss, K. C. Land, A. C. Michalos, M. Peterson, A. Sharpe, J. Sirgy & J. Vogel (2001): Quality of Life Indexes for National Policy: Review and Agenda for Research. Social Indicators Research 20 (9), 225-40.

Hamer, D. H. (1996): The Heritability of Happiness. Nature Genetics 14 (2), 125-6.

Hobart, J., D. Lamping, R. Fitzpatrick, A. Riazi & A. Thompson (2001): The Multiple Sclerosis Impact Scale (MSIS-29): A New Patient-based Outcome Measure. Brain 124 (5), 962-73.

Hunt, S. M. (1999): The Researcher's Tale: A Story of Virtue Lost and Regained. C. R. B. Joyce, C. A. O'Boyle & H. McGee (eds.): Individual Quality of Life: Approaches to Conceptualization and Measurement, Amsterdam: Harwood.

O'Carroll, R. E., K. Smith, M. Couston, J. A. Cossar & P. C. Hayes (2000): A Comparison of the WHO-Quality of Life-100 and the WHO-Quality of Life-BREF in Detecting Change in Quality of Life Following Liver Transplantation. Quality of Life Research 9, 121-4.

Kahneman, D., E. Diener & N. Schwarz (1999): Preface. Kahneman, D., E. Diener, & N. Schwarz (eds.): Well-being: The Foundations of Hedonic Psychology, New York: Russell Sage Foundation.

Kind, P., R. Rosser & A. Williams. (1982): Valuation of the Quality of Life: Some Psychometric Evidence. M. W. Jones-Lee (ed.): The Value of Life and Safety, Amsterdam: Elsevier.

Latour, B. (1992): Where are the Missing Masses? The Sociology of a Few Mundane Artifacts. W. Bjiker, & J. Law (eds.): Shaping Technology, Building Society: Studies in Sociotechnological Change, Cambridge, Mass.: MIT Press.

Leplege, A. & S. Hunt (1997): The Problem of Quality of Life in Medicine, Journal of the American Medical Association 278, 47-50.

Lukes, S. (1986): Power, Oxford: Basil Blackwell.

Lykken, D. & A. Tellegen (1996): Happiness is a Stochastic Phenomenon. Psychological Science 7 (3), 186-9.

McDowell, I. & C. Newell (1987): Measuring Health, Oxford: Oxford University Press.

McGregor, J. A. (2000): A Poverty of Agency: Resource Management Amongst Poor People in Bangladesh (unpublished).

Michalos, A. C. (1985): Multiple Discrepancies Theory (MDT). Social Indicators Research 16, 347-413.

Michalos, A. C. (2001): Social Indicators Research and Health-Related Quality of Life Research. Plenary Session ISQOLS 2001 (unpublished).

Milde, F. K, L. K. Hart, P. S. Zehr (1992): Quality of Life of Pancreatic Transplant Recipients. Diabetes Care 15, 1459-63.

O'Boyle, C., H. McGee, A. Hickey, K. O'Malley & C. R. B. Joyce (1992): Individual Quality of Life in Patients Undergoing Hip Replacement. Lancet 339, 1088-91.

Ravallion, M. & M. Lokshin (2001): Identifying Welfare Effects from Subjective Questions. Economica 68, 335-57.

Rosser, R., M. Cottee, R. Rabin& C. Selai (1992): Index of Health-related Quality of Life. A. Hopkins (ed.): Measures of Quality of Life and the Uses to which such Measures May Be Put, London: RCP.

Ruta, D. A., A. M. Garratt, M. Leng, I. T. Russell, & L. M. MacDonald (1994): A New Approach to the Measurement of Quality of Life. The Patient Generated Index. Medical Care 32 (11), 1109-26.

Ruta, D. (1997): Managing Health and Measuring Health Outcomes. Paper presented at: Managing and Measuring Health Outcomes: From Policy to Practice, Canberra: University of Wollongong.

Ryff, C. D. (1995): Psychological Well-being in Adult Life. Current Directions in Psychological Science 4 (4), 99-104.

Sartorius, N., W. Kuyken (1994): Translation of Health Instruments. J. Orley & W. Kuyken (eds.): Quality of Life Assessment: International Perspectives, Heidelberg: Springer Verlag.

Schimmack, U., E. Diener & S. Oishi (2002): Life-satisfaction is a Momentary Judgement and a Stable Personality Characteristic: The Use of Chronically Accessible and Stable Sources. Journal of Personality and Social Psychology 70 (3), 345-84.

Schwarz, N. & F. Strack: Reports of Subjective Well-being: Judgmental Processes and their Methodological Implications. D. Kahneman, E. Diener & N. Schwarz (eds.): Well-being: The Foundations of Hedonic Psychology, New York: Russell Sage Foundation, 61-84.

Skevington, S. & K. O'Connell, K. (2003): Assessing the Importance of Quality of Life Using the WHO-Quality of Life-100: How can we Identify Poor Quality of Life? (in press).

Strategy Unit (2002): Life Satisfaction: The State of Knowledge and Implications for Government, London: Cabinet Office.

Veenhoven, R. (1996): Happy Life-Expectancy. Social Indicators Research 39 (1), 1-58.

Veenhoven, R. (2000): The Four Qualities of Life. Ordering Concepts and Measures of the Good Life. Journal of Happiness Studies 1, 1-39.

Ware, J. E., C. D. Sherbourne (1992): The MOS Short form 36-item health survey (SF-36): Conceptual Framework and Item Selection. Medical Care 30, 473-83.

WHO-Quality of Life Group (1995): The World Health Organisation Quality of Life Assessment (WHO-Quality of Life): Position Paper from the World Health Organisation. Social Science and Medicine 41, 1403-9.

WHO-Quality of Life Group (1998): The WHO Quality of Life Assessment (WHO-Quality of Life): Development and General Psychometric Properties. Social Science and Medicine 46, 1569-85.

Williams, J. I. (2000): Ready, Set, Stop and Standing. Journal of Clinical Epidemiology, 53, pp. 25-7.

5. TOWARDS ENHANCING THE QUALITY OF LIFE IN AFRICA

Challenges, Problems, and Prospects

Patrick A. Edewor
Olabisi Onabanjo University, Ago-Iwoye, Nigeria

ABSTRACT

That some countries are rich while others are poor is a well-known fact. While people in the developed countries of Europe and North America, for example, enjoy good water, good food, good housing, clothing, medical facilities and education, those in the less developed countries of Africa suffer without these basics for a decent quality of life. Even though there are spatial inequalities within countries, in the quality of life, the disparity between the industrialized countries and those of Africa is astonishingly wide. Differences in the quality of life are explored by comparing the Gross National Income Purchasing Power Parity Per Capita, life expectancy, literacy, infant and child mortality, access to safe water, and sanitary facilities. The persistently high fertility in the face of declining mortality and the consequent high rate of natural increase in the population of the countries of Africa as well as a high dependency ratio are noted as impediments to the realization of socioeconomic development goals and enhancement of the quality of life of the people. Provision of mass education, changes in the perceived value of children, improved use of modern contraceptives, and reduced fertility amongst others are major steps towards enhancing the quality of life of Africans.

INTRODUCTION

That some countries are rich while others are poor is a well-known fact. While people in the developed countries of Europe and North America, for example, enjoy good water, good food, good housing and clothing, medical facilities and education, those in the less developed countries of Africa suffer without these basics for a decent quality of life. Even though there are spatial inequalities within countries, in the quality of life, the disparity between the industrialized countries and those of Africa is astonishingly wide. Compared with the rest of the world, Africa, particularly Sub-Saharan Africa, remains the world's poorest region with average living standards lagging behind those of other parts of the world (USAID, 2003). As at mid-2002, Africa's population stood at 840 million with Sub-Saharan Africa having a population of 693 million (PRB, 2002). Almost half of this population of Sub-Saharan Africa lives on less than 65 cents a day (USAID, 2003).

At the current annual population growth rate of 2.5 %, reaching the Millennium Development Goal (MDG) of reducing poverty levels in Sub-Saharan Africa by 50 % by 2015 will require a 7 % annual growth rate in Gross Domestic Product (GDP) (USAID, 2003). Africa continues to lag far behind the rest of the world in

61

Wolfgang Glatzer, Susanne von Below, Matthias Stoffregen (eds.), Challenges for Quality of Life in the Contemporary World, 61-72.

investment in its people, particularly in the area of education. The region suffers from an average illiteracy rate of 41 %. With 61 % of boys and 57 % of girls enrolled in primary school, Africa is the only region of the world in which access to education has actually decreased in the last 20 years.

Using different indicators, as we shall soon see, there is ample evidence to show that Africans have very low quality of life, compared with persons from other parts of the world. The health of Africans, for example, remains unacceptable poor by any standard. Continent-wide, the rate of decrease in child mortality has declined in the past decade. For every thousand children born in Africa in 2003, 175 will die before their fifth birthday, compared with 100 in Asia and just 6 in the developed world. A woman's risk of dying from maternal causes is 1 in 15 in Africa, about 10 times higher than in Latin America and over 2000 times higher than in North America. Similarly, unlike other parts of the world, malnutrition rates are actually increasing in Africa (USAID, 2003).

The central thrust of this paper is to examine the challenges, problems and prospects on the path to enhancing the quality of life in Africa. To put the discussion in proper perspective, the paper first attempts a clarification of the concept of quality of life. Thereafter, quality of life indicators are examined and quality of life in Africa is discussed, using selected quality of life indicators. A comparative approach is adopted to bring into focus, how significantly the quality of life in Africa contrasts with those of other parts of the world. The challenges, problems, and prospects of enhancing the quality of life are then discussed before the conclusion.

QUALITY OF LIFE DEFINED

The concept of quality of life has been variously defined. For example, Mendola and Pelligrini (1979) defined quality of life as an "individual's achievement of a satisfactory social situation within the limit of perceived physical capacity". Shin and Johnson (1978) conceived quality of life as "the possession of resources necessary to satisfy individual needs, wants and desires, participation in activities enabling personal development and the satisfactory comparison between oneself and others". On the other hand, Donald (2001) sees quality of life as "a descriptive term that refers to people's emotional, social and physical well being, and their ability to function in the ordinary tasks of living".

A group of researchers (Carr et al., 2001) was interested in knowing whether quality of life is determined by expectation or experience. They observed that "expectation may have a greater impact on quality of life than experience". In their opinion, based on the findings from their study, the perception of quality of life varies between individuals and is dynamic within them. They also noted that quality of life in relation to health is the gap between one's expectation of health and his/her experience of it. Persons with different expectations report a different quality of life even when the same clinical condition is present; and current measures for quality of life do not account for expectation of health.

Quality of life measures subjective experiences. In relation to health, it is not uncommon for patients and professionals to have different perspectives on what constitutes quality of life. These different perspectives pose a difficulty in the assessment of quality of life. Some further examples of varying definitions include the following:

"A measure of the optimum energy or force that endows a person with the power to cope with the full range of challenges encountered in the real world. The term applies to individuals, regardless of illness or handicaps, on the job, at home, or in leisure activities. Quality enrichment methods can include activities that reduce boredom and allow a maximum amount of freedom in choosing and performing various tasks" (Mosby's Medical, Nursing, and Allied Health Dictionary, 1998).

"Health-related quality of life represents the functional effects of an illness and its consequent therapy upon a patient as perceived by the patient" (University of Bergen, 2000).

"Quality of life of well-being is a composite of two components: (I) the ability to perform everyday activities, which reflect physical, psychological, and social well-being; (II) patient satisfaction with levels of functioning and control of disease and/or treatment-related symptoms" (Gotay et al., 1992).

Fallowfield (1993) has argued that quality of life focuses on four main areas; (I) psychological, including anxiety and depression as well as adjustment to illness; (II) social, including social relationships and intimate relationships; (III) occupational; and (IV) physical.

It is important to emphasize that what constitutes the quality of life is, in the final analysis, subjective: It has no right or wrong answer. Perceptions of quality of life may differ among individuals and may vary from place to place with differences in culture and societies. However, although everyone has a different perception of quality of life – a perception which is dynamic, the desire for a better quality of life is what makes us human. Quality of life is what makes us happy. The conventional measure of quality of life is defined in material and quantitative terms, for example, Gross Domestic Product (GDP). This conventional measure has some limitations. These derive from the realization that there is a cost/limit to extreme materialism: (I) destruction of nature; and (II) the fact that human fulfillment goes beyond materialistic needs. A perennial perspective is that there are three facets of quality of life for complete human fulfillment: material, intellectual and spiritual. An ideal measure of quality of life should be dynamic in the sense that it should be indicative of potential development. In addition, it should be accommodative of changing human perceptions of development. It should also take into account, major driving forces of change such as information and communication technologies (Sharriffadeen, 2000).

QUALITY OF LIFE INDICATORS

We need some measures to compare differences in quality of life among countries. Evidently, it takes wealth to acquire some of the things needed for a high quality of life, such as good food, housing, and education. The most commonly used measure of a country's wealth is Gross National Product (GNP) per capita. Usually, the higher a country's GNP per capita, the better its quality of life. But owing to the fact that money has different purchasing power in different countries, GNP values are converted to a common value as if there was a common international currency. This is called Purchasing Power Parity (PPP), meaning that all money has the same purchasing power. We can then explore differences in quality of life among countries by comparing GNP PPP per capita.

However, other indicators such as infant and child mortality, availability of medical services and sanitary facilities, prevalence of child malnutrition, life expectancy, literacy and access to safe water may be equally or even more important. In addition to GNP PPP per capita, these indicators are examined to determine the quality of life in African countries and to compare them with those of the developed countries of the world , thereby bringing into sharp focus how significantly poorer the quality of life is in Africa. Table 1 (see below) shows these quality of life indicators for African countries and some selected developed countries.

QUALITY OF LIFE IN AFRICA

In discussing the quality of life in Africa, we wish to examine the infant mortality rate, the prevalence of child malnutrition, as well as child mortality and life expectancy at birth. In addition, other quality of life indicators discussed include access to sanitation, access to safe water, adult literacy as well as Gross National Income Purchasing Power Parity per capita (GNI PPP per capita).

Infant mortality is becoming widely accepted as the most objective criterion for assessing the overall quality of life across highly diverse societies and cultures (Brockerhoff & Brennan, 1997). Whereas infant mortality is as high as 86 per 1,000 live births in Africa, it is only 6 and 8 per 1,000 live births in North America and Europe respectively. Apart from Reunion, Seychelles, and Mauritius which have achieved low infant mortality rates (8, 10 and 13.7 deaths per 1,000 live births respectively) and Tunisia, Libya, Cape Verde, Egypt and South Africa that have somewhat averagely low infant mortality rates (26, 30, 31, 44 and 45 respectively), others have infant mortality rates of at least 50 deaths per 1000 live births. Infant mortality rates are highest in Sierra Leone (153), Western Sahara (140), Liberia (139) and Mozambique (135 deaths per 1000 live births) (see Table 1). The generally high level of infant mortality in African countries is indicative of the low quality of life in these countries.

Using infant mortality as an indicator, evidence shows that quality of life declines in big and growing cities in developing countries especially those of Africa (Brockerhoff & Brennan, 1997). Infant mortality trends reveal deterioration in places that grow too big and two rapidly. Today's big cities in Africa are not keeping pace with the improvements in child survival throughout the rest of Africa. Since the 1970s, infant mortality has fallen precipitously in towns and villages, with declines ranging from about 14 % in Sub-Saharan Africa to more than 50 % in North Africa and the Middle East. In contrast, the largest cities of Sub-Saharan Africa have experienced less than 5 % decline in infant mortality. Indeed, infant mortality has risen from 73 to 90 deaths per 1,000 live births in cities of tropical Africa containing 50,000 to 1 million people. A similar trend has been observed in countries of North Africa and the Middle East: infant mortality declines much more slowly in the largest cities than in the rural settlements. Consequently, infant mortality rates registered by big cities and small settlements have converged.

The slower decline in infant mortality in big cities is accompanied by low investment in social services for children as well as adults, with big cities having lower rates of school enrollment, poor health care, inadequate nutrition, and other deprivations as compared to smaller settlements. All these reflect less improvement in the overall well-being in big cities. Ironically, the cities are the areas in which high incomes and publicly financed services are presumably concentrated. The poor social conditions of the cities may be connected with the overwhelming effect of migration inflows and persistent high fertility rates, which have strained the carrying capacity of the cities.

Child malnutrition is prevalent in Africa. Whereas only 1 % of children under 5 years suffer from malnutrition in United States, 33 % of children under 5 years suffer from malnutrition in Sub-Saharan Africa. Of the 44 African countries for which we have data on child malnutrition, only 11 (25 %) have child malnutrition prevalence rates of less than 20 %, mostly in Northern Africa. Prevalence of child malnutrition is as high as 50 % in Niger, 48 % in Ethiopia, and between 35 and 44 % in Nigeria, Burundi, Eritrea, Madagascar, Angola, and Chad. The high prevalence of child malnutrition in Africa is associated with the level of poverty in the region. Northern African countries and countries like Mauritius, Zimbabwe, Gabon and South Africa with relatively lower prevalence rates of child malnutrition have higher Gross National Income Purchasing Power Parity per capita relative to other African countries and child malnutrition is virtually non-existent in the countries of North America and Europe which are much richer.

Whereas the child mortality rate is as low as 7 per 1,000 live births in Canada, 5 in Sweden, 6 in Germany and Italy, and 5 in Switzerland and Spain, Sub-Saharan Africa had a child mortality rate of 151 per 1,000 live births in 1998. USAID (2003) actually reports 175 per 1,000 live births in 2003. While child mortality rates range between 32 per 1,000 live births (Tunisia) and 61 per 1,000 live births (Morocco) in North Africa, Sub-Saharan Africa records much higher child mortality rates with Sierra Leone, Niger, Malawi, Mali, Mozambique, Burkina Faso, Rwanda, and Angola recording over 200 deaths per 1,000 live births, particularly Sierra Leone and Niger in which more than a quarter or as much as a quarter of the children born die before their fifth birthday.

Life expectancy at birth is still low in Africa. Whereas it is 74 years and 80 years for male and female respectively in North America and 70 years and 78 years for male and female respectively in Europe, it is 52 and 54 years respectively in Africa (49 and 50 years respectively in Sub-Saharan Africa) (PRB, 2002). Sub-Saharan Africa's average life expectancy reported by UNAIDS (2002) is 47 years. North Africa records relatively higher life expectancy than Sub-Saharan Africa, with Libya and Tunisia recording life expectancy of over 70 years. Compared with other countries in Sub-Saharan Africa, Reunion, Mauritius and Seychelles (in Eastern Africa) and Cape Verde (in Western Africa) also record relatively higher life expectancy.

Table 1: Quality of Life in Africa and Selected Developed Countries

	IMR	CM5	MR5	LEB ♂	LEB ♀	AS	AW	AIR ♂	AIR ♀	GNI PPP
Africa	86	-	-	52	54	-	-	-	-	1,960
Sub-Saharan Africa	91	33	151	49	50	37	45	32	49	1,540
Northern Africa	55	-	-	64	68	-	-	-	-	3,500
Algeria	54	13	40	68	71	-	-	24	46	5,040
Egypt	44	12	59	65	68	11	64	35	58	3,670
Libya	30	5	-	73	77	-	90	-	-	-
Morocco	50	10	61	67	71	40	52	40	66	3,450
Sudan	82	34	-	55	57	22	50	-	-	1,520
Tunisia	26	9	32	70	74	-	-	21	42	6,070
Western Sahara	140	-	-	-	-	-	-	-	-	-
Western Africa	87	-	-	50	51	-	-	-	-	1,030
Benin	85	29	140	53	56	20	50	46	77	980
Burkina Fa-so	105	33	210	46	47	18	78	68	87	970
Cape Verde	31	-	-	66	72	-	-	-	-	4,760
Côte d'Ivoire	95	21	143	44	47	54	72	47	64	1,500
Gambia	82	17	-	51	55	37	76	-	-	1,620
Ghana	56	27	96	56	59	27	56	22	40	1,910
Guinea	119	24	184	47	48	70	62	-	-	710
Liberia	139	-	-	49	52	-	-	-	-	-
Mali	113	27	218	46	48	31	37	54	69	780
Mauritania	74	23	140	53	55	-	-	-48	69	1,630
Niger	123	50	250	45	46	15	53	78	93	740
Nigeria	75	39	119	52	52	36	39	30	48	800
Senegal	68	22	121	52	55	58	50	55	74	1,480
Sierra Leone	153	29	283	38	40	11	34	-	-	480
Togo	80	25	144	53	57	22	-	28	62	1,410
Eastern Africa	97	-	-	47	48	-	-	-	-	880
Burundi	116	38	196	40	41	-	-	45	63	580

Table 1: Quality of Life in Africa and Selected Developed Countries (continued)

	IMR	CM5	MR5	LEB		AS	AW	AIR		GNI
				♂	♀			♂	♀	PPP
Comoros	86	-	-	54	59	-	-	-	-	1,590
Djibouti	117	-	-	42	44	-	-	-	-	-
Eritrea	77	44	90	53	58	-	-	34	62	690
Ethiopia	97	48	173	51	53	10	17	58	70	660
Kenya	74	23	124	47	49	77	53	12	27	1,010
Madagascar	96	40	146	53	57	3	29	28	42	820
Malawi	104	30	229	37	38	53	45	27	56	600
Mauritius	13.7	15	-	68	75	100	98	-	-	9,940
Mayotte	75	-	-	57	62	-	-	-	-	-
Mozambique	135	26	213	38	37	21	32	42	73	800
Réunion	8	-	-	70	79	-	-	-	-	-
Rwanda	10	29	205	39	40	-	-	29	43	930
Seychelles	10	-	-	67	73	-	-	-	-	-
Somalia	126	-	-	45	48	-	-	-	-	-
Tanzania	99	31	136	51	53	86	49	17	36	520
Uganda	88	26	170	42	44	57	34	24	46	1,210
Zambia	95	24	192	37	37	23	43	16	31	750
Middle Africa	100	-	-	48	51	-	-	-	-	1,000
Angola	122	35	204	44	47	16	32	-	-	1,180
Cameroon	77	22	150	54	56	40	41	20	33	1,590
Central African Republic	98	23	162	42	46	-	18	43	68	1,160
Chad	103	39	172	49	53	21	24	51	69	870
Congo	72	24	143	49	53	9	47	14	29	570
Democratic Republic of Congo	102	34	141	47	51	-	-	9	53	680
Equatorial Guinea	108	-	-	49	53	-	-	-	-	5,600
Gabon	57	15	-	49	51	76	67	-	-	5,360
São Tomé and Principe	50	-	-	64	67	-	-	-	-	-

Table 1: Quality of Life in Africa and Selected Developed Countries (continued)

	IMR	CM5	MR5	LEB		AS	AW	AIR		GNI
				♂	♂			♂	♂	PPP
Southern Africa	51	-	-	50	51	-	-	-	-	8,610
Botswana	60	27	105	39	40	55	70	27	22	7,170
Lesotho	84	16	144	50	52	6	52	29	7	2,590
South Africa	45	9	83	50	52	46	70	15	16	9,160
Swaziland	109	-	-	40	41	-	-	-	-	4,600
North America	6	-	-	74	80	-	-	-	-	33,410
Canada	5.3	-	7	76	81	85	100	-	-	27,170
USA	6.6	1	-	74	80	85	90	-	-	34,100
Europe	8	-	-	70	78	-	-	-	-	16,150
Sweden	3.4	-	5	77	82	100	-	-	-	23,970
Germany	4.4	-	6	75	81	100	-	-	-	24,920
World	54	30	75	65	69	47	78	18	32	7,140
Developed Countries	7	-	-	72	79	-	-	-	-	22,060
Less Developed Countries	60	-	-	63	67	-	-	-	-	3,580

Sources: PRB (2002), World Bank (1998), World Bank (2000/2001). IMR=infant mortality rate; CM5=prevalence of child malnutrition in % of children under 5 (1992-98); MR5=mortality rate under age 5 per 1,000 (1998); LEB=life expectancy at birth in years (2002); AS=access to sanitation in % of population (1995); AW=access to safe water in % of population (1995); AIR=adult illiteracy rate in % of population aged 15 and older (1998); GNI PPP=income in purchasing power parities per capita in US$ (2000).

A major factor that has contributed to the low life expectancy in Africa is the emergence of AIDS. The average life expectancy which is presently 47 years in Sub-Saharan Africa would have been 64 years without AIDS (UNAIDS Report, 2002). In Botswana, life expectancy has dropped to the level of 1950 due to AIDS. At the end of 2001, as much 38.8 % of the population aged 15 to 49 years in this country were with HIV/AIDS. The corresponding figures for Zimbabwe, Swaziland, Lesotho, Namibia, Zambia and South Africa were 33.7 %, 33.4 %, 31.0 %, 22.5 %, 21.5 % and 20.1 % respectively. The HIV/AIDS seropositive prevalence rates in these countries are devastatingly high. Consequently, life expectancy in these countries has declined to very low levels.

Unlike Europe where the populations of most of the countries have 100 % access to sanitation, the story is different in Africa. Only 37 % of the population in Sub-Saharan Africa has access to sanitation. With the exception of Mauritius, Tanzania, Kenya, Gabon and Guinea in which at least 70 % of the populations have access to sanitation, in the majority of the other countries, less than 40 % of the populations have access to sanitation with only 3 % and 6 % of the population of Madagascar and Lesotho respectively, having access to sanitation.

Similarly, the majority of Africans has no access to safe water. Only 45 % of the population of Sub-Saharan Africa has access to safe water. Aside from Mauritius and Libya in which 98 % and 90 % of the population enjoy access to safe water respectively, in the majority of the other countries, access to safe water is very low with Ethiopia, Central African Republic, Guinea-Bissau, and Chad recording as low as 17 %, 18 %, 23 % and 24 % respectively. The generally low level of access to sanitation and safe water has serious implications for health and well-being of Africans especially when one considers the fact that most tropical diseases are water-borne.

Illiteracy is still as high as 41 % in the African region. Adult illiteracy rate in Sub-Saharan Africa is 32 % for male and 49 % for female. Niger has adult illiteracy rate of 78 % and 93 % for male and female respectively; Burkina Faso, 68 % and 87 % respectively; Ethiopia, 58 % and 70 % respectively; Benin, 46 % and 77 % respectively; and Mozambique, 42 % and 73 % respectively. However, Southern African countries have somewhat lower rates of illiteracy than the rest of the sub-regions in Africa with rates for females which are unusually lower than those for male in Botswana and Lesotho or about equal in Namibia and South Africa. With respect to literacy, the scenario in Africa contrasts sharply with that in Eastern Europe and Southern Europe where illiteracy is virtually non-existent.

Given the fact that it takes wealth to acquire some of the things needed for high quality of life such as good food, housing, and education, let us examine the Gross National Income in Purchasing Power Parity (GNI PPP) per capita in the African region. GNI PPP refers Gross National Income converted to "international" dollars using a purchasing power parity conversion factor. International dollars indicate the amount of goods and services one could buy in the United States with a given amount of money (PRB, 2002). Africa remains the poorest of all the regions of the world. While GNI PPP per capita is US$ 33,410 in North America and US$ 16,150 in Europe, it is only US$ 1,960 in Africa and US$ 1,540 in Sub-Saharan Africa. GNI PPP per capita is highest in Southern Africa (US$ 8,610) and lowest in Eastern Africa (US $880) with Western Africa and Middle Africa having about the same (US$ 1,030 and US$ 1,000 respectively). Mauritius has the highest GNI PPP per capita (US$ 9,940), followed by South Africa (US $9,160), Botswana (US$ 7,170), Namibia (US$ 6,410) and Tunisia (US$ 6,070). GNI PPP per capita is US$ 800 or less in Guinea-Bissau, Mali, Niger, Nigeria, Sierra Leone, Burundi, Ethiopia, Malawi, Mozambique, Tanzania, Zambia, Congo, and Democratic Republic of Congo. These show the extent of poverty in Africa.

ENHANCING THE QUALITY OF LIFE: PROBLEMS AND PROSPECTS

How can the quality of life be enhanced in Africa? What are the problems on the path to enhancing the quality of life? What are the future prospects? To enhance the quality of life, the challenges for quality of life as discussed in the preceding section must be addressed. In other words, infant and child mortality as well as child malnutrition have to be reduced. It goes without saying that a reduction in mortality rates would automatically increase life expectancy at birth. By the same token, access to sanitation and safe water, literacy and GNI PPP per capita must increase.

To reduce infant and child mortality, there is the need to improve the existing services for the reduction of infant and child mortality. Efforts should be made to ensure increased utilization and coverage of such services. One of the major reasons why fertility is high in Africa is high infant and child mortality. It follows that parents will be more willing to have fewer children if infant and child mortality are reduced. It has been established that infant mortality declines less rapidly in the cities owing to the overwhelming effect of migration inflows and persistently high fertility, which strain the carrying capacity of African cities.

Evidence shows that compared to cities that have grown less than 3 % a year, cities that have grown at rates of more than 5 % annually have higher infant mortality levels, higher by 24 % in countries of North Africa and Asia, 28 % in Latin America, and 42 % in Sub-Saharan Africa (Brockerhoff & Brennan, 1997). These results imply a need for continued efforts to reduce the pace of city growth in African countries.

Life expectancy at birth would increase with a decline in infant and child mortality rates. However, for there to be any appreciable increase in life expectancy, aside from reducing infant and child morality, the AIDS pandemic has to be effectively controlled. In less than two decades, HIV/AIDS has become a development disaster: Infection rates in Africa have reached alarming proportions, with Botswana (38.8 %), Swaziland (34.4 %) and Lesotho (31.0 %), in Southern Africa as well as Zimbabwe (33.7 %), in Eastern Africa, being the worst affected (UNESCO, 2001; PRB, 2002). These figures represent the prevalence rates among populations aged 15-49 years in these countries.

HIV/AIDS is having negative impact on households, agriculture, firms, education and many other sectors. Women contribute to over 50 % of the food production in Sub-Saharan Africa. Food shortages and malnutrition is one of the consequences of female-headed AIDS affected households. Owing to the fact that the vast majority of people living with HIV/AIDS are between the age of 15 and 49 in the prime of their working life, the epidemic hits productivity mainly through increased absenteeism. Funeral costs are provided by a number of employers and these are rising sharply. As it relates to education, evidence shows that infection and death rates are high among the skilled, trained and educated, draining countries of their intellectual resources and the groups most vital for development. Up to 10 % of teachers are expected to die of AIDS in the worst affected African countries over the next five years (UNESCO, 2001). Without the control of HIV/AIDS, an increase in life expectancy will remain an illusion. Uganda was the first country in Sub-Saharan Africa to curb the spread of HIV with a very comprehensive HIV/AIDS program including awareness and promotion of safer sexual behavior. The rest of Africa, particularly Southern Africa, should emulate Uganda by intensifying efforts or embarking on very vigorous and aggressive HIV/AIDS awareness programs and also promote safer sexual behavior.

Improvement in access to sanitation and safe water does not yet occupy top positions in the development agenda of African countries and these are inevitable in the enhancement of quality of life. Countries like Madagascar and Lesotho in which access to sanitation is extremely low should make this a top priority. The same applies to Ethiopia, Central African Republic, Guinea-Bissau and Chad in which access to safe water is extremely low.

Given the important role of education in the developmental process, it is disturbing to know that Africa is the only region in the world in which access to education has actually decreased in the last 20 years. It is even more worrisome to know that AIDS is further exacerbating the situation by reducing the supply of experienced teachers by AIDS–related illness and death (Bollinger et al., 1999), causing children to be kept out of school because they are needed at home to care for sick family members or to work on the farm to augment household income or drop out of school because their families can not afford school fees due to reduced household income as a result of AIDS death (ibid.). One way to curb the decreasing access to education, therefore, is through curbing AIDS.

CONCLUSION

Continued high population growth rates in Africa undermine the best efforts to improve the quality of life. Although fertility rates continue to decline in some countries, particularly those with relatively higher incomes, fertility rates are still high in most African countries. Consequently, the annual population growth rate is still 2.5 %, the highest in the world. Owing to the high birth rates, the age structure of the populations in Africa is such that there is a preponderance of young persons and consequently, a high dependency ratio, which serves as an impediment to the realization of socioeconomic development goals and enhancement of the quality of life of the people. Contraceptive prevalence rates remain under 15 % in Sub-Saharan Africa, even though the majority of women say they desire fewer children. Even with the devastating effects of the HIV/AIDS pandemic, the population of Sub-Saharan Africa is likely to increase from 693 million at present to about one billion in 2020, further straining the social infrastructure. Provision of mass education, changes in the perceived value of children and improved use of modern contraceptives and reduced fertility, improved access to sanitation and safe water as well as reduction in infant and child mortality are major steps towards enhancing the quality of life of Africans.

REFERENCES

Bollinger, L., J. Stover & O. Nwaorgu (1999): The Economic Impact of AIDS in Nigeria. The Futures Group International in Collaboration with Research Triangle Institute (RTI), The Centre for Development and Population Activities (CEDPA).

Brockerhoff, M. & E. Brennan (1997): The Poverty of Cities in the Developing World. Policy Research Division Working Paper No. 96, New York: Population Council.

Campbell, M. & Layde (2000) in :What is Quality of Life?:
    http://web.nmsu.edu/˜lleeper/pages/Lx6/qol.htm.

Carr, G. & Robinson (2001) in: What is Quality of Life?:
    http://web.nmsu.edu/˜lleeper/pages/Lx6/qol.htm.

Donald, A. (2001): What is Quality of Life? Kent: Hayward Medical Communications:
    http://www.evidence-based-medicine.co.uk.

Fallowfield, L. (1993) in: What is Quality of Life?:
    http://web.nmsu.edu/˜lleeper/pages/Lx6/qol.htm.

Gotay, C., E. Korn, M. McCabe, T. Moore & B. Cheson (1992) in: What is Quality of Life?:
    http://web.nmsu.edu/˜lleeper/pages/Lx6/qol.htm.

Mendola, W. & R. Pelligrini (1979) in: What is Quality of Life?:
    http://web.nmsu.edu/`lleeper/pages/Lx6/qol.htm.
Mosby's Medical, Nursing, and Allied Health Dictionary (1998) in: What is Quality of Life?:
    http://web.nmsu.edu/`lleeper/pages/Lx6/qol.htm
Population Reference Bureau (PRB) (2002): World Population Data Sheet, Washington, D.C.: PRB.
Sharriffadeen, T. M. A. (1979): Addressing the Information Divide: Improving Quality of Life. Paper
    presented at the Second Global Conference held at Kuala Lumpur, March 7-10.
Shin, D. & D. Johnson (1978) in: What is Quality of Life?:
    http://web.nmsu.edu/`lleeper/pages/Lx6/qol.htm.
UNAIDS Report (2002): http://www.unaids.org.
UNESCO United Nations Educational, Scientific and Cultural Organization (2001): HIV/AIDS and Edu-
    cation. Paris: UNESCO.
United States Agency for International Development (2003): Africa: U.S. National Interests, Washington,
    D.C.
University of Bergen (2000) in: What is Quality of Life?:
    http://web.nmsu.edu/`lleeper/pages/Lx6/qol.htm.
World Bank (1998): World Development Indicators. Washington, D.C.: The World Bank.
World Bank (2000/2001): World Development Report. Washington, D.C.: The World Bank.

PART II:
MONITORING QUALITY OF LIFE

6. WORLD DATABASE OF HAPPINESS

Continuous Register of Research on Subjective Appreciation of Life

Ruut Veenhoven

Erasmus University Rotterdam, The Netherlands

ABSTRACT

The World Database of Happiness is an ongoing register of scientific research on subjective appreciation of life. It brings together findings that are scattered throughout many studies and prepares for research synthesis. The database stores research findings and presents these in standardized abstracts. This system differs from bibliographies that store publications and data-archives that store investigations. The system prepares for synthetic analysis by capitalizing on conceptual selectiveness, comparability, and completeness. As the method is new, there is no common word for it. It is called a *finding-browser*.

The database allows selection of findings by a) indicator used, b) public, time and place, c) methodology of the investigation. The correlational findings can also be found on subject.

The system prepares for synthetic studies, in particular for reviews and meta-analyses; it facilitates comparisons across time and nations. When applied on a well-defined field, it allows a better accumulation of available knowledge and a better focusing of new research.

The data-system serves to cope with the following problems of research integration, a) chronic confusion of tongues, b) growing mass of research findings, c) scattered publication of findings, and d) selective reviewing and retrieval of findings. The database is freely available on the web. The Internet address is: http://www.eur.nl/fsw.eur.nl/research/happiness.

INTRODUCTION

Happiness is defined as the subjective "enjoyment of one's life as-a-whole". In other words: how much one likes the life one leads. Current synonyms are "life-satisfaction" and "subjective well-being". This concept is delineated in more detail in the basic work "Conditions of Happiness" (Veenhoven, 1984) and more recently in a paper entitled "The Four Qualities of Life" (Veenhoven, 2002).

Interest in Happiness

Happiness as defined here is a highly valued matter. In utilitarian moral philosophy it ranks as the highest good, and recent survey studies also show high rankings in the value hierarchy of the general public. Consequently there is broad support for public policies that aim at greater happiness for a greater number.

The relevance of happiness as a goal of social policy is growing. The better we succeed in eliminating pressing problems such as hunger and plagues, the more we

75

Wolfgang Glatzer, Susanne von Below, Matthias Stoffregen (eds.), Challenges for Quality of Life in the Contemporary World, 75-89.

move to abstract goals such as happiness. Individualization and post-modern relativism also press for higher ranking of happiness. One of the manifestations of this development in health care is the growing emphasis on "quality-of-life", rather than mere quantity of life years.

The higher happiness ranks on the public agenda, the greater the demand for scientific information on the matter. To promote happiness we must know its main determinants. We must also have a view on consequences of happiness to detect possible self-destructive effects and to appraise synergy with other values.

There is also a rising interest among individual citizens. Because happiness is becoming ever more prominent in the personal life of many people, there is a great demand for explanation and advice. The number of "how to be happy"-books increases and the contents have shifted gradually from matters of morals and mental hygiene to the "art of living". The greater the choice of life-styles in modern society creates greater demand for solid information about the consequences for health and happiness.

RISE OF EMPIRICAL RESEARCH ON HAPPINESS

Over the ages the subject has absorbed a lot of thought. Happiness was a major theme in early Greek philosophy and gained renewed interest in the later West-European Enlightenment. The philosophic tradition has produced a lot of ideas, but little operational knowledge. In fact, philosophers have raised more questions than they have answered. Most of the controversies they have raised could not be solved by the logic of reasoning. Settlement on the basis of reality checks has long been encumbered by lack of adequate research techniques.

The advent of the social sciences promised a breakthrough. New methods for empirical research opened the possibility to identify conditions for happiness inductively and even to test theories. This instigated a lot of research, most of which has been embedded in the newly established specializations of "social indicators research" and "health related quality of life research".

In the 20th century more than 3,000 empirical studies have dealt with the matter; in the beginning mainly as a side issue in studies about health and aging, but currently also as a main subject. This stream of research is growing. Reviews can be found with Diener (1999) and Veenhoven (1995; 1997).

Intriguing Findings

This new line of research has produced several unexpected results, such as:
- Happiness is not relative. Enjoyment of life appears not to depend on comparison, in particular not on social comparison. This finding contradicts cognitive theories of happiness and supports affective explanations (Veenhoven, 1991; 1995).
- Happiness is not very trait like; over a lifetime it appears to be quite variable. This finding does not fit notions of stable personality in psychology (Veenhoven, 1994b; Ehrhardt et al., 2000).

- The majority of mankind appears to enjoy life. Unhappiness is the exception rather than the rule. This is at odds with the results of misery counting in sociology (Veenhoven, 1993).
- Happiness tends to rise in modern societies. This contradicts longstanding pessimism about modernization (Cummins, 2000).
- In modern western nations happiness differs little across social categories such as rich and poor or males and females. The difference is rather in psychological competence (Headey & Wearing, 1992). This result is at odds with current sociology of deprivation.
- Differences in happiness within nations (as measured by standard deviations) tend to get smaller. This contradicts notions about growing inequality in sociology. (Veenhoven, 2000c.)
- Liberalist intuition is confirmed in the finding that people tend to be happiest in individualistic society, but the socialist expectation that people will be happier in a welfare state is not corroborated (Veenhoven, 1999; 2000b).

Stagnating Progress

Still, all this empirical research on happiness has not yet crystallized into a sound body of knowledge. Preliminary questions about conceptualization and measurement are now fairly well solved, but the understanding of determinants and consequences of happiness is still very incomplete and tentative. There are several reasons why the growing stream of empirical research has not yet brought greater understanding. In addition to complexities in the subject matter, there are several practical problems.

Lack of overview: The first and most simple reason for the stagnation is lack of coordination. There is high redundancy in the research effort; the same issues are investigated over and over again, in the same way. As a result, the range of variables considered is still rather small and methodological progress slow. A related problem is that research findings are very scattered. Most observations are in fact bibliographically irretrievable. Consequently, many of the findings get lost.

Conceptual confusion: The second reason is the confusion of tongues. As there is no consensus on use of words, it is quite difficult to select the data that pertain to happiness as defined here. Moreover the matter is measured in different ways. Getting an overview of the research findings requires first of all selecting studies that measured happiness as defined here, and next a grouping by comparable indicators.

Little view on contingencies: A more basic reason for the stagnation lies in the dominant research approach. The bulk of empirical happiness studies consist of cross-sections in particular countries. Typically investigators try to identify universal conditions for happiness using their local correlates. For instance, the observation in American studies that the happy tend to have high incomes is seen to mean that money buys happiness everywhere and that the basic underlying mental process is social comparison.

Yet, conditions for happiness are probably not the same at all times and at all places. Neither are its consequences. Though there are obviously universal requirements for a happy life (such as food and possibly meaning), some seem to be contingent on characteristics of the person and situation. For instance, happiness correlates strongest to income in poor and socially unequal countries, and most so among materialistic persons. Usually, such contingencies cannot be detected in single studies in one country. They can be identified only if many studies are compared in a systematic meta-analysis. This requires first of all that the available findings be compiled.

No view on macro level: Further, correlational studies within nations cannot grasp macro-social conditions for happiness. As their focus is on differences in happiness within nations, they are blind to variation in happiness across nations. Therefore, current research has as yet little relevance for major political discussions such as the priority of continuous economic growth, preserving the welfare state or promoting social coherence. Investigation of such matters requires cross-national studies, preferably in a semi-longitudinal design. Such studies are scarce as yet, but we can do a lot by comparing the available one-nation studies. Again this requires compilation of the available findings.

Little view on causality: Lastly, correlations say little about cause and effect. If rich Americans tend to more happy, this does not prove that money buys happiness, because happiness can also boost earning chances. Separation of cause and effect requires panel studies and experiments. Such studies are scarce as yet, and the results difficult to retrieve. Progress requires at least that these scattered findings be brought together.

Growing Need for Research Compilation

A main priority is therefore to gather the available research findings on happiness and to present these in a comparable format. Without a complete and detailed view on the available data, there will be little cumulation of knowledge. This need for a focused catalog of research-findings becomes ever more pressing. The higher the pile of research reports, the greater the need for a good overview of findings.

Now more than 3,000 studies have been published on happiness, the heap of findings has grown too big to be handled by narrative research reviews. At the same time the stockpile becomes ever more suitable for quantitative meta-analysis. Yet meta-analysis requires much investment in gathering of relevant research and in homogenizing the findings. Investment is particularly high if one wants to cover all the world's research. Such investments are made in capital-intensive fields such as pharmacological research, but uncommonly in this field. The few meta-analyses of empirical happiness research are based on small collections, e.g. Stock et al. (1983). As yet, all have been one-time shots, leaving no common database to build on. Hence each new investigator has to make a new start. Not surprisingly few do so.

Aims of the Database

The World Database of Happiness is meant to overcome these problems. First of all its Bibliography of Happiness provides a fairly complete inventory of contemporary publications. This may help to get an overview of the field and to trace literature on specific issues. I hope this will reduce redundancy somewhat.

Secondly, the database provides two homogenous selections of research findings; a selection of correlational finding in the Catalogue of Happiness Correlates, and a selection of distributional findings in the Catalogue of Happiness in Nations. Both selections are based on the same concept of happiness and consequently on the same array of happiness indicators. The Catalogue of Happiness Correlates provides an assortment of comparable correlational findings that is ordered by subject matter. The collection provides a convenient overview of the available research and can serve as a basis for meta-analysis. Because the collection covers data from different nations and social categories, meta-analysis can reveal universal patterns as well as contingencies. The Catalogue of Happiness in Nations provides a collection of comparable observations about level and dispersion of happiness in nations. First of all, the data on the average level of happiness serves to identify the macro-social factors that mark off more and less livable societies. The data is also of use for monitoring progress and decline. The data on dispersion of happiness in nations can be used in comparative studies of inequality in life chances.

Thirdly, the cross-national analysis of these findings is facilitated by a database of societal characteristics of nations and change in these characteristics over time. Part of the findings on happiness in nations is already entered in that database called "States of nations".

Lastly, the Directory of Investigators lists addresses of scientists who have published on happiness. It is meant to facilitate communication in the field.

STRUCTURE OF THE DATABASE

Type of Source

This database differs from common bibliographies, abstract systems and data banks in that it provides direct access to the outcomes of empirical investigations. The core of this source is a collection of standardized descriptions of research findings. It is therefore called a "finding browser".

Inventories

The Database consists of five inventories, which are mutually linked: 1) a bibliography of scientific publications on happiness, 2) a directory of investigators in this field, 3) an inventory of acceptable measures of happiness (test bank), 4) an inventory of distributional findings yielded with these indicators (in general population samples in nations and among special publics), and 5) an inventory of correlational findings. The cross-national analysis of these findings on happiness is facilitated by an additional database of nation characteristics. Figure 1 depicts the way in which these inventories are linked.

Figure 1: Flow Chart

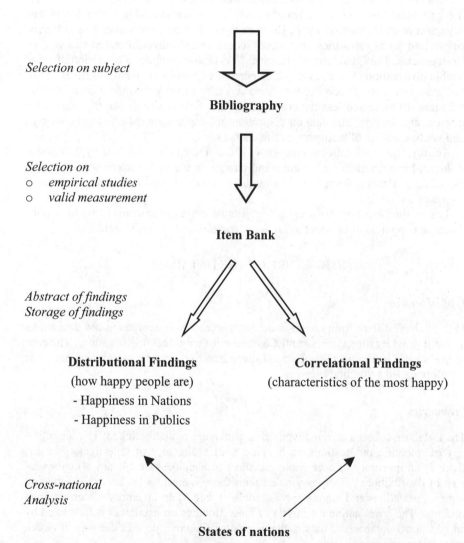

Literature on happiness

Selection on subject

Bibliography

Selection on
o   *empirical studies*
o   *valid measurement*

Item Bank

Abstract of findings
Storage of findings

Distributional Findings   **Correlational Findings**
(how happy people are)   (characteristics of the most happy)
- Happiness in Nations
- Happiness in Publics

Cross-national
Analysis

States of nations

Data Gathering

The data for these collections are largely drawn from publications on happiness in books and journal articles. However, this database is not limited to findings that reached "authorized" publications. Grey reports and mere data-files are included as well.

One reason for this strategy is that the original investigator does not publish many findings that may be relevant in a meta-analysis because they appeared not to be relevant in the context of his report. Another reason is that the publication process involves some systematic biases, one of which is under-report of non-correlations.

By deliberately including "unpublished" data this database allows a more realistic view of conditions for happiness. Therefore, meta-analyses based on this database can yield conclusions that differ from impressions based on narrative literature surveys.

Funding

This system was developed at Erasmus University of Rotterdam since 1984 and is also funded by the Dutch science foundation NWO.

BIBLIOGRAPHY OF HAPPINESS

All publications on happiness are entered in the "Bibliography of Happiness", which involves a detailed subject index. This listing allows an overview of the field and helps to trace literature on specific issues.

Most publications in the bibliography are books and journal articles; however, the collection is not limited to "authorized" publications. Grey reports are also included. The main reason is that the publication process involves some systematic biases, one of which is under-reporting of non-correlations. By deliberately including "unpublished" findings, this database allows a more realistic view of conditions for happiness.

Reports of empirical investigations are selected from this collection. Research reports are indexed by their methodological characteristics. This helps to single out suitable studies, for instance, to trace the scarce panel studies and experiments that bear information about causality. The next step is selection of investigations that used acceptable indicators of happiness. This selection is based on the above concept of happiness and consequently on an assortment of indicators that fit this concept. Results of the selected studies are entered in the research inventories.

Scope: Any research report that refers to the subjective appreciation of life-as-a-whole, even if this subject is only a side issue. Not included are related fields like "mental health", "social adjustment", "alienation", and satisfaction with "domains of life".

Coverage 1-9-2003: 3874 titles; almost complete coverage of the social-science literature up to 2000 in English, German, and Dutch; includes not only journal articles, but also books, dissertations, conference papers and unpublished research reports.

Contents: title descriptions involving: author, title, publisher or journal, year of publication, language of the report, type of study; subject classification (388 subject categories); data classification (empirical studies only): time frame: past/present/future/perceived change; variant measured: overall happiness/hedonic level/contentment; included or not in the finding catalogs ("Distributional Finding" or "Correlational Findings"), depending on whether the happiness measure fits our conceptualization.

Search facilities: search on co-author, on words in title; select on year of publication, on type of study, on data-type (time-frame, variant of happiness).

DIRECTORY OF HAPPINESS INVESTIGATORS

Names of interested scholars are stored in the "Directory of Happiness Investigators", which now contains 5,818 names, and some 3,000 recent addresses. The directory is linked to the bibliography, which is indexed by subject. Therefore one can easily select specialists. Because the bibliography is also indexed by year of publication, one can also identify the currently most active researchers.

The directory is available on request to peer researchers. In the last few years it has been of great help in creating research networks around this theme. Obviously it is also a good help for bringing this database to the attention of the field.

Scope: address data of scientists who have published on the subject of subjective appreciation of life. Includes most authors of works in the "Bibliography of Happiness". Research groups that focus on the quality-of-life.

Coverage at 1-9-2003: 6,938 names; about 2,500 recent addresses, of which some 1,100 with e-mail; mainly investigators who published after 1975; fairly complete up to 2003.

Contents: name; institution; address; year of publications on happiness; link to publications.

Availability: The addresses are available to peer-researchers for scientific purposes only. The list (or selection on subject, countries) is send on request as an E-mail attachment or paper print (labels). Investigators can be selected by subject or by nation.

Search facilities: search on name, years, institution; select on subject matter.

ITEM BANK

All the acceptable indicators are listed in an "item bank". This inventory orders the indicators by happiness-variant, time reference and method of assessment. It provides full text of questions and observation schedules, and summarizes the available psychometric data. The inventory links to the studies that used these measures, and thereby provides an easy overview of the scores yielded by the same indicators in different populations. The catalog is quite useful for selecting indicators and for comparison results afterwards. It is also a valuable tool for identifying instrument effects.

Scope: Valid measures of happiness.

Coverage at 1-9-2003: 689 measures, mainly single questions.

Contents: Full description classified by: happiness variant, time reference, method of observation, rating of responses, full text in English, occasionally in other languages; reference to observed distribution of responses, observed reliabilities.

Search facilities: search on word, select on variant, time reference, method of observation, and rating scale used.

DISTRIBUTIONAL FINDINGS

Findings about the distribution of happiness are recorded in an inventory that summarizes population and sampling and provides the full frequency distribution of responses, as well as means and standard deviations. Comparison is facilitated by additional transformation of means and standard deviations to a common 0-10 scale and by presenting the 95 % confidence interval around the central tendency statistics. The inventory can be searched on methodology of the investigation, for example one can easily get to the distributions observed with a particular indicator of happiness, or compare findings yielded with face-to-face interviews to self-administered reports.

Distribution of Happiness in Nations

This inventory has a special section for results of studies in representative nation samples. This "Catalog of Happiness in Nations" lists the distribution of responses to acceptable questions on happiness in nationwide samples. As such it provides a basis for an international statistics of happiness. The data are ordered by question type and by year and nation. Thus the catalog allows comparison across nations and trough time.

The data on *average happiness* serve to identify the macro-social factors that mark off more and less livable societies. These data are also of use for monitoring social progress and decline. The data on *dispersion of happiness* in nations can be used in comparative studies of inequality in life chances. The uses of these data are spelt out in more detail elsewhere (Veenhoven, 1993, chapter 8; Veenhoven, 2002).

Scope: distributions of happiness in nations, as observed in representative samples of the adult population, only findings based on survey questions that validly tap an individual's "overall appreciation of his own life-as-a-whole".

Coverage at 1-9-2003: 2,165 distributions in 112 countries between 1945-2002; time series for 15 countries of twenty years and more; mainly first world countries, but also data from some third and second world nations; fairly complete up to 2002.

Contents: standard abstracts of findings involving: happiness indicator: full description, statistics: frequency distribution in %, mean and standard deviation – comparison is facilitated by transformation of all scores to range 0-10, number of (non-) respondents, bibliographics: author, title, year of publication, page reference, survey name: name of survey program or institute, location of data file; summary reports of nation rankings and trends over time.

Search facilities: on nation and year, on happiness measure.

Distribution of Happiness in Special Publics

This inventory can be searched on characteristics of the population; for instance, one can easily select all the findings on happiness among handicapped people.

Scope: distributions of happiness in special publics, such as aged or handicapped people; only findings based on survey questions that validly tap an individual's "overall appreciation of his own life-as-a-whole".

Coverage at 1-9-2003: 772 studies in 97 nations between 1911 and 2000; 1,133 distributional findings in 149 different publics; mainly first world countries, but also data from some third and second world nations; fairly complete up to 2000.

Contents: happiness indicator: full description; statistics: frequency distribution in %, mean and standard deviation. Comparison is facilitated by transformation of all scores to range 0-10, number of (non-) respondents, bibliographics: author, title, year of publication, page reference; survey name: name of survey program or institute, location of data file.

Search facilities: select on public type, country, time and happiness query.

CORRELATIONAL FINDINGS

Next to these distributional findings, the database provides an inventory of correlational data. The research findings are condensed in standard abstracts, which provide detail about measurement, population and time. These abstracts are ordered by subject matter. For instance, there are 204 abstracts of research findings on the relation between happiness and "age". These abstracts are easily retrieved.

This collection of well comparable research findings provides a basis for synthetic analysis of past research. It facilitates both narrative reviews and quantitative meta-analysis. The collection also helps to guide future research, by marking white spots. As the collection covers data from different nations and social categories, it can reveal universal patterns as well as contingencies.

Scope: empirical research findings on co-variants of happiness; not only factors found to be statistically associated to happiness, but also non-correlates; only findings yielded by indicators that validly tap happiness as the "overall appreciation of one's life-as-a-whole"; all findings that could be traced, not only the ones that reached scientific journals.

Coverage at 1-9-2003: 772 studies in 97 nations between 1911 and 2000; 8,132 correlational findings.

Contents: standard abstracts of correlational research findings ordered by subject, country and time. The abstracts include details about: bibliographic source: author, year, page reference, study design: population, sample, number of subjects, year, co-variate: label, measurement, subject-category, happiness-measure: type, statistics: association, significance, elaborations of the statistical relationship; text reports of findings by subject category, such as "age" or "income". These reports are in pdf and can be downloaded.

Search facilities: search on keyword; select on subject class, happiness query, public nation and time.

STATES OF NATIONS

Comparative analysis of the above findings is facilitated by a data file that involves both findings on happiness and characteristics of the nations in which these results were found.

Scope: Characteristics of nations that are relevant for the cross-national analysis of findings on happiness.

Coverage at 1-9-2003: 78 nations, among which all Western nations and Latin American nations; time series from the 1960s on.

Contents: societal characteristics such as wealth, individualism and religiousness; findings on happiness in these nations, both distributional and correlational.

Availability: The codebook is available on the web and can be browsed with keywords. The SPSS data file is available on request.

WEBSITE

The database (www.eur.nl/fsw/research/happiness)is freely available on Internet. On this site you can browse the various inventories. You can also download text reports of findings. These are reports on distributional findings in nations and reports of correlational findings by category. These reports are refreshed periodically.

USES OF THE DATA-COLLECTION

The data-collection on happiness will first of all be used for scientific purposes, for a better understanding of happiness and related matters. The collection will also facilitate policy orientation and public enlightenment.

Scientific Understanding of Happiness

When all the results of the 20th century's research are entered, this database will be a true treasure trove: This collection of research findings can improve our understanding in the following ways:

Inductive Illumination

One way to understanding is to go through the facts and consider their theoretical relevance. This can be called a "drag-net method". In that metaphor the facts stand for fish and is the net the whole of explanatory notions. This method does not only detect the findings that fit preexisting theories; it also makes us aware of phenomena we cannot easily explain. A systematic application of this approach can be found in Veenhoven 1984.

This collection of findings is quite suited to this method. Firstly it provides a broader scope than separate primary studies can offer. Secondly, the abstracts of research findings provide more condensed information than most reports of primary studies do. Thirdly, the collection brings unexpected findings to light, often findings that were marginal in the original investigation and hence not saliently reported.

For example, if we go through the rich data on the relationship between happiness and age, we see easily that there is a universal pattern of non-difference in overall life-satisfaction. This is at odds with current theorizing about both age-deprivation and cultural specificity. At a closer look we can also see that contentment rises with age, while mood tends to decline. This bears an important suggestion about variability in the way we strike the balance of life.

Deductive Theory Testing
Another road to understanding is to derive predictions about happiness from a theory and then test these inferences. Such tests can be performed on the findings in this collection. An example is the above-mentioned test of the theory that happiness is relative. Ideally one might prefer tests on primary data that are especially gathered for a particular test, but practically test on such secondary data is often the best feasible, especially when the test requires costly comparison across time and nations.

Synthesis of Past Research
Both approaches figure in current techniques for research synthesis, in narrative review studies as well as in quantitative meta-analyses. The greatest problem for such studies are to get a focused view on all the relevant research, and that is precisely what this collection of findings provides.

Regular state-of-the-art reviews are essential for the cumulating of knowledge on happiness. Yet such studies have become scarcer over the years because the field is ever more difficult to oversee. This collection of research findings solves that problem largely, because it presents a complete overview of the available findings in a well-accessible format.

On several subjects the data are sufficiently rich and homogenous to allow quantitative meta-analysis. This is for instance the case with data on the relationship of happiness to "sex", "age" and "income". Meta-analytic techniques allow a better estimate of general tendencies and of differences across time, nation and social categories.

For these purposes it is important that the collection is complete and well indexed. If only half the available research is covered, reviewers still have to go through the entire literature. Completeness is also important for keeping sight of exceptional findings and of methodologically outstanding studies.

Comparative Studies
The data-collection is quite suited to grasp differences in happiness and its determinants across time and culture. Comparison of the many observations of average happiness in nations helps to identify macro variables that render society more or less livable. Comparison of the rich correlational data enables distinction between universal requirements for happiness and cultural specific conditions. Size and homogeneity of the collection are crucial for this purpose.

Orientation for New Research
Further the database will improve the yields of further research. Research will at least be more innovative, because the white spots are better visible, and research will be better comparable because investigators have a more complete view of the measures used in earlier research. Hopefully research questions will also be better focused as a result of improved understanding. Completeness of the collection is most important for this purpose.

Policy Information

Happiness is of relevance in various policy issues and gains an ever more prominent place on the agenda. In social policy, happiness is at least one of the goals. In some of the care domains it is even a quite important goal, for instance in palliative healthcare and in psychotherapy.

Social policy
Findings on happiness can serve social policy in several ways. First they can help to identify pockets of dissatisfaction that are not recognized in the political process, or reversed, dismiss the exaggerations of lobbyists. Secondly, the findings provide clues about the probable effects of interventions, such as income suppletion, job creation and housing schemes. Lastly, the findings bear information about the relative effectiveness of the policy regime as-a-whole. This use of the findings is discussed in more detail in Veenhoven 1993b; 1995; and 2000b.

Part of the research on happiness has been instigated for these reasons, but the use of the outcomes has been limited so far. One reason is that voiced demand still carries more weight than silent suffering. Another reason is that some policy makers are disenchanted with the results, for instance, that people thrive equally well in nations with modest social security. This does not mean that happiness is insensitive to all policy. The findings suggest that happiness is quite responsive to improvements in legal security, interest articulation and tolerance.

Though apparently unwelcome in some circles, the message is still relevant. Sooner or later the findings will find their way in the policy process, in particular when cuts in social expenditure requires real priority setting.

Therapy
Findings on happiness can also guide therapeutic interventions at the individual level, both in curative medicine and in psychotherapy. Happiness is also a criterion for evaluating the long-term effectiveness of treatments. The need for monitoring quality-of-life outcomes is now widely recognized in the therapeutic professions and has given rise to a broad stream of research, with its own journals and research associations. In that tradition quality of life is typically measured using multidimensional inventories. These inventories tap not just subjective enjoyment of life, but also performance status and that practice devoids the findings of a clear meaning. Therefore the field can profit very much from the selection of findings on hap-

piness in this collection. Though this selection comprises less than 10 % of the re-search effort, it is still considerable because this research is so voluminous.

Care
Happiness is a more prominent aim in the care professions and is particularly rele-vant when chances for autonomy and improvement are small. Hence happiness is an important outcome variable in this trade. At the individual level it can serve to moni-tor the treatment of particular patients. At the organizational level it informs about the performance of clinics and departments. In this field there is also an established tradition of quality-of-life monitoring, but again the measures used for that purpose lack a clear meaning. Again a lot of more focused findings on happiness can be plucked from this research. When made well accessible for professionals, that in-formation will give voice to the needs of clients.

Public Enlightenment
Journalists often use the collection and this use will probably increase in the future. As noted in the introduction, there is an increasing demand for information about happiness for personal clarification and for orientation in lifestyle choices. This demand materializes in a continuous stream of documentaries on happiness, both ego-documents and popularizations of scientific research. Such use of the collection will increase when its availability and accessibility is improved.

Wider Uses of the Data System

Though developed for the study of happiness, this findings-browser can also be used for synthetic studies on other subjects. The basic software can be applied in quite different fields, such as in medical research or in cross-cultural psychology. Field specific elements, such as the classification of indicators and the list of statistics can easily be adapted. When applied on related matters, such as depression or self-esteem, the current classifications can be largely copied.

Synthetic studies will yield ground in the future. As the pile of research data is growing, synthesis becomes ever more profitable. Consequently there will be a greater need for systems that prepare for that. In the practice of research synthesis the greatest problem is not in the analysis, but in the preparation of the data.

HOW TO INCLUDE YOUR WORK

This database is updated continuously. If you deem your work relevant to this bibli-ography of happiness, please send a copy to the address below. "Grey" papers are also welcome.

All scientific work on subjective appreciation of life-as-a-whole will be included in the bibliography. Results of empirical work will also be summarized in the cata-logs (Happiness in Nations, or Correlates of Happiness), provided that the measures of happiness used fit our validity demands. Not all the work eligible for the catalogs is entered at the moment. About 500 reports wait for extraction. You can speed up inclusion of your work if you enter the results on an electronic form. That form can be downloaded from the website. Send your work to: World Database of Happiness, c/o Prof. Ruut Veenhoven, Erasmus University Rotterdam, Faculty of Social Sciences, POB 1738, NL-3000 DR Rotterdam, Netherlands, e-mail: veenhoven@fsw.eur.nl.

REFERENCES

Cummins, R. A. (ed.) (2000): Happiness and Progress. Journal of Happiness Studies 1 (3), 3-5.
Diener, E. (1999): Subjective Well-being. Three Decades of Progress. Psychological Bulletin 125, 276-301.
Ehrhardt, J., W. E. Saris & R. Veenhoven (2000): Stability of Life-satisfaction over Time in a National Panel. Journal of Happiness Studies 1, 177-205.
Headey, B. & A. Wearing (1992): Understanding Happiness, a Theory of Subjective Well-being, Melbourne: Longman Cheshire.
Stock, W. A. et al. (1983): Age Differences in Subjective Well-being. A Meta-analysis. Evaluation Studies Review Annual 8, pp. 279-302.
Veenhoven, R. (1984): Conditions of Happiness, Dordrecht & Boston: Kluwer Academic Publishers.
Veenhoven, R. (1991): Is happiness relative? Social Indicators Research 24, 1-34.
Veenhoven, R (1993): Happiness in Nations: Subjective Appreciation of Life in 56 Nations 1946-1992, Rotterdam: Erasmus University Rotterdam.
Veenhoven, R. (1994b): Is Happiness a Trait? Tests of the Theory that a Better Society Does not Make People any Happier. Social Indicators Research 32, 101-60.
Veenhoven, R. (1995): Developments in Satisfaction Research. Social Indicators Research 37, 1-46.
Veenhoven, R. (1997) : Progrès dans la Compréhension du Bonheur. Revue Quebecoise de Psychologie 18 (2), 29-74.
Veenhoven, R. (1999): Quality of Life in Individualistic Society. Social Indicators Research 48, 157-86.
Veenhoven, R. (2000a): The Four Qualities of Life. Journal of Happiness Studies 1 (1), 1-39.
Veenhoven, R. (2000b): Well-being in the Welfare State: Level not Higher, Distribution not more Equitable. Journal of Comparative Policy Analysis 2, 91-125.
Veenhoven, R. (2002): Return of Inequality in Moderns Society? Trends in Dispersion of Life Satisfaction in EU-nations 1973-1996. Published in German in: W. Glatzer, R. Habich & K. U. Maier (eds.): Sozialer Wandel und gesellschaftliche Dauerbeobachtung. Festschrift für Wolfgang Zapf, Opladen: Leske & Budrich, 273-94.

7. COMPARATIVE SURVEY QUESTIONS ON QUALITY OF LIFE: THE "DYNAMIC INFORMATION CENTRE"

A Contribution to a User-friendly Online Infrastructure for the Social Sciences

Michaela Hudler-Seitzberger

Paul Lazarsfeld Society for Social Research, Vienna, Austria

ABSTRACT

The "Dynamic Information Centre" (http://www.plg.at/search), which informs about comparative national and cross-national survey questions and survey programs relevant to welfare and quality of life measurement, has been established by the Paul Lazarsfeld Society for Social Research in the world wide web as one objective of the TSER project "EuReporting" – financed by the European Commission within the 4th framework program. The "Dynamic Information Centre" compiles besides information about survey questions and surveys, as survey description, archive, location of available data, questionnaires, countries and periods covered, links to related websites as well as additional information or services and allows online searches across data provider such as archives or research institutes linked to the "Dynamic Information Centre". Furthermore related literature which illustrates and explores survey data with special emphasis on data quality, is provided via a data base covering literature-cites. The "Dynamic Information Centre" functions as a retrievable user-friendly information platform on comparative social-welfare surveys carried out in the 15 member states of the European Union, the Czech Republic, Poland, Hungary, Switzerland and Norway. Within this science based information system, survey questions on social welfare are indexed according to a theoretical concept developed within this project by our project partners from ZUMA-Mannheim. This paper will inform about the structure of the "Dynamic Information Centre" and show the functionality for researcher working on social welfare and quality of life.

INTRODUCTION[1]

The World Wide Web offers new possibilities for research institutes and data archives to present their holdings and services to an interested audience. There is an enlarging number of initiatives and projects which aim in developing user-friendly web-based information systems which inform about surveys, meta-information dataholdings as well as related literature. There is a need in sciences for comprehensive information on surveys, survey data as well as related information within an user-friendly information platform organized within a science based data base for comparative cross-sectional and cross-national research. Especially data quality issues have to be regarded by such a system. Social sciences need science based categorization schemes for indexing surveys and especially survey questions which

91

Wolfgang Glatzer, Susanne von Below, Matthias Stoffregen (eds.), Challenges for Quality of Life in the Contemporary World, 91-105.

zation schemes for indexing surveys and especially survey questions which is essential for comparative research.

The development of the Dynamic Information Center (DIC) can be seen as one step into the direction of a dream machine for social scientists.

OBJECTIVE

An objective of the subproject 2.4 *Stocktaking of Comparative Databases in Survey Research* headed by Rudolf Richter, Paul Lazarsfeld Society for Social Research, Vienna, within the project "EuReporting – Towards a European System of Social Reporting and Welfare Measurement" financed by the European Commission within the 4th framework program had been to take stock of comparative national and cross-national surveys on social welfare currently available in Europe, Poland, the Czech Republic, Hungary, Norway and Switzerland.

A user-friendly information platform which provides survey questions and meta-information on social-welfare surveys should be designed for the use of an interested audience. Although several European data archives already offer meta-information the aim of this project has been to base such an information platform on a science based categorization scheme and to provide survey question documentation as well as comprehensive information in an user-friendly way. The new approach within this study has been to organize thematic information of cross-sectional national and cross-national surveys in an appropriate database in which searches across survey questions are possible.

One goal of the subproject was to develop and implement the DIC as a retrievable data base which offers information on surveys and survey questions in the area of social welfare. Information about the institutes or archives where the surveys are stored and survey data are available, the countries covered (for purposes of comparison), the year when it was carried out, any meta-information documentation on the surveys, the survey questionnaires, and related links to services offered on the base of the data (online data analyses, searches across codebooks and questionnaires, etc.) can be received from the data base.

Another issue of interest within this project is the topic data comparability and quality of pre-existing survey data. Similar, the same or almost the same questions have been asked in many countries, using translated survey questions. However, it cannot be guaranteed that exactly the same issues are measured in the different countries by multi-lingual versions, or even that the words or the questions themselves have the same meaning to the people asked in the investigated countries. Despite regarding the different equivalencies in question wording, response scales in the original and translated version of a questionnaire, there can be no certainty that the data is really measuring exact the same construct. A multitude of factors and reasons can have an influence on data quality: familiarity with the survey, questionnaire format, questioning style and a multitude of other reasons. Cultural background and different survey-execution methods, sampling methods, and all other aspects of technical survey execution can cause serious effects on data quality and the comparability of data gathered in different countries. The DIC has been developed as a meta-information system but also as information center which allows searches across survey questions and will summarize relevant information of the surveys with special emphasis on data quality.

METHODOLOGICAL APPROACH

Within this project work can be seen as divided into two parts: an inventory study, which takes stock of comparative cross-national and national surveys on social welfare and the investigation of information about data quality of comparative surveys. In the following the survey-selection process and subproject documentation efforts will be described as well as an outline of the features of an ideal database for the social sciences. The indexing and categorization concerns as well as efforts to document data quality within the DIC will also be reported. Finally the structure and the purpose of the literature database, which offers data related literature cites, is presented in another section.

Inventory Study – Survey Recruitment

In a first step, comparative surveys on social welfare, both cross-national and national, currently available in online catalogues of data archives have been identified. To guarantee a certain quality standard and to safeguard quality control, only surveys which are stored in data archives meeting a set of quality standard in documenting survey meta-information, as well as in preparing survey data and providing data to users via online catalogues have been recruited. The time horizon, the year 1980 was pragmatically chosen, and in order to allow comparisons over time a repetition of the survey program a minimum of three times since then are required. The documentation includes surveys till 2000. The countries covered are the 15 member states of the European Union, Hungary, Poland, the Czech Republic, Norway and Switzerland. The keywords used for selecting the surveys and survey programs have been "quality of life", "welfare", and "standard of living".

As relevant to the project have been identified: the cross-sectional and cross-national *Eurobarometer Surveys* executed twice a year in the member states of the European Union; the *Central and Eastern Eurobarometer Surveys*, carried out in Central and Eastern Europe from 1990 to 1997, but no longer exist in this design. The *Eurobarometer Surveys* cover issues mainly related to the European Union, but they often include questions on social and economic trends and on special topics. *The International Social Survey Programme,* carried out annually with special social topics changing every five years, has also been identified as relevant. This survey program covers countries in Eastern as well as Western Europe.

The five waves of the *New Democracies Barometer Surveys* have been fielded in many Eastern European countries, investigating socio-economic and political matters which are of relevance for the project.

The *World Values Survey*, executed every decade since 1980 in various societies throughout the world (for a total of three times), is another survey program of interest for measuring welfare. The *World Values Surveys* investigates values in different areas of life.

The *International Crime (Victim) Survey*, had been in field for three times during the phase of observation. These surveys cover the topic public safety and crime.

The *International Social Justice Project*, which has also been considered to be relevant for the project has been conducted twice – and in some countries, three times. It deals with many issues concerning inequality and social exclusion. Data of the *International Social Justice Project* are available for Western as well as in Eastern European societies.

The comparative research programs listed below cover also issues relevant for the project have been identified as relevant for the project because they allow cross-national comparisons of results, though not longitudinal comparisons. The identified surveys have carried out once since 1980. The surveys are *Comparative Project on Class Structures and Class Consciousness, Reader's Digest Eurodata, Pulse of Europe, Dismantling of the Social Safety Net and Its Political Consequences in East-Central Europe, Social Stratification in Eastern Europe after 1989* and *Social Consequences of Economic Transformation in East-Central Europe.*

A further objective of the project was to look at longitudinal surveys with repeated cross-sectional samples (repeated at least three times since 1980). National comparative surveys have been recruited via online archive enquiries and expert consultations:

- *Great Britain and Northern Ireland*: British and the Northern Ireland Social Attitudes Survey;
- *Czech Republic*: Economic Expectations and Attitudes (EEA), Czechoslovak Social Structure and Mobility Survey, Ten Years of Social Transformation;
- *Finland*: Finnish Level of Living Survey, Finnish Social Thinking;
- *France*: Living Conditions and Aspirations of the French;
- *Germany*: German Welfare Survey, Social Survey (ALLBUS);
- *Netherlands*: Living Conditions in The Netherlands, Cultural Changes in The Netherlands;
- *Norway*: Norwegian Level of Living Survey;
- *Poland*: Polish General Social Survey, The Poles, Life Conditions and Aspirations, Social Structure and Consciousness of Polish Society;
- *Spain*: Latinobarometer, Centre for Research on Social Reality Survey;
- *Sweden*: Swedish Level of Living Survey, The Swedish National Survey of Living Conditions (ULF).

Within the DIC the survey question documentation is kept in English and German. If a questionnaire from a survey program has not been available in an official English or German version, the project could not cover these questions. There have been no financial and time recourses for professional science based translation.

However, in order to cover as many surveys as available, the principal investigators of all the surveys mentioned have been contacted and asked for any existing German or English version of questionnaires of the referring surveys. Only surveys, where such questionnaires have been offered, have been considered as relevant for the DIC and documented as described in the following section.

The surveys investigated in the inquiry cover social welfare using objective as well as subjective indicators to a different extent. The Scandinavian surveys investigate more or less objective indicators. *The World Values Surveys* apply mainly sub-jective ones. The survey questions documented within the DIC range from covering exclusively objective information to exclusively subjective information.

Within the DIC only surveys which have been carefully documented and de-scribed, and where data are available and documented by data archives or institu-tions for secondary analysis. This pragmatic decision guarantees a certain quality standard.

Because it is important for the DIC to get as many surveys as possible for docu-mentation and provide a comprehensive collection of comparative academic sur-veys. Therefore in a next step, our *EuReporting* partners – all well-known experts in the field of social reporting and welfare measurement – have been contacted and asked to provide social-welfare surveys of relevance to this project. It can be as-sumed that such a strategy will ensure that the project will obtain well-documented and high-quality surveys that are worth documenting down to the question level, as it is the intention of this project.

Following information has been collected by the team of this subproject:

- archives and institutions where the surveys and the survey data are avail-able,
- countries covered for comparative reasons,
- year carried out,
- meta-information documentation from the surveys (via link where avail-able),
- data-quality criteria,
- survey questionnaires (also via link where available),
- related links to services instituted on the basis of the data (online data analy-ses, codebook or questionnaire searches, etc.).

The DIC has been designed following the vision of an "ideal" science based data-base for the social sciences and intends to develop a user-friendly database with simple and visually clearly structured interface for searches and results, which offers quick and easy access to survey questions on social welfare, and to provide precise information the user is looking for, delivered as search results which also offer tips on where further information and data are accessible or where online analyses are offered.

In the following, an overview of the concept of a science based database cover-ing survey questions on social welfare will be described.

Concept of a Science-based Database Covering Survey – Questions on Social Welfare

The purpose of creating the Dynamic Information Center (DIC) has been to provide a science based databases for use by the scientific community, policy-makers and other users that covers questions relevant to welfare measurement of comparative cross-sectional surveys, meta-information, questionnaires, information on data qual-ity, related links and survey-related literature.

Within the project the general policy was that every information that is already available in the web and is essential for our project will be integrated into the database of the DIC via link. This policy guarantees that no duplication of effort and copyright violations will take place. In order to link already offered information to the DIC permission has been requested from archives and institutions offering such information and services. Only links, where those permissions have been received, are opened. The addresses of the other links are inactive, so that a user can copy and insert them into the command line. Links are opened within a separate window so that anybody can see that the link refers to a page in the www.

To realize the vision of an ideal database for the social sciences an option to carry out online analyses and to visualize results have to be offered. Data archives already provide such tools for online analyses therefore the project tries to develop a database which is compatible to the tools designed by archives so that the information stored within the database is compatible to the new tools like NESSTAR (Networked Social Science Tools and Resources), which allows online analyses and the visualization of results.

The database behind the DIC is established using the software Microsoft ACCESS and designed as an open system which can easily be transformed into a SQL database for the www.

The database of the DIC offers detailed searches across survey questions on questions covering different life domains asked in surveys carried out in the fifteen member countries of the European Union as well as in Norway, Switzerland, Hungary, Poland and the Czech Republic. In order to offer a *science-based database* for social welfare research, the keywords refer directly to the life domains listed in the *European System of Social Indicators* (henceforth called EUSI) developed by Berger-Schmitt and Noll (2000). Indexing took place at the question level.

Categories for Indexing Survey Questions

In general, for indexing clear, easy-to-understand and controlled science-based vocabulary should be used to enable quick and easy access to survey questions on social welfare.

The indexing process of survey questions is a crucial act. Especially within the multiple-search options intended by the project, to specific keywords enhance no result searches whereas to generous keywords do not produce exact results. After examining different thesauri which are offered by some institutions for special topics (ILO, UNESCO, etc.) and having a look the elaborated thesaurus HASSET (Humanities And Social Science Electronic Thesaurus) which is provided by the Data Archive in Essex (UK), the team decided to use these terms developed by Berger-Schmitt and Noll (2000) for indexing survey questions. The usage of common keywords over the three subprojects allows searches among the three subprojects.

The keywords closely related to EUSI which are used for indexing are the *life domains:* population, migration/foreigners, households and families, women and gender inequality, children and youth, older people, housing, transport, leisure, culture and communications, participation and social integration, education, employment and working conditions, income and consumption, poverty, health, environment, social security, public safety and crime. *In addition, the categories mentioned below are used:* values and attitudes, social inequalities as goal dimensions, social exclusion as measurement, sustainability, which is considered to represent a welfare concept in accordance with the theoretical concept developed within the project (see Berger-Schmitt & Noll, 2000). To guarantee the reliability of the categorization, questions were categorized by two rater.

For detailed searches across social-welfare survey questions, it has to be useful to introduce further selection criteria. It appeared necessary to differentiate between information raised at the objective level, according to the above-mentioned classification system, and subjective information. Therefore, it would be useful to introduce the following selection fields to ensure a proper classification:

-   *objective* (objective living conditions and demographic characteristics),
-   *objective/subjective* (questions indicating social status and social behavior),
-   *subjective/objective* (questions concerning the perception of one's situation in different areas of life), and
-   *subjective* (questions inquiring satisfaction in different areas of life, happiness and well being and attitudes towards persons, institutions, topics, services in various life domains) about social welfare.

Furthermore, more detailed keywords – for example according to a scientific categorization scheme as well as the introduction of free text searches could allow more precise searches and results. Unfortunately until now no such comprehensive indexing catalogue has been developed. An attempt has been made by the Data Archive in Essex.

The new approach of subproject 2.4 has been, that survey questions have been indexed. This is a new and innovative approach for survey documentation.

META INFORMATION OF SURVEYS ACROSS EUROPE

Meta information of social science surveys is online available via data archives or social science institutions. Although there are certain standards for meta information documentation the amount of information provided is different depending of the provider. There are no standards which information has to be to offer. Huge differences can be observed in the both quality and quantity of the information documented and presented.

Within the DIC meta information of project relevant surveys is integrated via links. Only meta-information from surveys which cannot be integrated via link has been published but only if the team has written authorization to do so. If the permission is given, additional services offered by certain institutions – such as downloading data, carrying out online analyses, searching for related literature, searching across codebooks – are linked to the database. The original-version of the questionnaires is also offered through the DIC, but only if they have already been published on the Internet and/or if the Paul Lazarsfeld Gesellschaft has been given authorization to publish the survey questionnaire.

Database Structure

The database of the DIC has been established in MS ACCESS and consists of several modules: a module covering survey questions, including question characteristics directly related to data quality, a module covering meta-information of surveys not stored in social-science data archives, a module covering meta-information of surveys stored in social-science data archives, a module covering publications or websites on data quality, a module covering survey related links, a literature database.

The survey question module offers a detailed description of each question indexed, according to the EUSI life domains (Berger-Schmitt & Noll, 2000). Based on the official English versions (of the basic questionnaires), the survey questions have been documented and categorized. Questions are described using the following categories: question header (introductory text of a question or battery of questions), question text (text of the question or item), interviewer instructions (those which the interviewer has to follow), filter text (stipulating that certain questions are only to be asked of certain sample groups), labels (response categories), type of information asked (agree/disagree, judgement, frequency), response scale characteristics, keywords related to EUSI life domains (Berger-Schmitt & Noll, 2000).

The fields type of information asked and response scale characteristics are both selection criteria for the survey question search option. Type of information asked, type of response scale and length of response scale are according to the research results of Saris et al. (1997) directly related to data quality.

The module presenting meta-information published by archives offers survey descriptions via link to the concerning data archives or institutions. In order to avoid duplication of effort and copyright violations, any archives and research institutes have been contacted for authorization to link their information published in the web to our database. Only the links to such information are active where the team obtained the permission to publish the information via the DIC, the other link addresses are also available but inactive. In that case, the user-friendliness of the DIC is not really given.

The module covering quality criteria posts, on the one hand, websites with information about data quality of the concerning survey data, and on the other, links providing access to papers dealing with quality of data in the corresponding surveys.

The module offering related links summarizes links to services and information provided by research institutes, principal investigators or data-storing organizations.

After the selection process, the following comparative cross-national and cross-sectional survey programs have been documented and the survey question categorized:

Eurobarometer, Central and Eastern Eurobarometer, International Social Survey Programme, World Values Survey, New Democracies Barometer, International Crime and Victim Survey, International Social Justice Project.

Several other cross-national and cross-sectional surveys have also been described within this data base. These surveys have been carried out only once since 1980 and are available in data archive. Special focus is put on those surveys which have been carried out in Central and Eastern Europe:

Social Costs of Transition, Pulse of Europe, Reader's Digest Eurodata 1990, Dismantling of the Social Safety Net and Its Political Consequences in East-Central Europe, International Social Justice Project 1991 (which has been replicated in several countries in 1995 and in 1999), Social Stratification in Eastern Europe after 1989.

Also national comparative survey programs which cover survey questions relevant to social reporting have been analyzed:

British and Northern Ireland Social Attitudes Surveys, Economic Expectations and Attitudes, Czechoslovak Social Structure and Mobility Survey, German Welfare Surveys, German General Social Surveys, Polish General Social Survey, Poles 1995, Swedish Level of Living Surveys, Swedish National Survey of Living Conditions, Ten Years of Social Transformation.

To describe surveys which are not documented in archives, the following fields have been used: survey name (title of the survey and, if applicable, program as well), survey type (an artificial grouping of national and cross-national survey programs, for comparative purposes), geographical coverage (countries covered by the survey/project), principal investigator (name of the researcher or institution responsible for the survey), research instrument (link to the original questionnaires), field-work period (period during which the survey was carried out), sample description (information on both the sample and the sampling strategy), sample size (number of respondents), data-collector (staff collecting data in the field), data-collection method (tells how the survey was carried out, e.g. as a face-to-face interview, self-competence survey, etc.), translation procedure (documents attempts to control translations; applies only to cross-national surveys).

The category "survey type" has been introduced as an artificial category for summarizing survey programs. The programs are grouped as follows:

International social surveys: *International Social Survey Programme;*

National social surveys: *German General Social Survey, Polish General Social Survey, British Social Attitudes Survey, Northern Ireland Social Attitudes Survey;*

International welfare surveys: *Euromodule;*

National welfare surveys: *German Welfare Survey, Swedish Level of Living Survey, The Swedish National Survey of Living Conditions;*

Eastern European transition surveys: *New Democracies Barometer, Social Consequences of Economic Transformation in East-Central Europe, Dismantling of the Social Safety Net and Its Political Consequences in East Central Europe, Social Stratification in Eastern Europe after 1989;*

Eurobarometer: *Eurobarometer, Central and Eastern Eurobarometer;*

Other international special-purpose social surveys: *World Values Survey, International Social Justice Project, International Crime and Victimisation Survey, The Pulse of Europe, Reader's Digest Eurodata;*

Other national special-purpose social surveys: *Economic Expectations and Attitudes, Ten Years of Social Transformation, Czechoslovak Social Structure and Mobility Survey, The Poles, Latinobarometer.*

Searches across questions are enabled by the following selection fields: survey name, survey program, survey type, keyword, time period, countries, type of information, type and length of the response scale (tells whether it is a verbal, numeral or line-producing scale and how many categories the response scale has).

Running a query as result of any search, the surveys, year, and question text will appear in the left navigation frame. By clicking on a question, full question documentation will appear in the right navigation frame. Also appearing is information on countries where the questions have been executed and information on data quality (translation procedures for cross-national surveys, if not included in the meta-information documentation). Additional information as survey-related meta-information provided by the archives where the studies are stored, as well as related links to services offered by the archives, e.g. codebooks or bibliography searches are also results of a search.

Another objective of the subproject has been to deal with data quality. Data quality in survey research is a very complex research field, even more so in comparative cross-national survey research. The subproject tried to provide information about data and data quality at different levels.

Approach towards Data Quality

In comparative survey research the question concerning equivalence of data and survey questions is an ever lasting. Does a single question measure the same concept in different societies? Does a question really measure what it ought to measure? How reliable and valid is this measurement? These are the questions of interest.

In many research approaches has been shown, that for example the optical design of questionnaires, question position, question formulation, response-scale character-istics and so on all have a significant influence on data quality. The well known errors like coverage, sampling, non-response and measurement errors lead to re-spondent bias, instrument bias, interviewer bias and mode bias.

The documentation of meta-information provided by archives give an overview of the technical and methodological issues related to data quality in survey research. The technical or methodological reports of the surveys include coverage (definition of the population), sampling, non-response, and mode of data collection. But unfor-tunately many documentations include only a small part of the information research-ers needs for their scientific work.

As mentioned above, question characteristics within survey questions can have an influence on survey results especially in cross-national research (Saris et al., 1997). In general, the project's approach towards data quality focuses on the reliabil-ity and validity of survey results.

Already published quality estimates of survey data have been entered into the da-tabase. Existing and published quality criteria – e.g. reliability, validity, internal consistency – are presented within the DIC database. To get access to information about quality of survey data the principal investigators of the surveys or the survey programs have been asked for information on the quality of their survey data. A small number of principal investigators replied and provided several publication titles and abstracts dealing with the data quality of their surveys. Many researchers informed us that there are no publications known to them where data quality has been analyzed more extensively than in archives in the technical descriptions. In many cases this information is included into the methodological reports of the sur-veys, and some informed us that there is no relevant information available in Eng-lish. For almost every survey technical or methodological reports provide common information on the design and fieldwork of a survey. But within such reports hardly any information could be found which refers to reliability or validity of survey data. Our approach of publishing information on data quality which is already available could maybe initiate further research on data quality, especially for comparative purposes.

To get as many information about data quality as possible, in a second step survey related publications offered online have been inspected. Some literature cites where data quality has been analyzed have been the result of the investigation. In the following some examples of data quality information which are given within the DIC are described:

Saris and Kaase (1997) examined the effect of the sample design, method of data collection and translation on data quality for a *Eurobarometer* survey.

In the framework of the *International Social Survey Programme* (ISSP) ZUMA-Mannheim established a special methodological working group. Some scales from the ISSP survey questionnaire have been analyzed concerning data quality. The research results have been in the *ZUMA Reports* and are also available via the *Zentrales Informations-Service* (ZIS), provided by ZUMA as an online information service which informs about quality of used scales. The information provided within ZIS is the description of each indicator of the scale, the response scale, development of the instrument, sample description, dimensionality of the scale, item characteristics, reliability, validity and data-analyzing instructions. Furthermore the theoretical background and literature cites of related publications are also published there. ZIS provides relevant data quality information included into for the DIC of following surveys: the *German General Social Survey* (ALLBUS), *International Social Survey Programme* (ISSP) and *International Social Justice Project* (ISJP).

Information on data quality of certain scales and surveys from the ALLBUS program is published online in ALLBUS working papers and several other working papers of the ALLBUS research team at ZUMA. In the frequently appearing *ZUMA News*, quality estimates can also be found. Within the DIC these reports are included via link.

ZUMA Special News deals with *Cross-cultural Survey Equivalence* (1998). A few items from the ISSP and *British Social Attitudes Survey* questionnaires have been analyzed for cross-cultural comparisons concerning data quality.

Kreuter (2000) deals with the effect of different response scales on data quality and comparability on the example of the *German Welfare Survey* and *International Victimization Survey.*

Quality analyses on the base of the *New Democracies Barometer* data have been carried out on comparable scales across time and countries, which will also be available within the DIC.

Besides many other influences, question characteristics have a relevant impact on data quality. Saris et al. (1997) analyzed the impact of different survey question characteristics and found out that each one of them causes deviations in validity and reliability estimates. Especially in order to provide a science-based approach, the team decided that the type of information requested and the type and length of a response scale – both considered by Saris et al. to have an impact on data quality – will be provided within the DIC as search fields.

Survey and survey data related literature cites of publications which are organized within a literature data base are also linked to the DIC in order to provide a comprehensive information service.

Concept of the Literature Database

Mainly "grey literature" deals with and explores survey data. This literature can hardly be accessed. The intention of the project team to establish a literature database was the assumption that anybody using the question database could also be interested in related literature based on data obtained by a certain survey. The literature databases documents categorized survey related literature. As indexing terms the science-based categories developed by Berger-Schmitt and Noll (2000) have been applied.

The cites have been selected from publications of the principal investigators with related references, web-sites of the studies or survey programs – including related papers – the information gathered from several online catalogues and from the descriptions of special surveys (for details, see Hudler & Richter, 2000a).

The literature hints have been categorized and entered into a ProCite database applying a common standard developed under the co-ordination of our project partners of subproject 2.5. Guidelines, style sheets, categorization topics and forms have been developed for entering the cites. The technical realization of implementing the literature database on the web has also been an issue of subproject 2.5.[2]

Data have been entered into the literature database during the life span of the project. Indexing has been based on abstracts of the publications when they have been available. In the case no abstract has been there, indexing has been based on the keywords of the title. Indexing has been controlled by indexing the same cites by two rater.

Within the literature, data base searches are possible across topics, year, country, survey type and survey name. In the following two charts, the mask as well as a search result can be viewed. The DIC can be seen as one attempt towards a user-friendly service for social scientists. Access to the information is free and the system is easy to handle.

DISCUSSION

Of course this attempt, described in the previous sections is a first step into the direction of a social-science's dream machine. The requirements which should be met by an ideal data base for the social sciences are much more elaborated as could be realized within the DIC.

How such a dream machine could look like as described also in the final report of the project is outlined in the concluding paragraphs.

Survey research on social welfare as well as the documentation has to be based on hard scientific data. The indicators, at the one hand based on traditional concepts or at the other on new developments, should be grounded on the basis of recognized social and economic theories.

In the future, given new developments in information and communication technologies, any documentation on social reporting activities needs to appear not only in printed but also in electronic form. Beside CD-ROMs, the web has become the new publishing media for scientific activity.

Information about surveys, survey documentation and data on social welfare have to be available world wide, easily accessible, fast and free.

Such documentation and information systems on the web have to be designed as open systems where already existing information can be integrated into new frameworks. The systems themselves should allow easy integration into other systems.

Comprehensive information systems on social-welfare data are required. Official statistics and cross-sectional survey data should be available in a common system including all relevant information and references.

Standardized and harmonized meta-information on a high standard should be provided within such information systems. There would also be a need that a user can identify high-quality data sets. As a minimum requirement can be seen a comprehensive meta information documentation, online question databases, links to related websites, links to data related articles, links to other sources, such as related web pages, e-mail addresses, databases, data-quality estimates, codebook searches, downloadable data, online data analysis (even advanced analysis), visualization of results, active intelligent clients, which help to select information on a certain topic. Filtering and ranking possibilities should be offered to obtain appropriate results and reduce server loads.

Quality has to be guaranteed at any steps in the searching process. This includes of course reliable results, as well as an efficient, scientifically well-grounded indexing system. Expert experience can be integrated into such a system.

Documentation systems need to be multi-lingual including comprehensive multi-lingual science-based categorization schemes. At the time English is the *lingua franca* for documenting surveys and related information. Searches should be possible but also search results have to appear optional in different languages. Language concerns should not be a barrier to get access to information and data. Translations have to be executed according to state-of-the-art scientific standards. Multilingual free text searches should also be implemented. The demand for a standardized multi-lingual science-based thesaurus to provide keywords detailed enough to find specific issues and open enough to include new concepts and developments. National as well as international issues have to be covered.

It is very important that the content and data of such a system are kept up to date. This means routinely updating the information and services.

The DIC can be seen as a very important first step in the context of knowledge management. The DIC offers information which survey questions have been asked in which states at which time and tells which information and services are available. It summarizes information provided by different sources.

For the purposes of comparative research and for producing time series in order to monitor or detect social changes and development, an inventory of previously asked questions can help when designing new questionnaires. It helps to contribute to data quality by increasing the quality of survey questions.

The DIC is intended as a meta-information platform which brings together relevant information, data, services and questionnaires from the important European comparative cross-national and national cross-sectional social-welfare surveys available in the www. Data quality as a precondition for data comparison is a special focus of this information collection.

NOTES

1   This paper has been drawn from the Final Report of the EuReporting subproject 2.4 delivered to the European Commission in 2001 by Rudolf Richter and Michaela Hudler-Seitzberger.
2   We would like to take this opportunity to thank the subproject 2.5 team.

REFERENCES

Berger-Schmitt, R. & H.-H. Noll (2000): Conceptual Framework and Structure of a European System of Social Indicators. EuReporting Working Paper No. 9, Mannheim.

Borgers, N. & J. J. Hox (2000): Reliability of Responses in Questionnaire Research with Children. Paper presented at the Fifth International Conference on Logic and Methodology, Cologne.

Groves, R. M. (1989): Survey Errors and Survey Costs, New York: Wiley.

Hudler, M. & R. Richter (2000a): State of the Art of Surveys on Social Reporting in Western and Eastern Europe. EuReporting Working Paper No. 7, Vienna: Paul Lazarsfeld Gesellschaft für Sozialforschung.

Hudler, M. & R. Richter (2000b): Source-book about Questions on Social Reporting in Cross-national and Cross-sectional Surveys - an Example on Questions Covering the Life Domain Education. EuReporting Working Paper No. 13, Vienna: Paul Lazarsfeld Gesellschaft für Sozialforschung.

International Labor Office (ILO) (1990): International Standard Classification of Occupations: ISCO 88, Geneva: ILO.

Kaase, M. & W. E. Saris (1997): The Eurobarometer - a Tool for Comparative Survey Research. M. Kaase & W. E. Saris (eds.): Eurobarometer: Measurement Instrument for Opinion in Europe, ZUMA Nachrichten Spezial Band 2, Mannheim.

Kreuter, F. (2000): Uncertainty in Capturing Uncertainty: Toward Measurement of Fear of Crime. Part I: Measuring Subjective Probability. Paper Presented at the ISQOLS Conference, Gerona, 2000.

Scherpenzeel, A.C. & W. E. Saris (1997): The Validity of Survey Questions. Social Methods and Research 25, 341-83.

Saris, W. E. (1997a): Comparability across Mode and Country. M. Kaase & W. E. Saris (eds.): Eurobarometer: Measurement Instrument for Opinion in Europe, ZUMA Nachrichten Spezial Band 2, Mannheim.

Saris, W. E. (1997b): Adjustment for Differences between Face-to-face and Telephone Interviews. M. Kaase & W. E. Saris (eds.): Eurobarometer: Measurement Instrument for Opinion in Europe, ZUMA Nachrichten Spezial Band 2, Mannheim.

Saris, W. E. & J. A. Hagenaars (1997): Mode Effects in the Standard Eurobarometer Questions.M. Kaase & W. E. Saris (eds.): Eurobarometer: Measurement Instrument for Opinion in Europe, ZUMA Nachrichten Spezial Band 2, Mannheim.

Saris, W. E. (1998): The Effects of Measurement Error in Cross-Cultural Research. Cross-Cultural Survey Equivalence, ZUMA - Spezial Nachrichten Nr. 3, Mannheim, 1998.

UNESCO (1997): International Standard Classification of Education ISCED 1997, Paris: UNESCO.

UNESCO (1999): Operational Manual for ISCED 1997, Paris: UNESCO.

Vogel, J. (1997): The Future Direction of Social Indicators Research. Social Indicators Research 42, 103-16.

Zenk-Möltgen, W. (2000): Deutsche nationale Wahlstudien 1949-1998. Available on CD-ROM. ZA-Information 47, Cologne.

REFERENCES ON THE WORLD WIDE WEB

Centre for the Study of Public Policy:
    http://www.cspp.strath.ac.uk
Danish Data Archive:
    http://www.dda.dk
Data Archive in Essex:
    http://www.data-archive.ac.uk
Digital Information System for Social Indicators (DISI):
    http://www.gesis.org/en/social_monitoring/social_indicators/Data/Disi/disi.htm

Humanities and Social Science Electronic Thesaurus (HASSET):
   http://biron.essex.ac.uk/searching/zhasset.html
Networked Social Science Tools and Resources (NESSTAR):
   http://www.nesstar.org
The Council of European Social Science Data Archives (CESSDA):
   http://dasun3.essex.ac.uk/Cessda/IDC
Zentraler Informationsdienst (ZIS):
   http://www.gesis.org/Methodenberatung/ZIS/Download/download.htm

8. AN EVIDENCE-BASED APPROACH TO THE CONSTRUCTION OF SUMMARY QUALITY-OF-LIFE INDICES

Kenneth C. Land

Duke University, Durham NC, USA

ABSTRACT

This paper commences with a review of some objectives for social indicators and quality-of-life research that were stated in the founding years of the social indicators movement. It then reviews the current state of the art in constructing objective social indicators and in studies of subjective well-being. Using recent work the author and associates have done on the development of a Child Well-being Index (CWI), it is demonstrated how the findings of studies of subjective well-being can be used to inform the construction of summary quality-of-life indices. In particular, it is shown how the CWI can be viewed as a well-being-evidence-based measure of trends in averages of the social conditions encountered by children and youths in the U.S. across recent decades. Several key properties of the CWI are discussed. Various empirical findings regarding child well-being in the United States are summarized. The presentation concludes with some developments in the CWI that are needed if it is to fulfill the founding objectives of the social indicators project.

INTRODUCTION[1]

When Wolfgang Glatzer, President of the International Society for Quality-of-Life Studies, asked me to prepare a presentation for the Opening Session of the Fifth Conference of ISQOLS, I commenced by collecting my thoughts about the purpose of "opening sessions" for conferences of scholarly societies. It became clear to me that these sessions function in many ways like the meetings of religious organizations. That is, what we have here at the Conference is a gathering of diverse people from many academic disciplines and many regions of the world, all of whom are united by their common interest in studying the conceptualization of the quality of life, how to measure it, and how to track changes therein over time and social space. What we need, therefore, in an opening session is for presenters to remind us of our common values and beliefs – those ideas and things which we hold in common, the paths our predecessors have broken, where we are today, and where we can hope to be in the bright tomorrow.

These, then, are the objectives of my presentation. I will begin with a review of the "holy words" of the founding documents and founders of the social indicators and quality-of-life movements of the 1960s and 1970s. You will see that these

Wolfgang Glatzer, Susanne von Below, Matthias Stoffregen (eds.), Challenges for Quality of Life in the Contemporary World, 107-124.

statements are ambitious indeed. Then I will take up the question: Where are we now? I will review the current state of our knowledge base with respect to the goals of the founding figures of our field. As an illustration of current practice, I then will use some recent work in which I have been engaged on the development of an index of child and youth well-being in the United States and on the measurement of trends therein over the past quarter century. I will conclude by raising the question: Can we do more? I will briefly sketch some of the possibilities for future work.

WHERE DID WE BEGIN 30+ YEARS AGO? A REVIEW OF THE FOUNDING GOALS OF SOCIAL INDICATORS AND QUALITY-OF-LIFE RESEARCH

To understand where we are today with respect to scholarly efforts to define and measure the quality of life and with respect to the development of social indicators for that purpose, it is useful to recall some key definitions from our predecessors. To begin with, the term *social indicators* was born and given its initial meaning in an attempt, undertaken in the early 1960s by the American Academy of Arts and Sciences for the National Aeronautics and Space Administration, to detect and antici-pate the nature and magnitude of the second-order consequences of the space pro-gram for American society (Land, 1983, p. 2; Noll & Zapf, 1994, p. 1). Frustrated by the lack of sufficient data to detect such effects and the absence of a systematic conceptual framework and methodology for analysis, some of those involved in the Academy project attempted to develop a system of social indicators – statistics, statistical series, and other forms of evidence – with which to detect and anticipate social change as well as to evaluate specific programs and determine their impact. The results of this part of the Academy project were published in a volume (Bauer, 1966) bearing the name *Social Indicators* and the following definition:

> "... *social indicators* – statistics, statistical series, and all other forms of evidence – that enable us to assess where we stand and are going with respect to our values and goals..." (Bauer, 1966, p. 1)

It should be noted that the appearance of the Bauer volume was not an isolated event. Several other influential publications commented on the lack of a system for charting social change and advocated that the U.S. government establish a "system of social accounts" that would facilitate a cost-benefit analysis of more than the market-related aspects of society already indexed by the National Income and Prod-uct Accounts (see, e.g., National Commission on Technology, Automation and Eco-nomic Progress, 1966; Sheldon & Moore, 1968).

The need for social indicators also was emphasized by the publication of the 101-page *Toward a Social Report (TSR)* on the last day of the Johnson administra-tion in 1969. Conceived of as a prototypical counterpart to the annual economic reports of the president, each of its seven chapters addressed major issues in an im-portant area of social concern (health and illness; social mobility; the physical envi-ronment; income and poverty; public order and safety; learning, science, and art; and participation and alienation) and provided its readers with an assessment of preva-lent conditions. In an appendix that addressed the question of how we can do better social reporting in the future, Mancur Olson, the principal author of *TSR*, put for-ward the following influential definition:

> "A *social indicator*... may be defined to be a statistic of direct normative interest which facilitates concise, comprehensive and balanced judgments about the condition of major aspects of a society." (USDHEW, 1969, p. 97)

In brief, *TSR* firmly established the link of social indicators to the idea of systematic reporting on social issues for the purpose of public enlightenment about how we are doing with respect to certain social conditions.

Another major pathway and avenue of exploration to the measurement of social indicators was opened in 1976 with the publication of a book entitled *The Quality of American Life: Perceptions, Evaluations, and Satisfactions* by Angus Campbell, Philip E. Converse, and Willard L. Rodgers. As signaled in the subtitle of the book, these social psychologists proposed to monitor the conditions of life by attempting to measure the experiences of individuals with the conditions of life, or as they put it:

> "... we propose... to 'monitor the *quality of American life*' ... our concern was with the experience of life rather than the conditions of life... [we] define the quality of life experience mainly in terms of satisfaction [with life and specific life domains]. (Campbell, Converse, and Rodgers 1976, pp. 7,9)

In brief, the key emphasis of this definition is on the measurement of human experiences of social conditions.

WHERE ARE WE NOW? A REVIEW OF THE CURRENT STATE OF THE ART IN CONSTRUCTING SUMMARY QUALITY-OF-LIFE INDICES – WITH A FOCUS ON CHILD WELL-BEING

Various observers (e.g., Land 2000; Noll 2002) have noted that these "founding definitions" of the social indicators and quality-of-life concepts have led to two major lines of development over the past 30+ years.

Objective Social Indicators

This line of development began with the Bauer (1966) volume and extends to the present. The emphasis is on the development of statistics that reflect important "social conditions" and the monitoring of trends in a range of "areas of social concern" over time. The key undefined terms here require the identification of:
- the "social conditions" to be measured, and
- the "areas of social concern" for which trends are to be monitored.

Since the 1970s, the primary approach to the identification and definition processes has been through the creation of "expert" panels of social scientists, statisticians, and citizens. These panels have applied a variety of approaches to their work, such as:
- the "indicators of social change" approach (Sheldon and Moore, 1968);
- the Swedish "level of living" approach (Erickson, 1974); and
- the "goals commissions" approach (e.g., the *U.S. Healthy People 2010* Goals; see USDHHS, 2000).

The key element of this approach is that the experts must achieve consensus. Specifically, as Noll (2002, p. 175) notes, there must be consensus on:
- the conditions and areas of concern to be measured;

-   good and bad conditions; and
-   the directions in which society should move.

These, of course, are strong requirements. And, in its reliance on "expert" panels, the objective social indicators tradition is always open to the criticism that the conditions identified have not been corroborated as relevant to how people actually experience happiness, life satisfaction, and subjective well-being. This criticism motivates the other major tradition of work on the measurement of the quality of life.

Subjective Social Indicators, Subjective Well-Being, Happiness, and Satisfaction

This line of development commenced with the Campbell, Converse, and Rodgers (1976) volume cited above and the Andrews and Withey (1976) volume, *Social Indicators of Well-Being: Americans' Perceptions of Life Quality* published in the same year. As noted above, the key element of this approach is on the use of various social science research techniques, including in-depth interviews, focus groups discussions, clinical studies, and samples surveys to study how people define their happiness and satisfaction with life and the social conditions of life that they experience on a day-to-day basis.

In the more than two decades since the publication of the path-breaking studies by Campbell, Converse, and Rodgers (1976) and Andrews and Withey (1976) volumes, many studies of subjective well-being have been conducted. To put it simply, we today are the beneficiaries of these many studies, and, as a result, we know a lot more about what makes people happy and satisfied with life today than in the early-1970s. In particular, Cummins (1996, 1997) reached the following conclusions about the quality of life based on comparisons of findings across numerous subjective well-being studies:

-   there is a potential for tremendous variety of assessments of satisfaction with life experiences, with individuals often differing in their ratings of importance of the key elements associated with their life satisfactions and happiness;
-   but, at the same time, the accumulation of findings across many studies shows that certain domains of well-being occur over and over again;
-   there also is a fairly high degree of similarity among individuals on the relative weightings given to these domains in determining overall life satisfaction;
-   and, perhaps most interestingly, there is a lot of similarity between the domains of well-being identified in subjective well-being studies and the areas of concern identified by expert panels in objective social indicators studies.

This naturally leads to the question: Can the empirical findings from subjective well-being studies about domains of well-being be used to inform the construction of summary quality-of-life indices? That is, can subjective well-being studies be used to make summary quality-of-life indices more *evidence-based* not only in the use of empirical data, but also in the selection of the domains of well-being and indicators used in their construction? Put more figuratively, can we bring these two social indicators/quality-of-life traditions into intersection so that we may construct summary social indicators that are more firmly grounded in what we have learned about subjective well-being over the past three decades. My answer to these rhetorical questions is "yes" and I will illustrate how this can be done by reviewing some of my recent work on the development of an index of child and youth well-being.

EXAMPLE: THE CHILD WELL-BEING INDEX

As an example of the possibility of using our current heritage of subjective well-being studies to construct better social indicators, consider the Child Well-Being Index (CWI) recently developed by Land, Lamb, and Mustillo (2001) to measure changes in child and youth well-being in the United States over the period from 1975 to the present. The Child Well-Being Index is:
- a summary measure of trends over time in the well-being of America's children and young people
- that consists of several interrelated summary indices of annual time series of numerous social indicators of the well-being of children and youth in the United States.

The general objectives of the CWI summary indices are to:
- give a sense of the overall directions of change in the well-being of children and youth in the U.S. as compared to two base years, 1975 and 1985.

The CWI is designed to address questions such as the following:

Overall, on average, how did child and youth well-being in the U.S. change in the last quarter of the 20th century and beyond?
- Did it improve or deteriorate?
- By approximately how much?
- In which domains of social life?
- For specific age groups?
- For particular race/ethnic groups?
- For each of the sexes?
- And did race/ethnic group and sex disparities increase or decrease?

Methods of Construction

Annual time series data (from vital statistics and sample surveys) have been assembled on some 28 national-level Key Indicators in seven quality-of-life domains:
- Material well-being,
- Health,
- Safety/behavioral concerns,
- Productive activity (educational attainments),
- Place in community (participation in schooling or work institutions),
- Social relationships (with family and peers), and
- Emotional/spiritual well-being.

These seven domains of quality of life have been well-established as recurring time after time in over two decades of empirical research in numerous subjective well-being studies (Cummins, 1996, 1997). They also have been found, in one form or another, in studies of the well-being of children and youths. The 28 Key Indicators used in the construction of the CWI are identified with brief descriptions in Table 1. A full description and justification for the use of the Key Indicators in the construction of the CWI is given in Land et al. (2001).

Table 1: Twenty-eight Key National Indicators of Child Well-being in the United States

Material Well-being Domain	1. Poverty Rate – all Families with Children
	2. Secure Parental Employment Rate
	3. Medium Annual Income – all Families with Children
Material Well-being* and Health Domains:	4. Rate of Children with Health Insurance Coverage
Material Well-being and Social Relationships* Domains:	1. Rate of Children in Families Headed by a Single Parent
Social Relationships Domain:	2. Rate of Children who Have Moved within the Last Year
Health Domain:	1. Infant Mortality Rate
	2. Low Birth Weight Rate
	3. Mortality Rate, Ages 1-19
	4. Rate of Children with very Good or Excellent Health (as Reported by their Parents)
	5. Rate of Children with Activity Limitations (as reported by their Parents)
	6. Rate of Overweight Children and Adolescents, Ages 6-17
Health and Behavioral Concerns* Domain:	1. Teenage Birth Rate, Ages 10-17
Safety/Behavioral Concerns Domain:	2. Rate of Violent Crime Victimization, Ages 12-17
	3. Rate of Violent Crime Offenders, Ages 12-17
	4. Rate of Cigarette Smoking, Grade 12
	5. Rate of Alcoholic Drinking, Grade 12
	6. Rate of Illicit Drug Use, Grade 12
Productivity (Educational Attainments) Domain:	1. Reading Test Scores, Ages 9, 13, 17
	2. Mathematics Test Scores, Ages 9, 13, 17

Table 1: Twenty-eight Key National Indicators of Child Well-being in the United States
(continued)

Place in Community* and Educational Attainment Domains:	1. Rate of Preschool Enrollment, Ages 3-4
	2. Rate of Persons who Have Received a High School Diploma, Ages 18-24
	3. Rate of Youths not Working and not in School, Ages 16-19
	4. Rate of Persons who Have Received a Bachelor's Degree, Ages 25-29
	5. Rate of Voting in Presidential Elections, Ages 18-20
Emotional/Spiritual Well-being	1. Suicide Rate, Ages 10-19
	2. Rate of Weekly Religious Attendance, Grade 12
	3. Percentage who Report Religion as Being very Important, Grade 12

Source: Land et al. 2001, p. 249f. A few indicators can be assigned to two domains. For these, the * denotes the domain-specific index to which the indicators are assigned for computation purposes. Explanations for the domain assignments are given in the text. Unless otherwise noted, indicators refer to children ages 0-17.

To calculate the CWI, each of the 28 time series of the Key Indicators is indexed by a base year (1975 or 1985). The base year value of the indicator is assigned a value of 100 and subsequent values of the indicator are taken as percentage changes in the index. The directions of the indicators are oriented so that a value greater (lesser) than 100 in subsequent years means the social condition measured has improved (deteriorated).

The 28 indexed Key Indicator time series are grouped into the seven domains of well-being by equal weighting to compute the domain-specific Index values for each year. The seven domain-specific Indices then are grouped into an equally-weighted Child Well-being Index value for each year. Hagerty and Land (2003) show that an equal-weighting strategy for summary indicators of well-being is privileged in the sense that it minimizes disagreement among all possible individuals' weights.

Since it builds on the subjective well-being empirical research base in its identification of domains of well-being to be measured and the assignment of Key Indicators to the domains, the CWI can be viewed as *well-being-evidence-based measure of trends in averages of the social conditions encountered by children and youth in the United States across recent decades.*

Some Empirical Findings Using the CWI

With the Child Well-Being Index defined and operationalized as described above, it can be used to measure changes in child and youth well-being as Land et al. (2001) have shown. In the following sections, a number of findings on these changes are briefly sketched.

(1) *A Domain-Specific Report Card for 2001.* To begin with, for each year for which we have complete data on all of the 28 Key Indicators in the CWI, we can compute a "report card" that shows how each of the seven domain-specific indices is changing relative to the base year of the Index. For instance, the year 2001 is the last year for which we have currently have complete data on all of the Key Indicators. With the data for 2001 in hand, we now can compare changes in the domain-specific indices from the year 2000 to 2001, with the changes taken as a percentage of the 1975 base year values of the Key Indicators. The report card is displayed in table 2:

Table 2: Report Card 2000/2001

Domain	Change from 2000 to 2001 as a % of Base Year 1975 Value
Material Well-being	-0.77
Health	-1.68
Safety/Behavioral	+4.17
Educational Attainment	No Change
Place in Community	-0.74
Social Relationships	+5.56
Emotional/Spiritual	+3.57

Source: Own calculations.

In brief, the material well-being domain index, which was affected by an economic slowdown/recession in 2001, declined by 0.77 percent from 2000 to 2001, where the changes are measured relative to 1975 base year values. The health domain and place in community indices similarly show slight declines in 2001. By contrast, the safety/behavioral, social relationships, and emotional/spiritual domain indices show substantial increases.

(2) *Trends in Child Well-Being from 1975 into the early 21st Century.* How do the domain-specific changes from 2000 to 2001, as shown above in the report card, combine to measure overall changes in child well-being in 2001, relative to the 1975 base year, and in comparison to other years since 1975? Figure 1 shows the overall summary Child Well-Being Index from 1975 to 2001 with projections for 2002. The projections are computed by modeling the time series behavior for each of the 28 Key Indicators and then projecting these one year beyond the year for which observed data on all of the indicators are available. The projected values of each of the Key Indicators then are averaged to compute the domain-specific summary indices

and these, in turn, are averaged to comprise the projected overall summary index for the projected year.

Figure 1: Summary Child Well-being Index, 1975-2001, with Projection for 2002

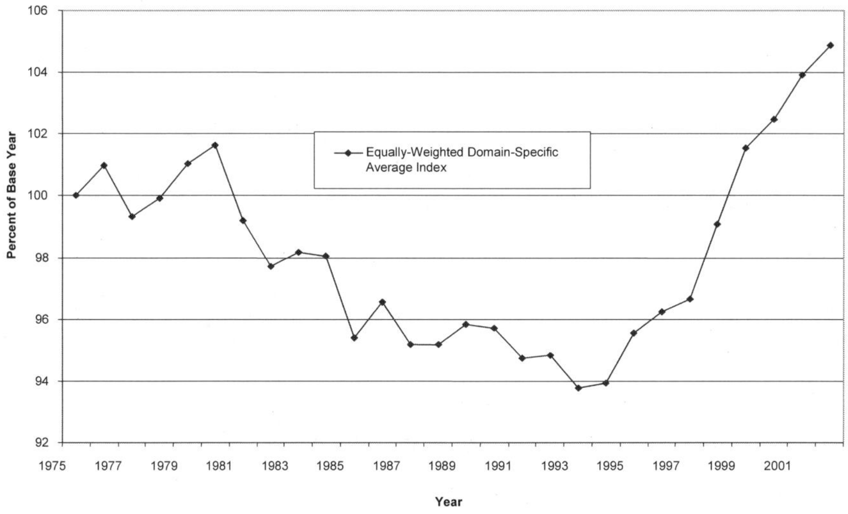

Source: Own calculations.

It can be seen from Figure 1 that the value of the Index for 2001 is about 104 – indicating that overall child well-being in the United States was a bit higher in 2001 than in 1975 (i.e., by about 4 %). By comparison, the Index was about 102.5 in 2000 and is projected to rise to about 105 in 2002. Overall, the CWI shows a decline in child well-being that began in 1982 and bottomed out in 1993. Since 1994, the Index has been in a sustained uptrend.

To understand these changes in the overall summary Child Well-Being Index, it is useful to examine trends over time in the domain-specific summary indices. These are shown in Figure 2.

Figure 2: Domain-Specific Indices of Child and Youth Well-being, 1975-2001, with projections for 2002

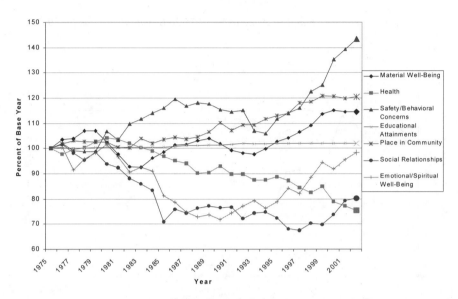

Source: Own calculations.

The domain-specific indices in Figure 2 show that much of the decline in child well-being in the early-1980s was due to downturns in the social relationships and emotional/spiritual domains of well-being. In the mid-1980s, there also was a decline in the safety/behavioral concerns domain. By comparison, the material well-being domain index shows the imprint of the economic recessions of the early-1980s and the early-1990s, and the health domain index shows a sustained decline since about 1980 (more about this below). Since the early-1990s, however, several domain indices, including the material well-being, safety/behavioral, place in community, and emotional/spiritual well-being domains, have shown fairly sustained increases. This movement, in concert, of these four domains of well-being is what accounts for the rise in the overall CWI shown previously in Figure 1.

As noted above, the health domain index has shown a general decline since the early-1980s. In an effort to understand this decline, Figure 2.1 reports the result of a sensitivity analysis. It shows the sensitivity of the health domain summary index to whether or not the obesity indicator – namely, the prevalence rate of overweight children and adolescents – is included in the domain index.

Figure 2.1: Health Domain with and without Obesity Indicator, 1975 to 2001, with Projections for 2002

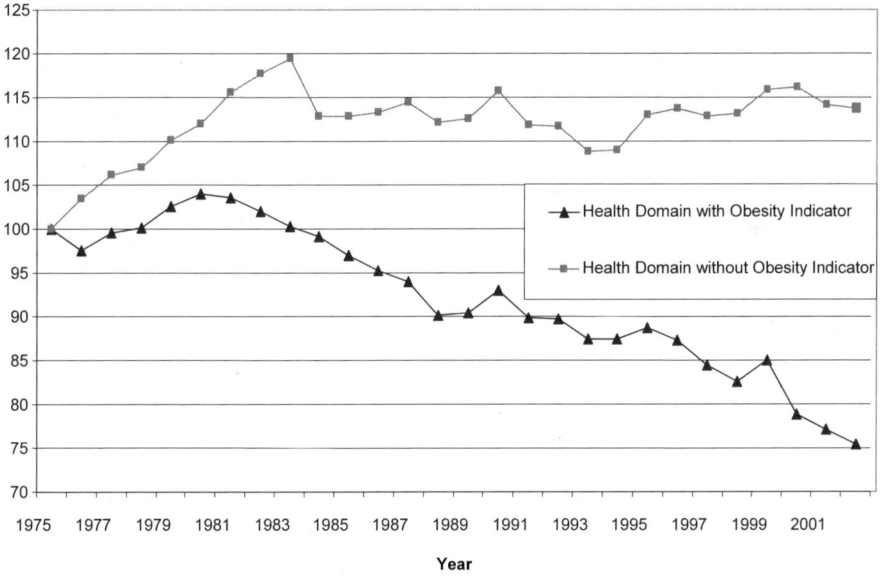

Source: Own Calculations.

In brief, Figure 2.1 demonstrates a relatively large impact of the inclusion/exclusion of the obesity indicator on the health domain summary index. Specifically, with the obesity indicator in the health domain, the index decreases by about 23 %from 1975 to 2001. By contrast, with the obesity indicator not included, the health domain index increases to about 15 percent above 1975 base year values by the mid-1980s and then shows fluctuations in the range of about 10-15 % above 1975 values through 2001.

The Key Indicators included in the CWI, as identified in Table 1, cover an entire age range of child and youth – from birth to young adulthood. Given this, another exercise in sensitivity analysis of the CWI consists of grouping the Key Indicators into smaller age ranges. Figure 3 shows the components of the CWI grouped into three age groups, namely, infants/preschoolers (ages 0 to 5), childhood (ages 6-11), and the adolescent/teenage years (ages 12-19). Correspondingly, Figure 3.1 displays the results of a sensitivity analysis for the childhood well-being index in Figure 3 – with and without the obesity indicator.

Figure 3: Age-Specific Summary Well-being Indices, 1975-2001

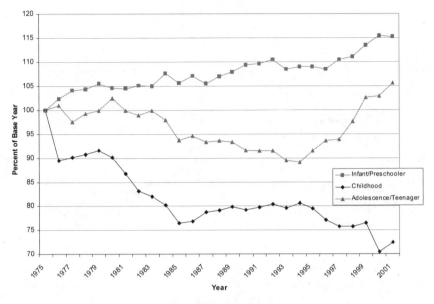

Source: Own Calculations.

Figure 3.1: Childhood Well-being Index with and without Obesity Indicator, 1975-2001

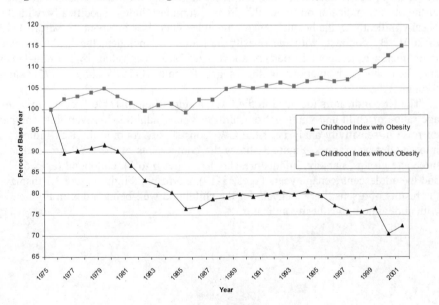

Source: Own Calculations.

In Figure 3, it can be seen that the well-being index specialized to the infant/preschool years shows a fairly steady increase over the years, up to about 15 % above 1975 base year values by 2001. By comparison, the well-being index specialized to the adolescent/teenage ages exhibits the impact of declines in the safety/behavioral and emotional/spiritual domain components of the index during the period from the mid-1980s to the mid-1990s. And still more differently, the well-being index specialized to the childhood years shows a fairly sustained decline from the mid-1970s to recent years. Again, in order to better understand the elements of the sustained decline in the childhood index, Figure 3.1 reports the impact of including or excluding the obesity indicator in the childhood index. It can be seen that excluding the obesity indicator leads to a very different conclusion about trends overtime in the health domain for the childhood index. In brief, except for the impact of the increasing prevalence of overweight children, the overall health of children has improved in the 25-plus years since 1975.

Figure 4 displays the graphs of trends in the CWI for children and youth grouped into three major race/ethnic categories: whites, blacks, and Hispanics. Because the Key Indicator data series used in the construction of the CWI are available specific to these race/ethnic categories only back to the mid-1980s, the indices graphed in Figure 4 use 1985 as their base year. Also, note that the race/ethnic-specific indices plotted in Figure 4 are measured within-groups, that is, relative to the values of the Key Indicators within each race/ethnic group as of the base year 1985. Therefore, the indices measure improvements or deterioration across the years in the overall child well-being of each race/ethnic group relative to its value of 100 for the base year.

Figure 4: Race/Ethnic Group-Specific Child Well-being Indices, 1985-2001

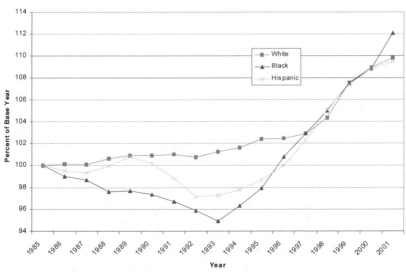

Source: Own Calculations.

Two main conclusions can be drawn from Figure 4. First, all three race/ethnic groups show improvements in child and youth well-being from 1993 to 2001 and all three groups have index values greater than those of the base year. This implies that overall child and youth well-being for all three groups is better in 2001 – by on the order of 10-12 % – than in 1985. Second, the downturn in child and youth well-being from the mid-1980s to the early-1990s was more severe for black and Hispanic children and youth than for white youth. In fact, for white youth, this period evidences a slowdown in improvements in well-being but not an actual decline.

Figure 5: Male/Female Child Well-being Indices, 1985-2000

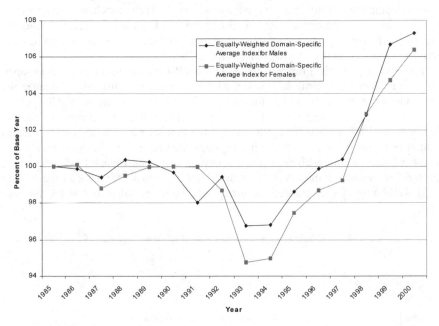

Source: Own Calculations.

Similar comparisons of trends in the CWI by sex are shown in Figure 5. Again, the Key Indicator data series used in the construction of the CWI are available specific to male and female children and youth only back to the mid-1980s. Therefore, the indices graphed in Figure 4 use 1985 as their base year. It can be seen that the trends in this overall summary index of child and youth well-being from 1985 to 2000 are roughly parallel. In fact, trends in the Key Indicator time series over this period of time show that females improved relative to their base year values at greater rates than males on some indicators of well-being and males improved better than females on others. But the summary indices plotted in Figure 5 show that neither sex improved at a greatly higher rate than the other over this 15-year period.

(3) *Summary of Findings on Trends in Child and Youth Well-Being.* In summary, the foregoing and related analyses of trends in the CWI (Land et al. 2001) show:

- The overall well-being of children and youth in the U.S. showed substantial improvements in the seven years from 1994 to 2000.
- Improvements continued in 2001, and likely in 2002, but at a slower pace.
- Child well-being in the U.S. deteriorated fairly steadily for a number of years in the 1980s and reached low points in 1992-94. They then began the upturn of the past several years.
- Recent increases in the CWI have pierced the 1975 base year level only in the past few years.
- The downturn in well-being that occurred in the 1985-1994 period was particularly severe for black and Hispanic children and youths.
- There have been overall improvements in well-being for both males and females since 1985, but there are some domains and indicators in which males have done better and some in which females have done better.
- Historical best-practice analyses (Land et al. 2001) using the best values on each of the component indicators of the CWI ever recorded for the U.S. show that the CWI could be 20 to 25 percent higher than its values in recent years.
- International best-practice analyses (Land et al. 2001) using the best values of the of the component indicators recorded in recent years by other nations show that the CWI could be 35 to 40 percent higher than its value in recent years.
- Sensitivity analyses of the CWI show that the Health domain sub-index is greatly impacted by the inclusion of the indicator for trends in obesity and this indicator also has a big impact on the childhood well-being index.
- The CWI also helps identify domains of well-being for which the data base needs to be improved (Land et al. 2001). Component indicators for the social relationships and emotional well-being domains are particularly weak.

CAN WE DO MORE? SOME GOALS FOR THE FUTURE

In the preceding sections, I have sketched the heritage of the social indicators and quality-of-life research traditions. In particular, I have:
- described the founding definitions and goals of the social indicators and quality-of-life movements of the 1960s and 1970s;
- reviewed the current state of the art with respect to the objective social indicators and subjective well-being approaches to the measurement of well being;
- cited the results of recent literature reviews of the findings of numerous studies in the subjective well-being research tradition with respect to domains of subjective well-being that consistently and repeatedly have been found to be related to happiness and life satisfaction;
- suggested that these two research traditions can be fruitfully intersected in the sense that the results of these literature reviews can be used to inform the selection of domains of well-being and indicators to be used in the construction of well-being/quality-of-life indices;

-   illustrated this process by describing how the Child Well-being Index of Land et al. (2001) is constructed; and
-   demonstrated how the CWI can be used to chart trends and produce a number of findings concerning child and youth well-being in the United States over the last quarter of the 20th century and into the early years of the 21st century.

In this final section, I will briefly outline some needed developments and possibilities for the future. Again, I will use the Child Well-being Index as a point of departure. For the CWI, there are two needed developments for the near future.

First, we need to bring the Child Well-being Index to levels of aggregation below the national level. In particular, we need to construct corresponding child well-being indices (insofar as databases permit) at the state and local levels. This involves the identification of the Key Indicators of the CWI for which there are suitable data bases at the state and local levels, the construction of indexed indicator time series from these data bases, the aggregation of these into domain-specific summary indices, and, finally, the aggregation of the domain-specific summary indices into summary indices of overall well-being.

Second, we need a further articulation and application of the teleological process described in Land and Ferriss (2002) to the Child Well-Being Index and its component indicators, as illustrated in Figure 6. That is, we need to develop the relationship of the Child Well-Being Index to a number of other products of social science research and policy formulation and analysis, as shown in Figure 6, which is adapted

Figure 6: Illustration of the Teleological Process Applied to the CWI

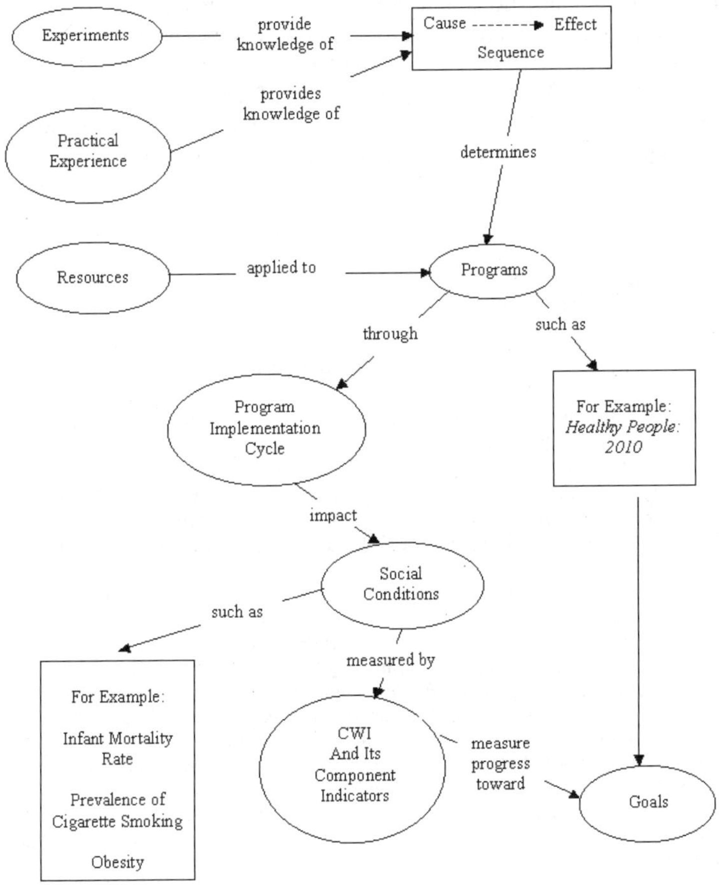

Source: Land & Ferriss, 2002.

from Land and Ferris (2002). For instance, we need to identify how the CWI and its component indicators relate to national and community goals, such as those identified in the *Healthy People 2010* report (USDHHS, 2000). Then we need to build the knowledge base of studies in the social sciences and epidemiology (experimental and nonexperimental) that help us to understand the causes and consequences of the trends we observe in the CWI and its component indicators. Such studies can be used in conjunction with the CWI and its indicators to develop policies and intervention programs designed to move the Index towards the goals that have been identified.

This is but a brief illustration of some of the possibilities for further work on the development of the Child Well-Being Index. If progress can be made along these lines, however, the Index can begin to fulfill the ambitious goals of the early social indicators movement – a statement of which began this essay. More generally, if similar developments can be fostered for other summary social indicators of well-being for other populations and aspects of the quality of life, then these ambitious goals can be achieved more broadly. That is, we can begin to achieve the promise and ambitions of the social indicators/quality-of-life movement of the 1960s and 1970s. Of course, this will not signal the end of our tasks. For these initial efforts no doubt will leave much to be desired, and there will be a need for improved conceptualizations, measurements and indicators for decades to come.

NOTES

1   The research on the Child Well-being Index reported herein was supported by a grant from the Foundation for Child Development.

REFERENCES

Andrews, F. M. & S. B. Withey (1976): Social Indicators of Well-being: Americans' Perceptions of Life Quality, New York: Plenum.

Bauer, R. A. (ed.) (1966): Social Indicators, Cambridge, Mass.: MIT Press.

Campbell, A., P. E. Converse & W. L. Rodgers (1976): The Quality of American Life: Perceptions, Evaluations, and Satisfactions, New York: Russell Sage Foundation.

Cummins, R. A. (1996): The Domains of Life Satisfaction: An Attempt to Order Chaos. Social Indicators Research 38, 303-28.

Cummins, R. A. (1997): Assessing Quality of Life. R. I. Brown (ed.): Quality of Life for Handicapped People, London: Chapman & Hall.

Erikson, R. (1974): Welfare as a Planning Goal. Acta Sociologica 17, 273-88.

Hagerty, M. R. & K. C. Land (2003): Constructing Summary Indices of Social Well-being: A Model for the Effect of Heterogeneous Importance Weights. Revision of a Paper Presented at the Annual Meeting of the American Sociological Association, Chicago, IL, August 16-19, 2002.

Land, K. C. (1983): Social Indicators. Annual Review of Sociology 9, 1-26.

Land, K. C. (2000): Social Indicators. E. F. Borgatta & R. V. Montgomery (eds.): Encyclopedia of Sociology, Revised Edition, New York: Macmillan, 2682-90.

Land, K. C. & A. L. Ferriss (2002): Conceptual Models for the Development and Use of Social Indicators. W. Glatzer, R. Habich & K. U. Mayer (eds.): Sozialer Wandel und gesellschaftliche Dauerbeobachtung. Festschrift für Wolfgang Zapf, Opladen: Leske und Budrich, 337-52.

Land, K. C., V. L. Lamb & S. Kahler Mustillo (2001): Child and Youth Well-being in the United States, 1975-1998: Some Findings from a New Index. Social Indicators Research 56, 241-320.

National Commission on Technology, Automation and Economic Progress (1966): Technology and the American Economy, Vol. 1, Washington, D.C.: U.S. Government Printing Office.

Noll, H.-H. (2002): Social Indicators and Quality of Life Research: Background, Achievements and Current Trends. N. Genov (ed.): Advances in Sociological Knowledge Over Half a Century, Paris: ISSC, 168-206.

Noll, H.-H. & W. Zapf (1994): Social Indicators Research: Societal Monitoring and Social Reporting. I. Borg & P. P. Mohler (eds.): Trends and Perspectives in Empirical Social Research, New York: Walter de Gruyter, 1-16.

Sheldon, E. B. & W. E. Moore (eds.) (1968): Indicators of Social Change: Concepts and Measurements, New York: Russell Sage Foundation.

U.S. Department of Health, Education, and Welfare (USDHEW) (1969): Toward a Social Report. Washington, D.C.: U.S. Government Printing Office.

U.S. Department of Health and Human Services (USDHHS) (2000): Healthy People 2010, Second Edition. With Understanding and Improving Health and Objectives for Improving Health. 2 Vols., Washington, DC: U.S. Government Printing Office.

9. THE SOCIAL STATE OF THE NETHERLANDS

*A Model Based Approach to Describing Living Conditions
and Quality of Life*

Jeroen Boelhouwer and Theo Roes
Social and Cultural Planning Office, Den Haag, The Netherlands

ABSTRACT

The "Social State of the Netherlands" (SSN) provides a systematic overview of the quality of life and living conditions of the Dutch population. The report describes various domains like income, work, education, health, crime, housing, participation, and leisure. In addition, there is a domain-crossing chapter describing the living conditions with one comprehensive index: the Living Conditions Index (LCI).

The SSN is a monitor which is based on a causal model centering around the living conditions of the citizen. For realizing good living conditions resources, like income and education, are available: the more resources at a person's disposal, the greater the chance of good living conditions. In the model attention is also paid to the (physical and social) environment.

The model is not only about the *actual situation* in which people find themselves, but also provides information about the way people *rate* their living conditions and the extent to which people are more or less happy.

A NEW REPORT: SOCIAL STATE OF THE NETHERLANDS

With the "Social State of the Netherlands" (SSN), the Social and Cultural Planning Office (SCP) describes the living conditions and quality of life of the Dutch population. Every two years the SCP will seek to describe and analyze living conditions systematically. A series of fields is covered, namely income, employment, education, health, leisure activities, participation, mobility, crime and safety, housing, and the residential environment. The SSN is a relatively new report, though it is the sequel to the Social and Cultural Outlooks, the final edition of which appeared in 1999.

The most important target groups of the publication are the Lower House and the Cabinet. The report provides them with information on the social situation in the Netherlands. There are other target groups as well. In the case of policy-makers who are already well informed the SSN provides a framework in which the developments in their particular field can be placed. The SCP is also seeking to reach the socially-interested public with this publication. The SSN provides information that is expected to be useful for the social debate.

Each of the chapters of the report describes the developments in a particular area over the past ten years. The data have been divided into various social categories –

Wolfgang Glatzer, Susanne von Below, Matthias Stoffregen (eds.), Challenges for Quality of Life in the Contemporary World, 125-138.

like sex, age and education – wherever possible and relevant. Furthermore the main objectives of government policy are briefly formulated in the introductions to the various chapters, while the concluding remarks contain summary information on the extent to which these goals have been achieved. In addition to these domain chapters the SCP presents a summary yardstick, the living conditions index (LCI), with which developments may be followed over time and the situation in various social categories can be readily compared. A description of the trends in public opinion concerning the welfare state and the action taken by the government completes the SSN.

With the SSN the SCP is reflecting the renewed international interest in social monitoring.

SOCIAL MONITORING

Following changes in political power and the revival of the economy, governments in various European countries have strengthened their input in the social field. Not only the fight against poverty but also combating social exclusion is an important topic.. The most frequently used instruments for achieving these objectives are improving the level of education of the population and the creation of employment. The governments formulate goals in the various fields, the attainment of which is closely monitored.

In the context of the implementation of the Maastricht Treaty and the Amsterdam Treaty, the European Union has taken a series of initiatives in the social field in relation to such topics as the improvement of living conditions, social security, equal opportunities and social exclusion (or lately social inclusion). In order to monitor the developments in these fields the Commission has also introduced periodic reports. One example is *The Social Situation in the European Union 2003*, a publication by Eurostat and the European Commission (Eurostat and the European Commission, 2003). This is a report with key figures on social developments in the countries of Europe.

The objectives of social monitoring instruments and also of the SSN may be formulated as follows:

- the provision of an overview of the living conditions of the population as a whole on the basis of key figures in a number of socially and politically relevant fields;
- the provision of systematic information on developments among various groups in society and in the various areas of the Netherlands;
- the provision of information on developments over time;
- the identification of social problems and disadvantages for political/policy purposes on the basis of that information;
- the analysis of the backgrounds to as well as causes and consequences of these problems;
- the provision of information on the extent to which the policy objectives are being attained.

The SSN therefore sets out to be more than a summary of key indicators in a number of selected fields. An additional value is achieved by means of the systematic analysis of social developments.

Theoretical Framework

The SSN is a monitor centering around the living conditions of the citizen. In terms of designating the content, the concept of "living conditions" is neutral. Related terms are living standard, quality of life, welfare, livability, social exclusion, and social cohesion. Many countries and international organizations have each developed their own standards and have constructed specific measures in order to objectify these types of concepts (Hagerty et al., 2001). The multitude of monitoring instruments and indicators sets which are based on them all address the same questions (see Berger-Schmitt & Noll, 2000):
- is the individual or the collectivity central?
- does the monitor record objective or subjective phenomena instead?,
- is it concerned with social opportunities or with realized welfare?, and
- how can the range and level be standardized?

The question of collectivity vs. individual depends primarily on the objective of the monitoring instrument. Living conditions research within countries is usually concerned with individuals or households; and so is the SSN.

Then there is the question of subjective and objective indicators. The subjective approach is based on people's needs, especially satisfaction and people's happiness in general and/or satisfactions concerning the various aspects of the living conditions (like family and friends, health, work and education). In this view these types of factors determine the extent to which a life situation can be designated as "good". In contrast to this the objectifying approach is based on the concept of living standard. This is defined as access to resources that are capable of influencing one's own living conditions. Examples include income and education, which can be employed in the various domains of life in order to make social progress. At issue therefore are indicators for objectively determining factors that are decisive for a person's living conditions. This approach is heavily oriented towards monitoring in the interests of social policy. The Scandinavian countries in particular follow this approach (Vogel, 2002).

The preference for objectively determinable living conditions is prompted by the policy-oriented nature of the monitoring system: the provision of information on phenomena that can be influenced by means of policy and feeding the public debate on social progress. As such the SSN largely presents primary *output or situational indicators*. Until recently most of government policy was formulated in terms of objective aims. However, since September 11th and some national tragedies (like the murder of a Dutch politician) more attention has been paid to perceptions and subjective opinions, maybe not in policy but at least in politics.

The answer to another question – social opportunities or realized quality of life – calls for a discussion concerning the question as to whether social policy is concerned with equal opportunities or actual social equality or inequality. In most welfare states social policy is no longer confined to the provision of opportunities for people but goals are also formulated in terms of realized life-chances. In the Netherlands the government not only wants to provide citizens with equal opportunities to e.g. appropriate housing but also ensures that all citizens are in principle able to occupy good quality and affordable housing. In doing so the government regulates the supply of (affordable) housing and provides additional financial resources in the form of individual rent relief.

The final important questions concern the scope of the monitor and the way in which a particular outcome is labeled good or bad. Living conditions is a multidimensional concept. Most monitoring systems include indicators for a number of life domains (see Hagerty et al., 2001). The choice of domains is prompted by policy considerations or is based on empirical research. In practice this is dealt with pragmatically but prevailing political and policy considerations must be discounted in the system of indicators if the SSN is to fulfill an identifying and policy-evaluating function. The level problem – i.e. where does the boundary between positive and negative values lie – may also be approached in various ways. Generally, however, minimum norms, that have been determined politically or in policy terms, apply in certain domains. These may then be taken as the starting point.

As for the time-horizon of the report a period of ten years is selected. This period is long enough for there to be various points of measurement in the different fields and for changes to be observable.

The Social Model

It is against the background of these considerations that the SCP has set up the SSN, thereby fleshing out the concept of living conditions. A broad approach has been adopted, under which the various types of data have been presented as an interrelated whole. The SSN is based on the causal model shown in figure 1.

Figure 1: The Social Model

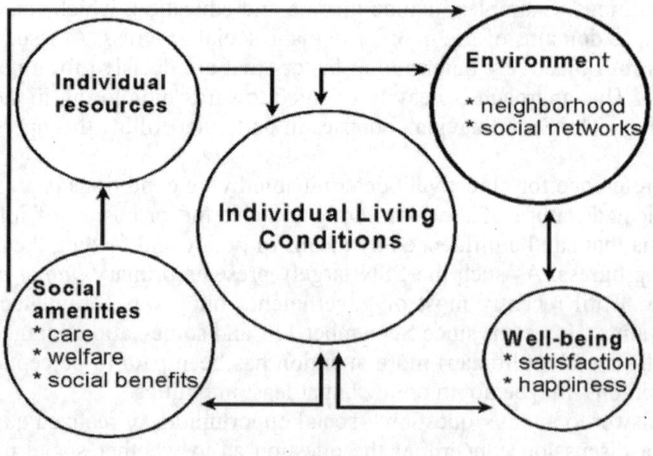

Source: SCP (2001).

Citizens dispose over individual resources in order to achieve good living conditions. In present-day society this primarily concerns education, employment and income. As we use a sociological approach, the resources are about social goods instead of mental constitution or other psychological factors. The model is based on a causal relationship between resources and living conditions: the more resources at a person's disposal, the greater the chance of good living conditions. The government, which tries to create as much equal opportunities as possible, exercises influence over the availability of such resources. It redistributes income and helps citizens to acquire social resources through public provision. The government therefore plays a supporting role in helping prevent social disadvantage. Where the social process and personal choices according to the norms of the community result in disadvantage, the government will compensate for this as far as possible. This is shown in the "social amenities" part of the model at the left corner.

The physical and especially the social environments are also important conditions for the living conditions of the individual citizen. In the SSN attention is paid to a number of physical characteristics of the residential environment and the correlations between the physical quality and social characteristics, such as crime and population structure. With social environment a wide variety of social networks is meant, like family, friends, neighbors, but also being a member of church or social organizations.

Somewhat different from the *actual situation* in which people find themselves is the way that people *rate* their living conditions and the extent to which people are more or less happy. Where the data are available, within each domain the relationship between the (objectively measured) living conditions and their subjective assessment is established.

Although the social model provides a certain frame of reference for ordering and selecting from the numerous possible topics, it does not help greatly in the practical choice of domains and associated indicators which best represent the social state.

Choice of Indicators

With regard to selecting the indicators, empirical research, drawing as it does on public opinion concerning what is important for the welfare and standard of living of citizens, provides a guide for determining what is usable and for making a selection. The SCP has a solid tradition in reporting on social trends and living conditions. The choice of concrete indicators for the SSN is accordingly based to a significant extent on previously conducted empirical research. In addition the SCP has been guided by the report Kerngegevens leefsituatie (Key life situation data) of Statistics Netherlands (CBS), which, with the aid of experts, surveys key indicators of the life situation in the Netherlands (CBS, 2000).

In addition prevailing political and policy considerations have played a role in the selection. These must be discounted in the system of indicators if the SSN is to fulfill an identifying and policy-evaluating function. Also there are long-term goals in the various policy areas. These have also acted as a guide in the selection of indicators. The main objectives of government policy have therefore been briefly formulated in the introductions to the various chapters, while the concluding remarks contain summary information on the extent to which goals have been achieved.

The third consideration in the selection of indicators relates to the agreements reached on social policy in the context of the Maastricht and Amsterdam Treaties. The European Union (EU) and the member states have undertaken to promote employment, to improve working and living conditions, to offer social security, to develop human capital and to combat social exclusion. By virtue of the decision taken at the EU summit on employment in November 1997, Eurostat (the European Bureau of Statistics) has developed a set of indicators in collaboration with the statistical bureaus of the European countries in order to monitor developments in these fields (Eurostat, 1998). The domains in question and the indicators that have been developed have wherever possible been taken into consideration when deciding upon the arrangement of the SSN.

Finally, a number of practical considerations have played a role in the determination of the domains and indicators. Needless to say the availability of relevant research data is of decisive importance. In particular there need to be databases with information on a large number of aspects of the living conditions.

The (causal) relationships presented in the model are not all identified for each domain. Sometimes that is because the relations are not relevant and sometimes there simply are no data available to do the analysis.

At the core of the model, however, is the living conditions index. This index provides a means of exploring the relations more systematically. Before turning to the living conditions index, we will present some other results of the 2003 report.

The Social State of the Netherlands, 1990-2002

As said, in the first part of the report various domains are described separately. In this part nine domains are covered: income, employment, education, health, leisure activities, participation, mobility, crime and safety, and housing. We will now describe the main results of each chapter briefly, starting off with the resources.

The level of education has risen, more people found work and income improved. The economic growth at the end of the nineties has even reached traditionally deprived groups like the elderly and ethnic minorities: their living conditions improved.

In the second part of the nineties average purchasing power increased by 8 %. Since 1990 labor market participation grew from 59 % to 68 %. The labor market participation of women grew from 44 % to 57 % and of people aged 55-64 from 27 % to 38 %. Besides, there were more double-income couples and fewer people on relief.

So, due to economic growth the material aspects of the living conditions improved. Next to the above described developments, car ownership grew in the nineties (75 % of the households nowadays owns at least one car) and housing conditions improved (bigger houses and more homeownership).

The other domains are more concerned with the social dimension. This dimension however shows a less clear picture. Though the level of education has risen, still too many people drop out of school and education arrears disappear very slowly.

Between 1990 and 2002 life expectancy increased for women by 0.5 years (to 80.6) and for men by 1.7 years (to 75.6). But on the other hand socio-economic health differences increased, though slightly.

In the nineties more people are sporting, but societal and cultural participation remains on the same level. That is only because of the growing participation of the elderly: the youth shows a lack of interest. And even more: the diversity of participation lessens.

And last but not least, the still increasing crime rate is alarming.

In short, one could say that developments of the Social State are positive, but that the worries grow at the same time, even more with the economic recession which nowadays urges governments to cut down expenses to a great extent.

The expected decline of purchasing power is 1 % in 2003. Unemployment grew by 40 % between spring 2002 and spring 2003. Unemployment is particularly high amongst the youth, women, less educated people and ethnic minorities. These are the groups that profited the most in the last decade. Earlier research has shown that these groups will most likely suffer the most from the economic recession: They showed the greatest decline in living conditions during the crisis of the eighties.

That the living conditions improved in the nineties can be shown by summing up the developments in all included domains, as we just did (and as we do in the report), but that is just one way to describe the overall social state of the Netherlands. Another way is by means of the Living Conditions Index (LCI).

Summarizing the Social State: The Living Conditions Index

With the living conditions index we can explore the relations of the social model (between the domains of living conditions and with other individual characteristics) more systematically, because all data stems from one source. We can analyze for example that improvement in one domain together with decline in another can lead to better living conditions all together (or, indeed, to worse living conditions).

The index combines indicators on eight domains. Most of the domains are covered in separate chapters of the SSN as well: housing, health, social participation, leisure activity, sport activity, mobility, vacation, and consumer durables.

There are several possibilities to integrate the indicators into one single index, like consulting experts or use political priorities. One other method is counting the trends in a relative simple way, using pluses and minuses in each domain or to take the sum of changes in percentages for each indicator. For example, in a certain year, 25 % of the people own a car and 30 % participate in an organization. In the next year of measurement, 50 % own a car and 35 % participate in an organization. A combined index will rise from 100 to 115 [that is: $100 + ((50-25) + (35-30)/2))$].

Yet another way is to start off with defining minimum needs. The extent to which these are met is then a percentage of the minimum. This method is used for example by the UNDP for their Human Development Index (United Nations Development Programme, 1998).

As there is no all-embracing theory available for combining the indicators, we opted for a different solution to do so. The starting point is the common dimension of the indictors, which all contribute positively or negatively to the living conditions. This is not a measured notion, so we cannot use the regression coefficient for example.

Because we are interested in good and bad, in deprivation and well-being, a single indicator which correlates better with the others should get a greater weight. Furthermore, the result has to be an individually based index as we are not only interested in developments of the country as a whole, but for different groups in society as well. We decided to statistically construct the index and let the statistical program weight the indicators. We use nonlinear canonical correlation analysis for constructing the index. This in factis a variation of principal component analysis, which calculates the weights so as to maximize the sum of the item-total correlations. Other advantages are that we can define the clusters not only theoretically, but in the analysis as well; it even does not matter if the one cluster has much more indicators than another. Secondly, not only indicators, but also categories of the indicators re-

---

ceive weights, enabling us to compare them, too, and indicators do not have to be measured at interval level.

What then does the composite index on living conditions tell us about the social state of the Netherlands?

Figure 2: Development of the Living Conditions of the Dutch Population and some Groups

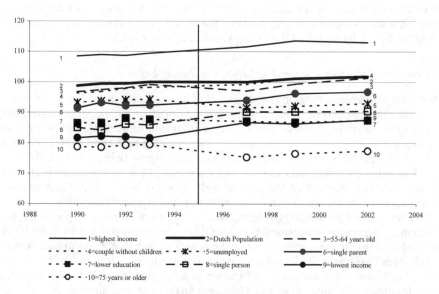

Source: SCP (2003).

The Social State Measured by the Living Conditions Index

Overall the living conditions improved from 1990 till 2002 (see figure 2). In the last five years the living conditions improved above average for deprived groups which before stayed behind, like the elderly, people with low income or those without employment, ethnic minorities and people living in the biggest cities (the last two groups are not in the figure).

Between 1999 and 2002 the material domains improved the most; due to the economic growth more people were able to buy more durable goods, such as cars and houses (see table 1). Besides, more people went away on holiday trips. On the other hand there was a decline in sport- and leisure activities.

Looking more into depth at the three groups that profited the most, reveals that their development is not equal with respect to the different domains (see figure 3):

- For people living in the four biggest cities the situation improved on *all* domains and on all domains more than national average.
- For people aged between 65 and 74, social isolation decreased and they were more active in volunteer work.

- For the lowest income group health get worse which is in line with the increased socio-economic health differences.

Table 1: Changes in Domains of the Living Conditions (1997=100 for each Domain)

	1997	1999	2002
Housing	100	100	102
Leisure Activities	100	101	100
Social Participation	100	100	100
Sport	100	100	98
Holiday	100	101	102
Consumer Durables	100	103	107
Mobility	100	101	101
Health	100	99	99
Overall Living Conditions Index	100	101	102

Source: SCP (2003).

Because the government tries to create equal opportunities and chances for everyone in society an important question is whether inequality increased or decreased. Inequality in terms of living conditions increased in the nineties when we look at the resources. The gap between low and high education became wider, as did the gap between working versus non-working people (see table 2).

Figure 3: Development of Domains of Living Conditions for the 3 Groups that Profited the Most between 1997 and 2002

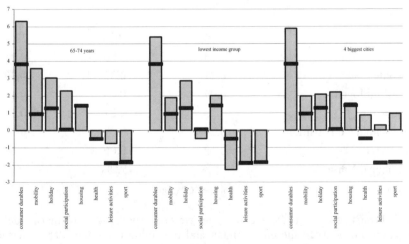

Source: SCP (2003).

The gap between the lowest and highest income groups became smaller. This has to do with developments on the labor market together with the growing economy. More people found jobs and thus got higher income. Especially the lower educated were the left-overs of the labor market and are still jobless. However: For all three groups inequality decreased between 1999 and 2002.

Table 2: Inequality in Terms of Living Conditions for Some Groups (Index Scores 1990-2002)

	1990	1999	2002
Lowest Income	82	87	88
Highest Income	108	114	113
Difference	25	27	25
Low education	86	87	88
High Education	105	109	109
Difference	19	23	22
Unemployed	93	92	93
Employed	103	106	107
Difference	10	14	14

Source: SCP (2003).

As said, a causal relationship between resources and the living conditions is posited. Multivariate analysis reveals this holds true: having a high level of education, a paid job and a good income causes better living conditions (see table 3). Age also plays an important role in the level of living conditions. The shown individual background characteristics together explain for about 55 % of the variance in living conditions.

Table 3: Influence of Resources and other Background Characteristics on the Living Conditions, 1993-2002 (Anova-analysis, ß-Coefficients)

	1990	1999	2002
Age	0.15	0.26	0.25
Income	0.21	0.32	0.30
(Un)Employed	0.04	0.10	0.11
Education	0.25	0.27	0.27
Household Composition	0.28	0.09	0.13
Source of Income	0.12	0.06	0.07
Explained Variance	48 %	57 %	55 %

Source: SCP (2003).

This brings us back to the social model we use. Another part of that model is the relationship between the environment and the living conditions. The environment has a social and a physical component. The social environment relates to the social network people belong to and the social contacts they have. Two indications of the social networks are in the index itself. These are a scale of social isolation and voluntary work. These indicators tell us something, but not all about the social contacts people actually have. That is why we relate the living conditions to the frequency of contacts with family, friends and neighbors. The relationship is clear: the more contacts people have, the better the living conditions are. This holds true not only for the network indicators within the index, but for all domains of living conditions.

The physical environment relates to the neighborhood people live in. This is one of the newest additions to our analysis of the living conditions index. There is a relationship between the individual living conditions and (social and physical) neighborhood characteristics. People with relatively bad living conditions live in neighborhoods with more rented apartments, lower rents, more elderly people and more people with low income than in neighborhoods were people with good living conditions live. All together: People with good living conditions live in a better-off environment than people with bad living conditions do.

To look at the broader physical environment of people we constructed an index for residential environment quality. In this index indicators are combined about rubbish on the streets, annoyance about noise and smells, crowding, and level of daily-used services. There is a relationship with the living conditions: The better the residential environment quality, the better the living conditions are (see figure 4).

Figure 4: Living Conditions for Levels of Residential Environment Quality

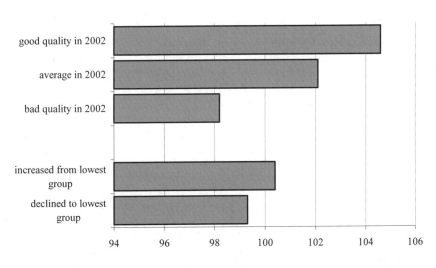

Source: SCP (2003).

This relationship does not answer the question which is more important for the living conditions: do individual characteristics add more to the living conditions than neighborhood characteristics do? We analyzed this question using multi-level techniques. The results show very clear that the individual characteristics like income and education are much more determining for the living conditions than neighborhood characteristics are. In fact, there is only a very limited influence of socio-economic deprivation of the neighborhood on the living conditions, i.e., in deprived areas the living conditions are slightly worse than one would expect on the basis of individual characteristics.

The Objective Social State versus Subjective Evaluations

The last part of the social model we studied is the relationship between the objective living conditions and subjective evaluations and happiness. This analysis shows that the happier someone finds himself, the better the living conditions are (see table 4). We did a first and rough analysis about a causal relationship between the living conditions index and happiness. The analysis showed that the very small influence of the index on happiness that we found at first sight disappeared almost completely when other subjective satisfactions were added to the model. By far the best explaining variable for happiness is subjective health.

Table 4: Some Figures about the Relationship between Subjective Evaluations and the Living Conditions Index

Domains of Living Conditions	Mean Report Grade (1-10)		Mean Living Conditions, 2002		
	1999	2002	Grade <5	Grade 6-8	Grade 9-10
Housing	7.9	7.9	88	102	104
Friends and Acquaintances	7.7	7.9	86	102	104
Housing Environment	7.7	7.7	93	102	104
Education	7.0	7.2	91	103	102
Dutch Society	6.6	6.4	97	103	95

	% 1999	% 2002	Mean Living Conditions, 2002
Happiness			
(Very) Happy	88	88	104
(Very) Unhappy	3	3	82
Subjective Health			
(Very) Good	77	77	105
(Very) Bad	10	5	86

Source: SCP (2003).

This is hardly surprising, as indicators of "the same kind", like subjective indicators as happiness and subjective health, can explain more of each other than a mix of (subjective and objective) indicators does.

Still, the results tell us something about the usefulness of subjective indicators for policy purposes. That is: Because of the lack of knowledge about what influences the subjective evaluations (other than personal characteristics, of which government has nothing to say) they cannot be used in a meaningful sense for changing policy. The best they can do is help us to get some clue about how people evaluate policies.

Looking at satisfactions with domains of the living conditions shows the same relationship: The more satisfied someone is, the better the living conditions are (see table 4). Over the years there has been hardly any change in these relationships. Not even after the tumultuous periods of the last years. For example: September 11th did not effect the happiness of the Dutch people in the long run. We have no data for the period shortly after 9-11, but looking at 2002 compared to 1999 shows the same amount of unhappy and very happy people.

In the Netherlands, too, there were a couple of tumultuous events, of which the most important one was the murder of a Dutch politician (Pim Fortuyn), who was winning the election polls. The elections afterwards (in the year 2000), shook our political landscape to a great extent. Still, comparing the opinion of the Dutch in 2002 with 1999, these events did not seem to have influenced the satisfactions with their personal environment. Figures of satisfaction with dwelling, residential environment, friends, education or financial possibilities did not alter. The one thing that has changed is satisfaction with society as a whole and with the administration, which decreased a lot. In 2000 77 % of the population were satisfied with the administration; in 2002 this was only 59 %. Satisfaction with the performance of government decreased from 65% in 2000 to 35% in 2002.

CONCLUSION AND DISCUSSION

In a new Dutch report on quality of life (called the "Social State of the Netherlands") a social model is used. The model is centered around the living conditions of Dutch citizens. Each chapter of the report describes a separate domain of the living conditions. Furthermore: In every chapter we try to include all relations described by the model. In addition to these domain-chapters the living conditions are monitored by means of a composite index. With this index the relations of the social model can be analyzed in a more systematic way.

Looking at the conclusions of the domain chapters showed a very diverse picture of the quality of life in the Netherlands. There have been improvements in some domains (particularly the more material or economic domains) whereas in other domains the situation was declining (crime and social participation). The index proved to be very helpful to describe the overall development of the living conditions. The conclusions of the report were easier drawn after the conclusion on developments of the index was known. The domain chapters showed such a diverse picture that it was very difficult to see the leading thread.

One of the things that need to be improved in the next version of the report is the link between social policy and social outcomes. There is nowadays a shift within the Dutch government from input oriented evaluation to output and outcome evaluation of policy. With this goes the call for measurable policy aims. The better these aims can be measured, the better we can tell in the report whether the policy has been successful.

REFERENCES

Berger-Schmitt, R. & H.-H. Noll (2000): Conceptual Framework and Structure of a European System of Social Indicators. EuReporting Working Paper 9, Mannheim: Centre for Survey Research and Methodology (ZUMA), Social Indicators Department.

CBS (2000): Main Indicators for Quality of Life (Kerngegevens Leefsituatie), Voorburg: Centraal Bureau voor de Statistiek.

Eurostat (1998): Living Conditions in Europe. Selected Social Indicators, Luxembourg: Official publications European Community.

Eurostat & the European Commission (2003): The Social Situation in the European Union 2003, Luxemburg: Official publications European Community.

Hagerty, M. R., R. Cummins, A. L. Ferris, K. Land, A. C. Michalos, M. Peterson, A. Sharpe, J. Sirgy & J. Vogel (2001): Quality of Life Indexes for National Policy Review and Agenda for Research. Social Indicators Research 55, 1-99.

Social and Cultural Planning Office (2001): The Social State of the Netherlands 2001 (De Sociale Staat van Nederland 2001), SCP, The Hague (SCP-publication 2001/14).

Social and Cultural Planning Office (2003): The Social State of the Netherlands 2003 (De Sociale Staat van Nederland 2003), SCP, The Hague (SCP-publication 2003/12).

United Nations Development Programme (1998): Human Development Report 1998, New York: Oxford University Press.

Vogel, J. (2002): Strategies and Traditions in Swedish Social Reporting: A 30-Year experience. Social Indicators Research 58, 89-112.

10. BIOGRAPHICAL ANALYSIS OF QUALITY OF LIFE PROCESSES IN MIGRATION

Maria Kontos

Institute of Social Research at the Johann Wolfgang Goethe-Universität, Frankfurt am Main, Germany

ABSTRACT

In this paper I attempt to develop a concept of quality of life that takes into account the processuality of social life and the agency of social actors. Starting point is the quality of life concept that is organized around the capabilities and the free choice of life options, as developed by Amartya Sen. I argue that the aspect of free choice highlights the polarity of internationality versus conditionality of action, as developed in the biographical research, as well as the processuality and sequential organization of social life. Assessing quality of life would mean to take into account, except of the relevant aspects of functionings, the ability of the individual to act intentionally and to realize own biographical plans. Functionings would be assessed in the framework of biographical plans, resources and strategies that are dependent on family relations, gender specific and generational social conditions. In the last part of my paper, I apply this concept to the case of labor migration. I propose to regard migration as a phenomenon closely related to the realization of biographical plans and choices and with these, to quality of life processes. Migration is to be regarded as an active and autonomous movement of people in the space towards the improvement of their own quality of life and the quality of life of their own family, whereas life in migration is frequently accompanied by constraints that can deprive migrants temporarily or in the longer term of the ability to act intentionally.

INTRODUCTION[1]

This paper pursues a twofold target. First, I try to bring together the capabilities concept of quality of life developed by Amartya Sen with the biographical perspective. With this, I aim to develop further the quality of life concept in its dimension of processuality and to offer a proposal on the operationalization of the concept. In this way, the static and distributive character of the objective and subjective concepts of quality of life will be enriched with the processuality of the social action paradigm. Second, I will try to apply this biographical quality of life concept on the case of migration and develop hypotheses on quality of life in migration. In the first part I will present shortly the capability concept. Then I will outline the points in which this concept converges with the biographical perspective. In the third part I will discuss problems of the operationalization of the concept in relation to family structures, gender and generational positions and finally I will discuss this concept in the case of migration.

The paper is an outcome of current discussions in the framework of the EU project "The Chances of the Second Generation in Families of Ethnic Entrepreneurs.

139

Wolfgang Glatzer, Susanne von Below, Matthias Stoffregen (eds.), Challenges for Quality of Life in the Contemporary World, 139-149.

Intergenerational and Gender Aspects of Quality of Life Processes" and reflects a collective work in progress.

THE CAPABILITY APPROACH TO THE QUALITY OF LIFE

For a long time, the quality of life discussion has been characterized by a split between objective and subjective factors of quality of life which reflect the broader sociological discourse and theoretical traditions on social inequality as well as the reflection of this discourse in the sphere of policy making and the split between liberal and welfare societies.

a)   The Scandinavian/Swedish "level of living approach" emerged in the socio-political discourse tradition and is organized around the concept of resources. Quality of life is defined as the "individual's command over, under given determinants, mobilizable resources, with whose help he/she can control and consciously direct his/her living conditions" (Erikson, 1974, p. 275; Erikson, 1993, pp. 72 ff.). Individual resources are understood as income, assets, education, social capital, mental and physical energy. Aspects of the conditions which cannot be influenced by the individual, such as the natural environment, health, and infrastructure are thought of as determinants of the quality of life. A further component is the aspirations of the individual, which together with the resources and determinants govern his or her well-being (Erikson, 1974, p. 275).

b)   The "American approach" (Noll, 2000) to quality of life-research is oriented towards subjective perceptions and self-evaluation processes. Subjective indicators such as contentedness, happiness, etc. have been developed, focusing on the experience of life, rather than on the conditions of life (Campbell, Converse & Rodgers, 1976, pp. 7ff.). In line with this approach, non-material components have been considered in connection with a change of values in western societies (Inglehart, 1989).

A prominent synthesis of the two approaches has been put forward by the Finnish sociologist Erik Allardt (Allardt, 1973; Allardt, 1993) with a broad concept of the quality of life based on three basic needs:

Having: material dimensions of life such as economic resources, living conditions, employment, work conditions, health, education, and the environment;

Loving: needs for belonging and social relationships, in the neighborhood, family, friends, participation in associations, etc.;

Being: options for participation and self-realization such as political participation, possibilities of influence, the possibility of exercising a meaningful professional occupation, and free time activities.

These approaches and their objective and subjective social indicators have set the ground for empirical research on quality of life for the past two decades (Glatzer & Zapf, 1984; Noll, 2000). Quality of life has been thought of in these concepts rather statically, as an expression of the state of a person in a synchronic moment.

A development of the individual quality of life concept has been achieved by Amartya Sen (1995) who under the title of capability called for attention for the aspect of "opportunity". It was not welfare alone that Sen thought people should have, but also the opportunity to achieve. The capability approach has been developed in the framework of the „human development" discussion, focusing, among other things, on the "free and autonomous choices of the individuals", i.e. the capacity of the subjects to realize what they consider important for their well-being (Sen, 1995) as a central aspect of quality of life (ul Haq 1999, p. 20).

> "(Sen) ....drew attention to the condition of a person (e.g. his level of nutrition) in a central sense captured neither by the stock of goods (e.g. his food supply) nor by his welfare level (e.g. the pleasure or desire satisfaction he obtains from consuming food). [...] (He) proposed two large changes of view: from actual state to opportunity, and from goods (and welfare) to what he sometimes called 'functionings'" (Cohen 1995, p. 10).

But what are functionings? Sen understands functionings as parts of the state of a person. They are things the person manages to do or be in leading life. We have to differentiate between elementary functionings like to be nourished and in good health and more complex functionings like having self-respect and being socially integrated.

Capability is "a person's ability to do valuable acts or reach valuable states of being [...] The capability approach to a person's advantage is concerned with evaluating it in terms of his or her actual ability to achieve various valuable functionings as a part of living" (Sen, 1995, p. 30).

Capability of a person represents the various alternative combinations of beings and doings of which the person can choose. Capability refers thus to a space of alternative combinations of functionings from which the actual set of functionings has been chosen. The quality of life is related to the ability to choose relevant functionings. In this way, the issue of freedom, thought of as the range of choices a person has (Sen, 1995, p. 34), becomes central in the quality of life concept. By introducing the aspect of capability, Sen emphasizes what a person can get, as opposed to (just) what he does get.

THE CAPABILITY APPROACH AND
THE BIOGRAPHICAL ACTION PARADIGM

Through the processuality inherent in the notion of choice this concept converges, more than the other quality of life concepts, with the social action paradigm of current sociological debates (Schütz, 1971). The opportunity as possibility that is highlighted by the quality of life concept of Amartya Sen can only be reasonable when thinking of social action as the core aspect of human life, and agency as an integral part to the social action paradigm. Quality of life appears to be a precondition and a result of human action. Person's overall goals are discussed as central in analyzing quality of life as "agency achievement" and "agency freedom". In contrast, the mere "well-being achievement" and "well-being freedom" is referring to the "standard of living". Sen's concept overcomes in this way the static and distributive character of the objective and subjective concepts in the quality of life debates enriching the Quality of Life concept with the dimension of the social action, the ability to act and agency.

Indeed, in the social action paradigm the possibility, ability, but also the need for choice is central. Ulrich Oevermann (1996) explicitly conceptualized in the framework of the social action paradigm this centrality, stressing that social action is structured as a sequentially ordered series of possibilities and choices among these possibilities. Social action means decision for an option and the subsequent ground-

ing of the choice. Therefore it seems more adequate to refer to quality of life processes instead of quality of life as a describable static state of being.

The ability to choose related to social processes is central for the biographical
analysis. In terms of the social action paradigm that is also central for the biographical analysis, the ability to choose is related primarily to the ability of the person to
act intentionally, to develop own action schemes and biographical plans, and to realize these plans in exchange with the social constraints deriving from the social structure. In contrast, the loss of the ability for intentional action means the confinement
of the individual in a biographical trajectory. The notion of „trajectory" has the
meaning that the individual having lost the ability to act intentionally is "delivered"
to outer social or natural powers and can only react to the processes that she/he is
exposed to. In this case, the individual's action is understandable only as conditional
(determined through the conditions) (Schütze, 1981; Riemann & Schütze, 1991;
Strauss & Corbin, 1991 (1964); Strauss, Fagerhaugh et al., 1991 (1964); Schütze,
1995). However, the intentional and conditional action should rarely be thought as
exclusive, as the intentional acting can bear unintended outcomes that can produce a
situation of merely conditional acting.

CONSIDERATIONS ON THE OPERATIONALIZATION OF THE CAPABILITY CONCEPT OF QUALITY OF LIFE

According to the aforementioned, the main indicator for quality of life would be the
ability of the person to act intentionally, as it is discussed in the biographical research. A first operationalization of the quality of life concept would be to detect the
empirical material for intentional versus conditional activity. Intentional acting is
acting towards reaching valuable functionings, while conditional acting as a mode of
acting is connected with the loss of valuable functionings. The contrast between
intentional and conditional acting is however not exclusive, as the outcomes of intentional acting can be contrastive to the intentions (Merton, 1936; Leung, 2003) and
can lead in the extreme case to the loss of the ability to intentionally act. At the same
time, the individual never looses entirely the ability to intentionally act. The analysis
of biographical trajectories shows that the individual develops strategies and intentional acting in order to overcome the trajectory and regain the ability to act (Riemann & Schütze, 1991). Besides of this fundamental difficulty in discriminating
between intentional and conditional acting, there are further problems arising by the
effort to capture empirically the capability concept of quality of life some of which
have already been discussed by Amartya Sen. In the following I will present some of
the operationalization problems and suggestions for overcoming these problems
through the biographical method.

The first problem Sen discusses is the problem of evaluation by the act of selecting a class of functionings in the description and appraisal of capabilities. The functionings are evaluated on the basis of concerns and values that are decisive for some
functionings to be important and others to be trivial and negligible. The first question here is what are the objects of value; the second is the value ranking, e.g. how
valuable are the respective objects. The identification of the objects of value speci-
fies the evaluative space. Investigating the quality of life concept would mean, beyond the analysis of the ability to act intentionally or the confinement of the person

in a biographical trajectory, to identify the value-objects and to reconstruct the evaluative space in terms of functionings and capabilities to function.

I suggest that the problem of the identification of values and the evaluative space of the person can be solved by using the method of the biographical narrative interview.

a)   The analysis of the biographical narration can reveal the (biographically given) social situation that constitutes the range of choices a person has as well as the range of choices that the person had and the choices that he/she has made in the past.

b)   It delivers criteria for the assessment of values and preferences that are at the basis of a person's choices and will thereby help to assess the freedom of a person to make choices.

c)   It allows reconstructing the emergence of values in the framework of biographical processes and the specific ranking of the values in the evaluative space of a person.

d)   It enables the reconstruction of the processes of choice on the cognitive and emotional level, and the process of developing capability by choosing among possibilities of doing and being.

e)   It enables the assessing of the outcomes of choices and their impact on the values and the evaluative space of the person, thereby allowing to reconstruct the processual character of the capability of a person and with that his/her quality of life.

The problem of specifying the evaluative space by evaluating functionings and their value ranking becomes even more complicated if we leave the perspective of the (male) adult individual and proceed by considering individuals as embedded in family relations and belonging to different sexes and generations. Amartya Sen has criticized this in the economic discussion, while society is viewed as a collection of adult individuals, family does not appear at all (Sen, 1984). However, family structures and family relations have a relevant impact on the quality of life of family members, which has moreover to be considered as interdependent. Functionings can refer to other family members so that the social situation and the functionings of family members can have a considerable impact on the functionings of other family members. To illustrate this consideration: The failure of functionings of the children, for instance their educational failure, might mean the failure of the biographical plan of the parents and might decrease the quality of life of not only the child itself but also of the parents. Therefore, the analysis of the quality of life of the members of a family has to be analyzed in relation to each other. Quality of life has to be discussed in relation to the social unit of family; however the focus is on the quality of life of the individual members of the family while their interrelationships within the family have to be taken into account.

However, if we follow the capability concept, in relation to quality of life families are a field of considerable differences. Family is a field in which choices are not met equally (Sen, 1984). Quality of life in relation to the social field of family has to be discussed under the aspect of unequal positions deriving from a gender and generational context of relationships, as the problem of the evaluation in the process of selecting a class of functionings in the description and appraisal of capabilities has serious implications in relation to gender and generation. In the following I will present some of the arguments deployed in the debate on equality, justice and quality of life in relation to gender.

The functionings are evaluated on the basis of concerns and values that are decisive for some functionings to be important and others to be trivial and negligible. These values are related to cultural notions on gender relations. There are cultural divisions between men and women in all known societies. Social institutions divide up kinds of activity between the sexes, while women and men see their lives differently. There seem to be two actual norms for human life. Sex may close some options entirely or merely make them more difficult. Gender always makes a difference to what options there are in life as a whole. In traditional societies the two norms for the lives of men and women produce a strongly enforced actual division of activities and ways of living. In more liberal societies this division is weakly enforced. Because of the different options there will be gender specific differences in the answer of the question what are the objects of value and how they rank in the evaluative space. There need not be laws that forbid women to hold certain jobs; customs suffice by making parents reluctant to "waste" resources for the education of daughters. Furthermore, it has been an adaptive strategy of women to adapt their desires according to circumstances and options that they perceive to be open to them. Therefore it is not possible to assess quality of life according to the satisfaction with the own life. The two norms "generate deep problems when we ask about the quality of individuals' lives". Annas (Annas, 1995) argues that it is not the self-evaluation but only the notion of a common human nature that enables an evaluation of values and capabilities in relation to the gender differences.

Onora O'Neill (O'Neill, 1995) considers family relations as relations of power and domination and she regards the problems of assessing the quality of life of women as problems related to the assessment of the quality of life of the weak, the marginalized and the exploited. Typical family structures would illustrate the gulf between

> "ideally independent agents [...] and actual powerlessness. These structures often draw a boundary between 'public' and 'private' domains, assign women (wives and daughters) to the 'private' domain, and leave them with slender control of resources, but heavy commitments to meet others' needs. They may lack adequate economic entitlements, effective enfranchisement, or access to sources of information or debate by which to check or challenge the proposals and plans of the more powerful. [...] Family structures always limit independence, and usually limit women's independence more. A woman who has no adequate entitlements of her own, and insecure rights to a share in family property or income, will not always be coerced, but is always vulnerable to coercion" (O'Neill, 1995, p. 320).

This vulnerability has an impact on the possibility of women to negotiate rules related to family life:

> "If she were an ideally independent agent, or even had the ordinary independence and opportunities of those who have entitlements adequate for themselves and their dependants, she could risk dissent or at least renegotiate proposals put by those who control her means of life. Being powerless and vulnerable she cannot readily do either. Hence any consent that she offers is compromised and does not legitimate others' proposals" (ibid., p. 321).

Similar to the case of gender, the quality of life concept involves some difficulties when applied to children. Freedom of choice as a core aspect applies to adults but bears a range of difficulties when applied to children. In the quality of life discussion, society is viewed as a collection of adult individuals, whereas, children come out as "anomalies". Implicit notions about human nature want children to be not yet morally fully developed, but having to be educated in order to become full members of society, with civil and political rights. There are some similarities and parallelities in the historical development of the rights of children and the development of the rights of women, in so far as norms producing inequalities are in both cases legitimized by the implicit notion of human nature. Social movements deconstructed norms on the differences between men and women as rationalizations thereby improving the social and political rights of women. A similar development can be observed, on a smaller scale, in the increase of children's rights in modern societies (decrease of the age for the right to vote, etc.).

The parents-children relationship is characterized by an imbalance concerning social competency and social power. Parents are acting as socializing agents for their children and as their legal representatives. By law they bear responsibility for the activities and well being of their children. Not the children but their parents are subject of choices that are related to the children's present and future well being. This acting on behalf of the children decreases as children grow older and become successively fully socialized social actors. The power imbalance between parents and children varies culturally, as the power between the sexes does. The notion of the ability of children to make choices for themselves is culturally determined. In liberal societies, in contrast to traditional ones, socialization practices aim at transmitting early to the children the possibility of choices, because of the principle of the development of an autonomous personality, a central value in socialization practices.

Nevertheless, childhood as socialization time is a phase in which the quality of life of the later adult is build up. In the center of this process lay

a)   the intergenerational transmission of norms, among others also of gender roles that determine options and values about functionings, and

b)   the development of the personality and the intergenerational transmission of immaterial (psychic/human and cultural) and material (i.e. inheritance) resources that determine the ability to choose among a range of functionings that means the capability of the person.

From this point of view, the quality of life of children can be assessed in a double perspective, as the perspective of the present, i.e. the actual/present living conditions, and the perspective of the future, i.e. the accumulation of resources (but also constraints) for the future quality of life. The biographical narrative interview offers the possibility to detect the latent dynamics that affect the quality of life of the family members and moreover, the dynamics of exchange, and negotiations that make the quality of life of family members interdependent.

Summarizing, we can state that regarding the operationalization of the freedom of choices as a core aspect of quality of life processes we are confronted with the fact that choices and evaluation spaces are related to social norms that are constraining options open to individuals especially in relation to women and children. We assume that with the method of the biographical interview we are able to reconstruct the self-reflexive dealing with social norms and the adaptation strategies that are developed according to the options that are left open to the individual. This procedure can diminish the residual uncertainty about the range of socially determined options. Furthermore, the biographical narrative interview allows not only to assess the valued functionings that a person has reached, and with this the present quality of life in relation to the past, but also the valued functionings in relation to the future, as the biographical narrative relates the present with the past and the future i.e. future plans, and options.

APPLYING THE CAPABILITY APPROACH ON THE CASE OF MIGRANTS

According to the biographical perspective developed above, quality of life would be assessed in relation to the capability to reach valuable functionings, to meet own choices and to realize life plans. Migrating can be regarded as an activity closely related to the realization of life plans and choices and with this in relation to the improvement of the quality of life. Migration is to be regarded as an active and autonomous movement of people within space towards the improvement of their own standard of living and the standard of living of their family (Rodrigues dos Santos & Marié, 1972). Migration is a step for reaching valuable functionings, for instance income, economic independence, freedom from oppressive political regimes, and educational chances for the own children.

On the other side, migration is accompanied by the loss of valuable functionings like being a full member of the society, having political rights, and living with the own family. These losses are either realized, or they can hit the migrant unexpectedly. Moreover, migration is frequently accompanied by unexpected difficulties and constraints that could not be foreseen and which can deprive migrants, temporary or for a longer term, of the ability to act intentionally (Apitzsch, 1996). Conditions and situations in the unfamiliar social, economic and cultural context can rarely be assessed properly before migration, there can be more constraints and hindrances than the migrant expected. In this sense, the intentional action of improving the quality of life through migration can turn to its opposite, whereas the intentional action can collapse under the burden of the unintended outcomes. Therefore, I suggest considering migration as a field in which the striving for valuable functionings meets with the loss of other valuable functionings. Migration emerges to be a field of struggle for quality of life.

Another issue touching upon the quality of life of migrants is the changes in the family relations and family structures through migration. We can recollect that family for migrants is a central resource for reaching ones own goals , as migration research has highlighted in many studies on ethnic business and migration networks. Research on migration has stressed how important ethnic networks and family solidarity are for overcoming the problems of integration and for stabilizing the own social position in the new society. Family can be the center of migration networks and it can bear a great deal of the ethnic resources that are central for starting up businesses in migration. Although gender and generation relations interfere with the distribution of family resources among the family members (Anthias & Boahene, 2003), this increases the meaning of family for the well being of migrants, their capacity to act intentionally, and the realization of their life plans. Furthermore, family is a place for developing valuable functionings like belonging that is denied by the host society. Because of this, in migration, the social field of family is more important for the quality of life of the individual than family is for non migrants.

While the relevance of family structures increases for the quality of life of migrants, the vulnerability of family relations through migration also increases considerably. Family relations and structures are affected by the process of migration. In most cases, migration leads to a temporal or definitive fragmentation of families. Either migrants migrate as representatives of a family in order to fulfill a concert task for the whole family, as the theory of household in migration has worked out, or migration can be family migration or individuals establishing a family in migration. Separation of family through a fragmented migration of its members becomes a strategy for achieving economic goals, implying the subsequent struggle for family reunion.

A further strain on migrant families is the problem of the harmonization of life options and life plans. The complexity of the inner and outer social environment for families is increasing in migration. Especially the range of disparity of life plans related to space, such as choices for moving or staying are impacting the family in migration stronger than non-migrant families. The fragmentation of family through migration is not only real, as outlined above, but also a steady option that is maintained and nourished by the multiplicity of options in migration. Thus, migration can mean a high risk to family cohesion. Through migration, family bonds are over-strained because of the opening of options that have not existed in the non-migration setting and which can threaten the family unity, such as the options of remigration or staying. Aspects of life which are normally self-evident, staying where someone is, loose their self-evidence and become one option among many. More options are possible which means a more complex strain for the family. This can be illustrated by the option of returning. The migration decision frequently implies the project of return of the whole family. Second generation migrants, however, might develop their own plans of migration and stay. Therefore, one main problem of the family as a general social system, namely, to harmonize the life plans of the family members becomes more critical in migration (Kupferberg, 2003).

Moreover, the interplay of the dynamics of family cohesion in migration with individualization processes reveals a further dimension of the instability of quality of life in migration. Such individualization processes are among others related to integration processes in the host society as they arise especially among the second generation of migrants as well as among migrant women irrespective their belonging to a certain generation.

SUMMARY

In this paper I presented some considerations related to the affinity of the capability version of the quality of life concept with the processual thinking of the social action paradigm and the biographical perspective. I have referred to the solution of problems of operationalization through the utilization of the biographical method. Finally I have discussed how this quality of life concept can be applied to the field of migration, referring to an interpretation of migration as a complex field of struggle for quality of life. Migration has to be thought of as a step towards improving the own quality of life and the quality of life of the own family, whereas, the migration process as such is entailing the possibility of loss of valuable functionings and with that a reduction of the quality of life. Especially concerning the quality of life in migration I have shown, that migrating can lead to high risks for family cohesion and the loss of family resources, and with that to high risks for the quality of life of migrants. The precarity of the quality of life in migration is further stressed through the specific gender and generation problems of the quality of life of members of a migrant family. The method of the biographical narrative interview seems to have the capacity to reveal the complex structures and layers of experience implied in the capability version of the quality of life concept.

NOTES

1   Central ideas of this paper emerged during preparing the proposal for the EU-project "The Chances of the Second Generation in Families of Ethnic Entrepreneurs: Intergenerational and Gender Aspects of Quality of Life Processes". I would like to thank Prof. Dr. Ursula Apitzsch, University of Frankfurt a.M., scientific coordinator of this project, for valuable inputs to this paper. I would also like to thank Dr. Maggi Leung, The Chinese University of Hong Kong for constructive comments and suggestions.

REFERENCES

Allardt, Erik (1973). About Dimensions of Welfare. Research Group for Comparative Sociology. Research Report No 1. Helsinki: University of Helsinki.
Allardt, Erik (1993). Having, Loving, Being: An Alternative to the Swedish Model of Welfare Research. M. C. Nussbaum & A. K. Sen (eds.): The Quality of Life, New York: Oxford University Press, 88-94.
Annas, J. (1995): Women and the Quality of Life: Two Norms or One? M. C. Nussbaum & A. K. Sen (eds.): The Quality of Life, New York: Oxford University Press, 279-302.
Anthias, F. & A. Boahene (2003). Refining the Research Concept of the EthnoGeneration Project. Paper presented at the 1st Workshop of the RTD Project "The Chances of the Second Generation in Families of Ethnic Entrepreneurs", 18-20 July 2003, in Frankfurt am Main.
Apitzsch, U. (1996): Biographien und berufliche Orientierung von Migrantinnen. R. Kersten et al. (eds.): Ausbilden statt ausgrenzen. Jugendliche ausländischer Herkunft in Schule, Ausbildung und Beruf, Frankfurt/M.: Haag und Herchen, 133-47.
Campbell, A., P. E. Converse & W. L. Rodgers (1976): The Quality of American Life, New York: Russell Sage Foundation.
Cohen, G. A. (1995). Equality of What? On Welfare, Goods, and Capabilities. M. C. Nussbaum & A. K. Sen (eds.): The Quality of Life, New York: Oxford University Press, 9-29.
Erikson, R. (1974): Welfare as a Planning Goal. Acta Sociologica 17, No. 3, 273-288.
Erikson, R. (1993): Descriptions of Inequality: The Swedish Approach to Welfare Research. Martha Nussbaum & A. K. Sen (eds.): The Quality of Life, New York: Oxford University Press, 67-83.
Glatzer, W. & W. Zapf (eds.) (1984): Lebensqualität in der Bundesrepublik. Objektive Lebensbedingungen und subjektives Wohlbefinden, Frankfurt/M./New York: Campus.
Inglehart, R. (1989): Kultureller Umbruch. Wertewandel in der westlichen Welt, Frankfurt/M./New York: Campus.
Kupferberg, F. (2003). Refining the Research Concept of the EthnoGeneration Project. Paper presented at the 1st Workshop of the RTD Project "The Chances of the Second Generation in Families of Ethnic Entrepreneurs", 18-20 July 2003, in Frankfurt am Main.
Leung, W. H. Maggi (2003). Quality of Life in Migration: A discussion of Concepts and Research Results. Paper presented at the Fifth Conference of the International Society for Quality-of-Life Studies "Challenges for Quality of Life in Contemporary Societies", 20th to 24th July 2003, Frankfurt am Main.
Merton, R. K. (1936). The Unanticipated Consequences of Purposive Social Action. American Sociological Review 1, 894-904.
Noll, H.-H. (2000): Konzepte der Wohlfahrtsentwicklung: Lebensqualität und "neue" Wohlfahrtskonzepte. Berlin WZB-Discussion-Paper P00-505: WZB.
O' Neill, O. (1995): Justice, Gender and International Boundaries. M. C. Nussbaum & A. K. Sen (eds.): The Quality of Life, New York: Oxford University Press, 303-35.
Oevermann, U. (1996): Theoretische Skizze einer revidierten Theorie professionalisierten Handelns. A. Combe & W. Helsper (eds.): Pädagogische Professionalität. Untersuchungen zum Typus pädagogischen Handelns, Frankfurt am Main: Suhrkamp, 70-182.
Riemann, G. & F. Schütze (1991): Trajectory as a Basic Theoretical Concept for Analysing Suffering and Disorderly Social Processes. D. R. Maines (ed.): Social Organization and Social Process. Essays in Honor of Anselm Strauss, New York: Aldine De Gruyter, 333-57.

Rodrigues dos Santos, J. & M. Marié (1972): Wanderungen und Arbeitskraft. G. Széll (ed.): Regionale Mobilität, München: Nymphenburger Verlagshandlung, 251-62.

Schütz, A. (1971). Gesammelte Aufsätze, Den Haag: Nijhoff.

Schütze, F. (1981): Prozeßstrukturen des Lebenslaufs. J. Matthes, A. Pfeifenberger & M. Stosberg (eds.): Biographie in handlungswissenschaftlicher Perspektive. Kolloqium am Sozialwissenschaftlichen Forschungszentrum der Universität Erlangen-Nürnberg: 67-156.

Schütze, F. (1987): Das narrative Interview in Interaktionsfeldstudien: Erzähltheoretische Grundlagen. Teil I: Merkmale von Alltagserzählungen und was wir mit ihrer Hilfe erkennen können. Hagen, KE 1 FB Erziehungs-, Sozial- und Geisteswissenschaften, mimeo.

Schütze, F. (1995): Verlaufskurven des Erleidens als Forschungsgegenstand der interpretativen Soziologie. H.-H. Krüger & W. Marotzki (eds.): Erziehungswissenschaftliche Biographieforschung, Opladen: Leske & Budrich, 116-57.

Sen, A. K. (1984): Resources, Values and Development. Oxford: Blackwell.

Sen, A. K. (1995): Capability and Well-Being. M. C. Nussbaum & A. K. Sen (eds.): The Quality of Life, New York: Oxford University Press, 30-53.

Strauss, A. & J. Corbin (1991): Trajectory Framework for Management of Chronic Illness (1964). A. Strauss: Creating Sociological Awareness. Collective Images and Symbolic Representations, New Brunswick & London: Transaction Publishers: 149-56.

Strauss, A, S. Fagerhaugh et al. (1991): Illness Trajectories (1964). A. Strauss: Creating Sociological Awareness. Collective Images and Symbolic Representations, New Brunswick & London: Transaction Publishers: 157-76.

ul Haq, M. (1999): Reflections on Human Development. Oxford: Oxford University Press.

PART III:
ECONOMIC CHALLENGES
FOR QUALITY OF LIFE

11. MONETARY STABILITY AND QUALITY OF LIFE

Heinz Herrmann

Deutsche Bundesbank, Frankfurt am Main, Germany

ABSTRACT

The paper starts out by considering in what sense quality of life can be seen as an economic term and what is meant by monetary stability. We continue by discussing why evaluating the standard of living depends on the correct measuring of price developments resp. price stability, and which problems may exist in this field. The following sections discuss why price stability is seen as a mean to foster the standard of living and other components of quality of life. We refer to surveys, economic theory, and empirical studies. The paper concludes with some consequences for monetary policy.

INTRODUCTION [1]

From the perspective of an economist, "Monetary stability and quality of life" is a very broad topic. In fact, one might argue that this subject encompasses everything in monetary economics and central banking. For researchers in the field of quality of life this statement may give the impression that monetary economics is a rather narrow field. However, I hope this paper will give an insight into the fact that seemingly simple matters can, in reality, be rather complex and that the behavior of central banks responsible for the development of the price level in an economy is of great relevance to our quality of life.

First of all, I will try to establish a definition of quality of life which suits an economist (section 2). Afterwards, I shall describe several links between the quality of life and monetary stability:
- monetary stability in a concept for measuring the quality of life (section 3);
- monetary stability and its consequences for income or the standard of living (section 4);
- monetary stability and further aspects of the quality of life (section 5).

The final section mentions some aspects of European monetary policy and offers some conclusions.

DEFINING THE TERMS

"Quality of life" seems to be a rather ambiguous concept. As far as I understand it, this is also a view shared by other researchers (see, for example, Noll, 2000). In my opinion, it is a subjective term. It has many aspects and only some of them are accessible to traditional economic analysis.

153
Wolfgang Glatzer, Susanne von Below, Matthias Stoffregen (eds.), Challenges for Quality of Life in the Contemporary World, 153-164.
© *2004 Kluwer Academic Publishers. Printed in the Netherlands.*

It is quite natural to start out by asking people what seems to be relevant to their quality of life. At first glance, this approach is quite straightforward; it does, however, involve a lot of difficulties. Comparing only a few surveys, one gains the impression that designing the questionnaire is an art in itself. The specific form in which a question is raised, as well as timing and method applied foreshadow the answers to a large extent.

To demonstrate this I have compared the findings of only four questionnaires: Cantril (1965) as quoted by Easterlin (2000), Habich, Noll, and Zapf (1999), Shiller (1996), and Easterly and Fischer (2001). These surveys differ in many respects and caution has to be exercised when comparing them. However, one result is striking: In two surveys which include inflation explicitly as a potential problem, people mention this phenomenon as a major concern, whereas it is not mentioned at all in the other two surveys.

It may well be that, responding to surveys which do not ask for inflation, people use a substitute to express their concerns about this problem. On the other hand a concern about inflation may well represent something else. I shall come back to this point later on.

This makes me a bit skeptical about this approach. In my view, surveys can be helpful, particularly if they are designed carefully. However, we have to be aware of their limitations and we should use them in conjunction with other analytical tools. The standard of living is an important – if not *the* most important – aspect of the quality of life in modern societies. A natural candidate for measuring the standard of living is real income or wealth.[2]

According to a table by Cantril (1965), which is based on a survey undertaken in several developed countries (including Germany) as well as in several less developed countries, the standard of living is the most relevant category, followed by family and health. Other categories mentioned are job/work, social and political. From Habich, Noll, and Zapf (1999) one learns that, in Germany, health, family, love, and affection are the most important components. These are no economic categories. However, it is tempting to make the point that these components may well have an economic background. They may be the "output" of a production function with income as an "input". Health, for example, is not independent of income. Life expectancy is highly correlated with the standard of living in any given country. In this survey, income is a separate item which also ranks rather highly.

If one attempts to translate all of this into traditional economic terms, welfare would seem to be the closest equivalent. Economists normally confine themselves to welfare which results from market processes. Sometimes people tend to see this as a very narrow spectrum of real life. This may be a misperception. The concept of welfare does not only include goods in the usual sense but also encompasses factors such as leisure and may well include the quality of the environment. The term "family" as an element of the quality of life may for example mean that people give a high priority to leisure in order to care for their children, etc. This can easily be integrated into a neo-classical framework of economics. Nevertheless, I do not pretend that all components of the quality of life can be discussed here. Most of this paper deals with monetary stability and the standard of life in a rather narrow sense, namely real income. However, towards the end we shall also go into further aspects in particular monetary stability and income distribution.

Turning to monetary stability, an economist is on safer ground. Nevertheless, it should be added that defining and measuring monetary stability has its problems too. Finding an appropriate approach depends to a large extent on the intention. For the moment, let us assume that monetary stability is something like a stable price level or a low inflation rate. It certainly does not mean fixing the prices of individual goods.

MONETARY STABILITY IN A CONCEPT FOR MEASURING THE STANDARD OF LIVING

As an initial step, a very down-to-earth issue will be discussed. How can price developments be used to measure the standard of living respectively its change? This question has various practical and theoretical aspects. Economic data are normally of a nominal nature. On the other hand, welfare – or the quality of life – depends on real variables, such as goods or leisure available to households. Measuring price developments correctly is a precondition for translating developments in nominal variables into real terms.

A very practical example may help to illustrate the issue. Measuring price developments correctly is important if nominal amounts of transfers to households are calculated on the basis of a given price index. Using a distorted index has immediate effects on the welfare of the recipient of the transfer. If the index underestimates inflation, in real terms the recipient is worse off than before. Such questions played a role when measurement problems were under discussion in the US some years ago (see Advisory commission, 1996).

A good starting point is the idea that monetary stability describes a situation where consumers can maintain their standard of living at a constant level by spending a fixed amount of money. Obviously, this does not mean that all individual prices are fixed. It does not even mean that individual price movements level themselves out. Assume that one has only two goods which can be substituted to a certain extent. If the price of one good increases and the other decreases, households will normally shift their consumption from the one that is now more expensive to the less expensive one. However, their welfare may be the same as before. The bundle of goods they buy has changed. In other words, in order to calculate a reasonable price index one has to look not only at changes in prices but also at changes in amounts consumed.

Economists have developed the concept of a cost of living index that measures the change in consumption expenditures required to maintain a constant standard of living. Although this idea seems simple and obvious, most official price indices as calculated by statistical offices obey this principle only within certain limits. In most cases, consumer price indices rely on what is known as the Laspeyres index, according to which – at least for a while – the basket of goods considered is kept fixed. If such a "conventional" price index overstates inflation – or, to put it another way, if consumption expenditures are deflated by such an index –, the increase in the welfare of the consumers will be underestimated.

This problem is known as a substitution bias in the literature on inflation measurement. However, one should add immediately that such an error is only of limited relevance in real life. For Germany, Hoffmann (1998) has estimated that the annual inflation rate may be overstated by a mere 0.05 percentage point owing to this bias.

One reason for this is that the statistical office holds the basket fixed only for a limited period. Furthermore, in normal times we do not observe dramatic changes in relative prices.

However, there exist other problems with price measurement if the principle of the cost of living index is adopted. Such problems are often related to the question of which goods should be included in our price index and the weight that should be given to them. The debate on the price effects of the changeover from national currencies to the Euro is interesting in this respect. In Germany, this became famous as the "Teuro" debate (which resembles the German expression for expensive). Following the introduction of the Euro in many European countries, people complained about sharp price increases. Such increases were not corroborated by the official statistics, however. According to the official statistics, the effects of the changeover on the inflation rate was, if anything, moderate.

One explanation of this phenomenon could be that consumers care more about the prices of some of the goods they buy than they do about others, whereas the weighting scheme of the statisticians reflects the weight of the individual goods in the goods basket of representative households. For example, people were very sensitive about price increases in restaurants, which really did increase more than the average, while they did not take into account that rents for flats were more or less stable. The share of rents in the goods basket of households is, however, much higher than the share of money spent on food in restaurants. As a consequence one may observe that perceived inflation and actual inflation showed a remarkable divergence (see figure 1). Although this episode shed some light on the deep question as to whether welfare is a an objective or subjective concept, the practical relevance of this experience should not be exaggerated.

Another issue is how to deal with goods which are consumed but which, for good reasons, are not included in our basket of goods. An increase of our consumer expenditures should be an indication of more welfare or of inflation if our price index aims to evaluate welfare. Now, take the safety of housing, for example. Let us assume burglary becomes more of an issue and people therefore spend more money on protecting their houses. Welfare has not increased compared to before. So, are such higher costs a sign of inflation? Another example is illness: If we spend money to cure some health problems, should this be reflected in inflation rates? Most people would hesitate to accept such an interpretation.

A final complication is the fact that a large part of the goods we buy serve not only our present-day welfare but are consumed over a period of time. Take clothes, cars or houses, for example. Should we consider the full price or only the services from these goods in the current period? Furthermore, goods change their quality. How much does an air bag in my car increase my welfare? Is a new price "justified" by a new brake system or is it due to inflation? This kind of question has been studied over the past few years.

Without going into further detail, it becomes clear that the principle of using a price index to evaluate the (change of) welfare of households is not always easy to implement and it is quite understandable why statisticians often shy away from such an approach and are usually much more modest. One has to accept that price indices used in real life are not entirely satisfactory as a theoretical concept for measuring welfare or the standard of living. Nevertheless, we hold the view that these problems are normally of limited quantitative relevance.

Figure 1: Price Perceptions, Price Expectations, and Actual Inflation

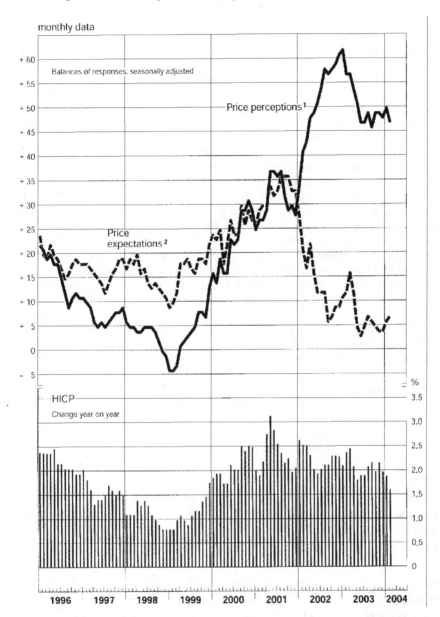

Source: European Commission Consumer Surveys. 1 = Price developments over the past 12 months. 2 = Price developments over the coming 12 months.

MONETARY STABILITY AS A TOOL FOR IMPROVING
THE STANDARD OF LIVING

Up to now, we have discussed price stability and the standard of living in the same way as we use a thermometer to measure temperature. Certainly, a good thermometer is a valuable item in itself. However, this is not the most important aspect of weather. For example we do not believe that the thermometer has an influence on the weather and welfare. A similar argument can be made with respect to measurement problems and inflation. Although some people think that price measurement has fewer defects in a low-inflation world, nobody believes that to be an important reason for disliking inflation.

However, inflation is obviously a matter of deep concern to the general public. The "Teuro" debate in the Euro area is only a recent example of how sensitively consumers react to inflation or, in this specific instance, even to inflation which is largely imagined and non-existent. Easterly and Fischer (2001) and Shiller (1996) conducted surveys to discover more about the relevance of inflation or price stability to the well-being of people. Easterly and Fischer use a large international sample of households. Furthermore, they are able to differentiate according to the households' standard of living, education and age. This enables us to draw some conclusions not only about different classes but also about possible motives why people dislike inflation. Shiller's sample includes responses from only three countries (Germany, USA, and Brazil). However, he goes more directly into the question of why people fear inflation.

The two papers agree on the most important point: inflation is seen as a major problem. According to Easterly and Fisher, it ranks third after unemployment and crime, but before drug abuse, corruption or environmental corruption (see table 1).

Table 1: Percentage of Responses that Mentioned Given Problems as among the Top two or three Problems, by Country

	Inflation and High Prices	Crime	Recession & Unemployment	Drug Abuse	Govmt. Corruption	Environmental Pollution
Australia	4	17	13	6	8	12
Austria	7	16	9	8	6	11
Belgium	10	13	18	10	12	5
Brazil	7	17	10	9	14	4
Canada	10	18	17	6	6	7
Chile	5	10	8	19	7	7
China	25	13	10	1	15	8
Colombia	9	15	11	10	10	9
Czech Republic	14	26	4	7	11	12
Denmark	3	12	10	3	3	15
Finland	4	21	24	5	9	8

Table 1: Percentage of Responses that Mentioned Given Problems as among the Top two or three Problems, by Country (continued)

France	4	12	21	6	6	4
Germany	8	21	16	7	6	12
Greece	9	13	20	15	6	8
Hong Kong	11	12	14	6	3	7
Hungary	19	17	10	2	9	8
India	13	14	14	7	9	6
Indonesia	12	24	24	11	5	4
Ireland	4	18	15	17	6	5
Italy	6	10	22	2	13	11
Japan	6	9	20	2	21	17
Mexico	17	13	18	7	15	4
Netherlands	3	23	12	7	5	7
Norway	2	19	12	11	4	11
Philippines	12	24	12	10	10	9
Poland	11	22	12	7	11	10
Russia	22	28	13	1	8	5
Singapore	23	12	9	4	2	10
Spain	7	6	18	13	10	6
Sweden	5	20	15	11	4	13
Switzerland	6	15	15	10	5	10
Taiwan	11	13	8	11	18	13
Thailand	5	23	12	10	8	10
Turkey	19	8	12	4	11	8
Ukraine	22	26	9	3	10	4
United Kingdom	5	19	14	9	6	7
USA	7	24	6	11	6	4
Venezuela	16	16	11	11	13	2
Sample Average	10	17	14	8	9	8

Source: Easterly and Fisher (2001), pp. 164f.

According to Shiller between 80 % and 90 % of the general public in the three countries under consideration perceive the control of inflation to be one of the most important missions of economic policy (see table 2).

A second important point on which there exists agreement is that people fear inflation will have a negative impact on their real income. Related to this is the finding that older people are more concerned about inflation than younger people are. From an economic point of view, this makes sense: older people who typically have more financial assets in their portfolios encounter greater difficulties in shielding themselves against inflation, whereas younger people with more human capital may be less vulnerable to inflation.

Table 2: Do You Agree with the Following Statement: "The Control of Inflation is one of the Most Important Missions of US/German/Brazilian Economic Policy."

	1	2	3	4	5	N
	Fully Agree		Unde-cided		Compl. Disagree	
US All	*56 %*	*28 %*	*7 %*	*7 %*	*2 %*	*123*
born before 1940	69 %	13 %	11 %	4 %	2 %	45
born after 1950	44 %	38 %	2 %	13 %	2 %	45
Germany All	*76 %*	*18 %*	*5 %*	*1 %*	*0 %*	*174*
born before 1940	90 %	8 %	1 %	1 %	0 %	77
born after 1950	51 %	40 %	7 %	2 %	0 %	55
Brazil	*56 %*	*32 %*	*2 %*	*4 %*	*7 %*	*57*

Source: Shiller (1996), p.18.

However, there are also some aspects of the two papers which are more difficult to reconcile. According to Shiller, households seem to give greater weight to unemployment than to inflation. This is not corroborated by Easterly and Fisher. Furthermore, Shiller's finding does not support the notion that people who have suffered from high inflation have a clearer perception of its problems, whereas Easterly and Fisher's finding conforms with that view. These differences may result from the fact that Shiller's sample of only three countries raises some problems. In fact, Brazil, which is meant to represent high-inflation countries in Shiller's paper, is an outlayer according to Easterly and Fisher.

Shiller does offer other insights, however. His article reveals that there is a lot of uncertainty about the inflation phenomenon. People have only a vague notion of the reasons for rising prices. Unfortunately, the survey did not include any questions on falling prices. Deflation was not an issue at that time. If Shiller is right, we should expect that people would be happy to see prices fall. However, this stands in stark contrast to the view of economists, who emphasize the problems of deflation.

Given the problems raised by the survey approaches under discussion, it would seem to be the obvious thing to use other, more "indirect" methods to shed light on these questions. Economists have used various approaches for explaining the welfare costs of inflation. One argument centers on the fact that inflation makes cash management more expensive. One simple example is known as the "shoe leather effect". In order to avoid the costs of holding money in an inflationary world, households try to minimize their cash. This comes at a cost. Stories from hyperinflation countries are well known. Wage earners hurry to spend their income before prices rise further. But even in less dramatic situations these costs become clear when we observe how much time and effort people invest in avoiding non-remunerative assets.

In recent years the costs of inflation have been analyzed carefully in models of general equilibrium. The idea behind these models may be summarized in the following way: Households maximize their utility by demanding and supplying goods (including labor). Prices are the coordination mechanism. As long as prices fully reflect demand and supply, they will guarantee the optimal solution in terms of welfare. This is the situation in a world of flexible prices. Now, let us assume that only some agents in the economy are free to change prices in a given period. Several theories, which are not discussed here, can be cited to justify this assumption. The sticky price model reflects a real-world phenomenon. We know that prices are not adjusted every day. In addition, such a model can explain why monetary policy has short-term real effects, as we observe from empirical studies. In an inflationary world, those who are free to adjust their prices will choose new ones; the rest have to keep prices stable for the time being. In the end, we shall see some distortions in the allocation of goods. Such distortions can be avoided only if those who are free to adjust choose the old prices (or prices we would see in a world with a stable price level). In other words, monetary policy has the task of establishing conditions we would observe in a world with fully flexible prices, and that means the task of establishing a stable general price level.

Certainly, we shall witness some deviations from this very simple model in the real world. However, it can be demonstrated that this finding is robust with respect to many modifications, such as incomplete competition. Indeed, the facts of real life even strengthen the point. For example, taxation of nominal income adds further arguments in favour of stable prices.

The economics profession has not only considered the case of inflation theoretically. Many empirical papers study the costs of inflation. There is overwhelming evidence that such costs exist. However, depending on the models used, the benefits of reducing inflation vary. One example is provided by Tödter and Ziebarth (1999). An exercise in calculating the benefits of reducing inflation in Germany by 2 % leads them to the conclusion that this would result in a year-on-year increase in GDP of more than 1 %. Others come to less dramatic conclusions but the negative implications of inflation, at least above a certain threshold, are not in dispute.

There is an ongoing debate on whether the costs of inflation show a linear increase with inflation. There are good arguments for assuming that inflation below a certain limit is of no relevance, whereas the costs of two-digit inflation (and more) are very high. For example, the Chairman of the Federal Reserve Board, Alan Greenspan, used to say that inflation is only a problem if people take it into account in their decisions. This is, on the one hand, true but, on the other, not always a very useful definition. Today, there seems to be a broad agreement, at least among central bankers, that an annual inflation rate below 2 % is not incompatible with price stability. Problems of inflation measurement, as discussed to some extent above, are one reason why central bankers are ready to accept some positive but small inflation rates. Another argument may be that deflation is seen as an even worse evil than inflation and one should avoid this risk even at some costs.

MONETARY STABILITY AND FURTHER ASPECTS
OF THE QUALITY OF LIFE

As mentioned earlier, "quality of life" is probably a broader concept than just the standard of living. Sometimes political, social and international concerns are mentioned (see Easterlin, 2000). According to the survey by Shiller, many people in the US and Germany expressed the view that inflation would create political chaos and would lower their country's international prestige. A further concern articulated in the survey is that inflation will be used by opportunists to exploit others. Sometimes the keyword "solidarity" appears. One possible interpretation of these arguments is that members of the public are not neutral with regard to the consequences of inflation for income distribution – some because they belong to the class of low income earners, others because they fear the negative consequences of a more uneven distribution of income.

A relevant question in this context is whether stable prices improve the position of the poor or not. This line of inquiry has two aspects: the impact of inflation on the income of the poorest in absolute terms and its impact on their relative position, that is income distribution. The answers to that may have implications for the quality of life of members of the general public.

Economists know much less about the relationship between inflation and income distribution than they do about the relationship between inflation and income in general. Certainly, one may have some prior awareness of why inflation is good or bad for the poor. The poor have fewer assets, which means they are less affected by the potential adverse consequences of inflation for real interest rates. On the other hand, they may have less sophisticated strategies for protecting their wealth and/or income against inflation or they may be more dependent on transfer income which is not (fully) indexed. Furthermore there are some indications that the wages of unskilled workers are more sticky than other types of income with negative consequences for their real income under inflation.

When analyzing whether the well-being of the poor is more affected by inflation than the well-being of the rich, one may pursue the two strategies described above: asking people directly or using statistical facts. Easterly and Fisher apply both strategies. Their survey data give a clear message: poor, less well-educated, and older members of society dislike inflation more than rich, well-educated and younger people do. The pattern is very consistent: aversion increases monotonically with decreasing income. Although Shiller casts doubt on how far people really know what inflation does, it may be reasonably stated that those who are less able to protect themselves against inflation are the ones who fear its consequences most.

Next, it should be asked whether this conclusion is supported by the statistical data. Easterly and Fisher use several measurements to find out whether inflation hurts the poorest more than the average. This indeed seems to be the case. Easterly and Fisher state, for example, that - over a decade - the income share of the bottom quintile of a country's population is reduced by high inflation.

Similar calculations have been made by C. and D. Romer (1998). The focus of their analysis is also on the long- term relationship between inflation and the income of the poorest. Such a long-term perspective makes a lot of sense. Although an expansionary monetary policy with accelerating inflation rates may have positive effects in the short run, these effects will be reversed (and possibly overcompensated) in the following period when central banks try to stabilize prices again or, at least, try to avoid an accelerating inflation rate.

Simple regressions as used by Romer and Romer are certainly a rough method and one should be cautious when drawing conclusions. They may be spurious and the causality is not at all clear. Keeping these caveats in mind, we report the results presented by Romer and Romer: Taking a sample of 66 countries, there is a negative relationship between average inflation and the income of the poorest fifth of the population. This negative relationship can be confirmed for the sample of industrialized countries (Romer & Romer, 1998 p. 187).

Furthermore, Romer and Romer report a positive result for regressions between the Gini coefficient and inflation: in other words, the higher inflation is, the more dispersed is income. Although it seems that this finding is less robust than the earlier one, it is significant for industrialized countries and also if we take all countries together. As mentioned, we have to be cautious in how to interpret the results. One possibility is that high inflation and inequality in income are a consequence of political instability, which may be seen as a third exogenous factor. However, it is also possible to make the point that inflation is a cause of political chaos (see above).

In spite of these caveats, one message seems to be clear: there are no indications that inflation can be used in the long run to improve the situation of the poor.

SOME CONCLUSIONS

In this paper, we have made three points. First, research on the quality of life and on monetary economics have common interests. Second, defining an appropriate measure of price development and price stability is a precondition for evaluating real income and the standard of living, which is an important aspect of the quality of life. Third, there is overwhelming theoretical and empirical evidence that price stability fosters the standard of living in an economy. There are indications that other components of the quality of life, such as the well-being of the poor, also benefit from stable prices.

These findings and the insight that inflation is a monetary phenomenon have led to many central banks nowadays being entrusted with the task of safeguarding price stability. The primary objective of the European Central Bank, as defined in the Maastricht Treaty, is to maintain price stability. Although the objective of the Federal Reserve System is less clear-cut, there appears to be strong support for this idea in the United States, too.

Nevertheless, consideration has to be given to the fact that most people dislike inflation but have only a very limited understanding of the underlying inflation process and its real costs. Furthermore, a loose monetary policy may have positive effects in the short run but inflationary consequences in the future. This makes it clear that we cannot take price stability permanently for granted. Central banks should not cease campaigning for price stability and, even in difficult times, need sufficient independence to do their job.

NOTES

1   This paper represents the author's personal opinion and do not necessarily reflect the views of the Deutsche Bundesbank.
2   The correct concept of "income" is no trivial question, but we shall not discuss this issue here.

REFERENCES

Advisory Commission to Study the Consumer Price Index (1996): Toward a More Accurate Measure of the Cost of Living, Final Report, Washington.
Cantril, H. (1965): The Pattern of Human Concerns, New Brunswick.

Easterlin, R. (2000): The World-wide Standard of Living since 1800. Journal of Economic Perspectives 14, 7-26.

Easterly, W. & S. Fischer (2001): Inflation and the Poor. Journal of Money, Credit and Banking 33 (2), 160-178.

Habich, R., H.-H. Noll & W. Zapf (1999): Subjektives Wohlbefinden in Ostdeutschland nähert sich westdeutschem Niveau. Informationsdienst Soziale Indikatoren 22, 1-6.

Hoffmann, J. (1998): Problems of Inflation Measurement in Germany, Discussion paper: Deutsche Bundesbank.

Noll, H.-H. (2000): Konzepte der Wohlfahrtsentwicklung: Lebensqualität und "neue" Wohlfahrtskonzepte: WZB Discussion Paper No. P00-505.

Romer, C. & D. Romer (1998): Monetary Policy and the Well-being of the Poor. Federal Reserve Bank of Kansas City (ed.): Income Inequality: Issues and policy options: Kansas City.

Shiller, R.J. (1996): Why do people dislike inflation? National Bureau of Economic Research, Working Paper 5539

Tödter, K. & G. Ziebarth (1999): Price Stability versus Low Inflation in Germany. An Analysis of Costs and Benefits. M. Feldstein (ed): The Costs and Benefits of Price Stability, Chicago, 47-94.

12. SEGMENTED QUALITY OF WORKING LIFE

Regular vs. Non-regular Workers in Korea

Byoung-Hoon Lee and Yoo-Sun Kim

Chung-An University and Korea Labor & Society Institute, Seoul, South Korea

ABSTRACT

During the past decade, the force of the market has become increasingly dominant in determining employment relations patterns on the global level. In the context of growing global competition, firms have tried to reshape the existing employment relations in the market-driven direction. In particular, management has taken a variety of actions to "unbundle" corporate structure and externalize employment relations by resorting to outsourcing, spin-offs, and the increased use of non-regular labor. Meanwhile, labor unions in most industrialized countries have experienced the shrinkage of their organizational base and political leverage under the pressure of globalization, and have become a more passive role-player in reforging employment relations schemes than ever, albeit a wide variance of unions' influence across countries.

Along with the proliferated use of non-regular labor (i.e. fixed-term workers, part-timers, temporary help-agency labor, on-call labor, and independent contractor), which can be viewed as a core part of the externalizing trend of employment relations, a new division line in the labor market has drawn attention of concern among academics and practitioners. In Korea, as a matter of fact, the total size of non-regular workforce has surpassed that of regular workers since the 1998 economic crisis, and the former's working conditions (i.e. wages, employment, corporate welfare, legal protection, and shop floor relations) have proven to be quite precarious and marginal, compared to the latter's. In this light, our paper intends to offer an analytical view on the segmented quality of working life, which has been further polarized between regular and non-regular workers in Korea. By drawing on the analysis of the government's official labor statistics and related surveyed data, we attempt to examine the growing trends and current employment conditions of non-regular workers, and to address some policy issues to tackle social problems, derived from this recent segmentation of national labor composition.

INTRODUCTION

The segmented labor market is not a new social phenomenon. Since Doeringer and Piore (1971) explored the segmentation of labor markets over thirty years ago, a pile of labor research literature has tried to clarify the trends, patterns, and rationale of labor market differentiation. As noted in Lee and Frenkel (forthcoming), recent years have witnessed a new division of labor markets, which is exemplified by the rapid proliferation of non-standard employment patterns, such as temporary or fixed-term labor, part-timers, temporary help agency or dispatched labor, on-call workers, contract labor, independent contractors, and home workers. This new fracture line that divides labor markets by workers' employment status (regular vs. non-regular) is commonly identified in industrialized countries, which have experienced

165

Wolfgang Glatzer, Susanne von Below, Matthias Stoffregen (eds.), Challenges for Quality of Life in the Contemporary World, 165-178.

intensified market competition fuelled by globalization, deregulation, and propelled technological breakthrough.

As a matter of fact, the growth of non-regular employment in Korea has been very remarkable, particularly in the context of the economic crisis which broke out at the end of 1997. The share of non-regular workers in the wage labor population of the country has exceeded that of regular (permanent and full-time) employees from 1999 onward. More importantly, the employment conditions of the former group of workers is quite inferior and more vulnerable, in comparison to the latter. As a consequence, two working class citizenships coexist in polarized labor markets – regular workers as the first-class citizens and non-regular workers as the second-class ones. Given the widening of the discriminatory schism in the employment status and condition of the two groups of workers, labor unions in Korea have launched organizing campaigns to represent those peripheral workers and have called for a more active governmental role, especially in terms of policies which will protect periphal workers both of which have been foiled by employers' strong opposition. Consequently, the new segmentation of the labor force by employment status becomes a core challenge to undermine the equitable quality of life for working people.

In this light, our paper aims to delineate the polarized quality of working life in Korea by comparing the employment conditions between regular and non-regular workers (chapter 3), and to discuss the causal background of the polarizing labor market (chapter 4). In comparing the quality of working life of the two worker groups, we focus on wages and working hours, social benefits, and legal protection. Prior to the comparison and causal analysis of the segmented Quality of working life (QWL), we present a brief sketch regarding the recent trends and peculiarity of non-regular employment in Korea. In conclusion, some policy implications to tackle the issue of polarized QWL are addressed.

NON-REGULAR EMPLOYMENT IN KOREA

As displayed in figure 1, the share of non-regular labor among the total wage labor force in Korea has grown since 1994, and sharply soared during the period of economic crisis (1997-1999). The proportion of non-regular workers in the wage labor force, estimated through the annual Economically Active Population Survey (EPS) by the National Statistical Office (NSO), increased from 43.2 % in 1996 to 51.6 % in 1999, thereby exceeding that of the regular workforce. As demonstrated in figure 1, both male and female non-regular employment shows an identical growth during this period. Yet, it should be noted that non-regular employment (66.4 % in 2002) among the female wage labor force is much higher than that (41.4 % in the same year) among the male wage workforce.

Table 1 notes the detailed composition of non-regular labor force by gender, which is estimated by the 2002 EPS – additional survey.[1] Among a variety of non-regular employment patterns, the share of temporary workers is over 70 %. It is also noteworthy that the vast majority of temporary workers is characterized as quasi-permanent, in that employers use them by renewing their short-term employment contract regularly in order to achieve a reduction of labor cost and numerical labor flexibility. Yet, those permanent temporary workers, termed by Tsui et al. (1995) and Way (1992), are observed to suffer from very insecure employment status, like other non-regular employment patterns, since the renewal of their contract can be arbitrarily refused by employers without legal constraint.

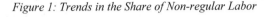

Figure 1: Trends in the Share of Non-regular Labor

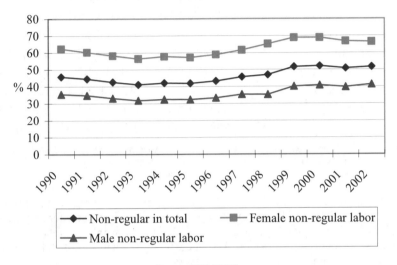

Source: KLI (2003).

When looking into the relative distribution of non-regular labor by age, we can find that there is a U-shape dispersion along age groups. As illustrated in figure 2, the youngest (15-19) and the oldest age (65 +) groups have the highest percentage of non-regular labor, while the age group of 25-34 shows the lowest level (48.1 %). This represents that the two age groups of 15-19 and 65+ are more likely to place themselves into the unstable job position of non-regular employment in labor markets, which might be linked to the former's low human capital and the latter's obsolete labor power.

Table 1: Composition of Wage Labor Force by Employment Status and Gender in 2002

	Total (1,000)	Male (1,000)	Female (1,000)
Regular Workers	5,922 (43.4 %)	4,780 (53.3 %)	1,642 (29.3 %)
Non-Regular Workers	7,708 (56.6 %)	3,752 (46.7 %)	3,956 (70.7 %)
Temporary Workers	5,404 [70.1 %]	2,738 [73.0 %]	2,666 [67.4 %]
Part-time Workers	565 [7.3 %]	172 [4.6 %]	392 [9.9 %]
On-call Workers	364 [4.7 %]	237 [6.3 %]	127 [3.2 %]
Independent Contractor	702 [9.1 %]	301 [8.0 %]	401 [10.1 %]
Dispatched Workers	88 [1.1 %]	42 [1.1 %]	46 [1.2 %]
Contract Workers	346 [4.5 %]	216 [5.8 %]	130 [3.3 %]
Home Workers	238 [3.1 %]	45 [1.2 %]	194 [4.9 %]

Source: The 2002 Economically Active Population Survey – Additional Survey. The figure in the paren-
thesis is the percent of total wage labor force, while that in the square bracket is the percent of total non-
regular employees.

Table 2 displays the relative composition of regular and non-regular workforce by
industry. The primary industry, including agriculture, fishery, and forestry, has the
highest proportion of non-regular labor, followed by the wholesale-retail-food-hotel
sectors and the construction sector. And, the wholesale-retail-food-hotel sectors employ the largest number of non-regular workers.

Figure 2: Relative Distribution of Non-regular Labor by Age in 2002

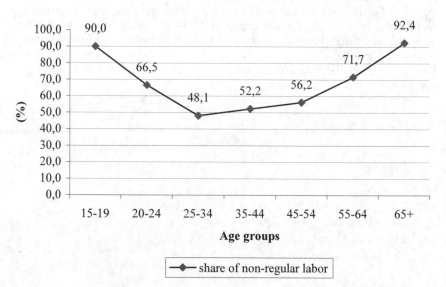

Source: The 2002 Economically Active Population Survey – Additional Survey.

The number of non-regular workers employed in the finance-real estates-renting business sectors is over 50 % of total employment in those sectors, while the manu-facturing (& mining) and the social and personal service sectors employ over 40 % of the labor force in the non-regular employment form.

The existing literature points out two notable features of non-regular workforce in Korea. First, according to Nam & Kim (2000) and Ryu (2001), both of which exam-ine the job transferability of non-regular workers by a time-series analysis of the EPS data, those peripheral workers in Korea are trapped into non-regular jobs, rather than being able to step into regular jobs. Nam & Kim (2000) note that only 1 % of non-regular workers succeed in being permanently transferred to regular jobs, while over 80 % of them, exiting from their marginal jobs, tend to return to non-regular employment status within two years. It can be inferred from these studies that the Korean labor market is completely segmented between regular and non-regular jobs.[2]

Secondly, a substantial portion of non-regular workforce in Korea is employed at this precarious job position against their will. That is, although many non-regular workers want to have regular jobs, they cannot but be involuntarily employed as disposable labor, due to employers' growing preference for the avoidance of regular employment on the labor demand side. This fact is evinced by Kim's analysis (1999) of part-time workforce, in which the share of involuntarily employed part-time workers grew from 23.8 % to 52.3 % between 1997 and 1998.

Table 2: Composition of Labor Force by Employment Status and Industry in 2002

Industry	Regular Labor (1,000)	Non-regular Labor (1,000)
Agriculture, Fishery, Forestry	6 (4.1 %)	140 (95.9 %)
Manufacturing & Mining	1,963 (57.8 %)	1,434 (42.2 %)
Electricity, Gas, Water Supply	40 (81.6 %)	9 (18.4 %)
Construction	301 (23.6 %)	974 (76.4 %)
Wholesale & Retail, Food, Hotels	547 (19.2 %)	2,305 (80.8 %)
Transport, Storage, Communication	548 (63.5 %)	315 (36.5 %)
Finance, Real Estates, Renting	419 (46.5 %)	482 (53.5 %)
Social & Personal Service	2,074 (50.2 %)	2,055 (49.8 %)

Source: The 2002 Economically Active Population Survey – Additional Survey. The figure in the paren-thesis is the percent of total employment in each industrial category.

The involuntary employment of non-regular workers is also exemplified by indus-try-level case studies regarding non-regular jobs. For instance, the Korea Metal Workers Federation (2003) reports that 61.6 % of surveyed contract workers in the metal industry have no chance to get regular jobs and, therefore, are forced to take up non-regular employment for their living. Another study on the banking industry presents a similar story: married women who have banking job experience and want to be re-hired after childbirth or childcare only have little chances of getting regular jobs, because most banks constrain those female job applicants from being re-employed as regular employees in practice. (Kwon, 1996) As a result, most of them are employed as temporary part-timers. Moreover, a KLI panel survey shows an interesting finding namely that the involuntary employment choice lowers job satisfaction for non-regular workers, with statistical significance (Ahn et al., 2001).

POLARIZED QUALITY OF WORKING LIFE BETWEEN REGULAR AND NON-REGULAR WORKERS

The polarized quality of working life by employment status is exemplified by a wide wage gap between regular and non-regular workers. As summarized in table 3, according to the 2002 EPS-additional survey, the average monthly wage of non-regular workers amounts to 96,000 won, which is only 52.7 % of regular workers' monthly wage. Although the monthly wage of non-regular workers has a slightly higher increase than that of regular workers between 2001 and 2002, the latter have earned nearly double the former's monthly wage during these years.

Figure 3 shows that independent contractors and dispatched workers earn relatively higher wages than the other non-regular employment patterns.

Table 3: Comparison of Monthly wages between Regular and Non-Regular Labor

Worker	Monthly Wage in 2001		Monthly Wage in 2002		Wage Increase
	Amount (1,000 Won)	Relative Ratio	Amount (1,000 Won)	Relative Ratio	
Regular	1,694	100 %	1,820	100 %	7.4 %
Non-Regular	891	52.6 %	960	52.7 %	7.7 %

Source: The 2001-2002 Economically Active Population Survey – Additional Survey.

Table 4 displays the comparison of weekly working hours between regular and non-regular workers. In general, the weekly working hours (45.5) of non-regular workers are a little longer than those (44.0) of regular workers. Particularly, the number of non-regular workers who are working over the statutory maximum limit of 56 hours reaches 1.84 million (23.8 % of total non-regular labor force), nearly twice the number of their regular counterparts (0.96 million, 16.2 %) in the same category. When considering specific employment patterns of non-regular labor, the working hour (50.3) by contract labor is longest, followed by dispatched labor (47.8) and permanent-temporary (46.7). Another remarkable point is that the weekly working hours of regular labor have been shortened by 1.9 hours between 2001 and 2002, which is almost double the reduced working hours for non-regular workers. This represents that regular workers have gained gain twice the benefit from the recent reduction of working hours (from 44 to 40) compared to non-regular workers.

Figure 3: Monthly Wages by Employment Patterns, 2001-2002

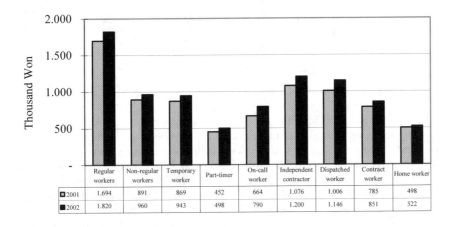

Source: The 2001-2002 Economically Active Population Survey – Additional Survey.

Table 4: Comparison of Working Hours between Regular and Non-regular Labor

Worker	Weekly Working Hours		Distribution of Working Hours, 2002 (%)				
	2001	2002	<36	36-44	45-50	51-56	>56
Regular	45.9	44.0	13.1	38.1	20.9	11.6	16.2
Non-regular	46.5	45.5	20.3	24.5	19.3	12.1	23.8

Source: The 2001-2002 Economically Active Population Survey – Additional Survey.

By taking working hours into account, we can compare the hourly wage between regular and non-regular workers. As shown in table 5, the average hourly wage of non-regular workers in 2002 amounts to 5,369 won, which is only 51.1 % of regular workers' hourly wage. During the recent two years (2001-2002), the relative ratio of non-regular workers' hourly wage divided by regular workers' has declined from 51.8 to 51.1. As noted above, this widening gap of hourly wages may be derived from the discriminatory reduction of working hours between the two groups. In the distribution of hourly wage, 62.6 % of non-regular workers (4.71 million) are paid an hourly wage of 5,000 won and below in 2002, whereas only 20.7 % of the regular labor force (1.16 million) is categorized as the same group of low hourly wage.

When delving into the distribution of monthly wage earnings by employment status, we can identify the notable distinction between regular and non-regular worker groups.

Table 5: Comparison of Hourly Wage between Regular and Non-regular Labor

Worker	Hourly Wage in 2001		Hourly Wage in 2002		Wage Increase
	Amount (Won)	Relative Ratio	Amount (Won)	Relative Ratio	
Regular	9,315	100.0 %	10,504	100.0 %	12.8 %
Non-regular	4,824	51.8 %	5,369	51.1 %	11.3 %

Source: The 2001-2002 Economically Active Population Survey – Additional Survey.

As demonstrated in figure 4, the number of non-regular workers who earn 1 million won and below on average per month is 5,386,000 (69.7 % of total non-regular employment), while that of regular workers in the same wage bracket is 1,193,000 (20.2 % of regular labor force). Similarly, regular workers whose monthly wage is 0.5 million won and below number only 29,000 (0.5 %), whereas their non-regular counterparts number 1,452,000 (18.8 %). As a result, one of every five non-regular workers is paid as very low a wage as 0.5 million won and below.

The official definition of the OECD sets low wage (or pay) as "equal to two-thirds of the median earnings of full-time, year-round workers". (OECD, 1998, p. 51) When applying this criterion to Korea, around 50 % of the entire wage labor force (48.6 %, 6,625,000) may be categorized as "low wage earners" of 1.05 million won and below.

Figure 4: Comparison of Wage Earnings Dispersion between Regular & Non-regular Labor

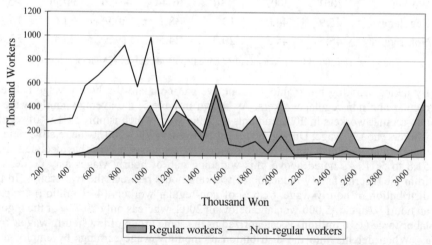

Source: The 2001-2002 Economically Active Population Survey – Additional Survey.

In specific, 70 % of non-regular employees (5,408,000) can be seen as belonging to the low wage worker group, while 20.6 % of the regular workforce (1,217,000) is placed under this category, as displayed in table 6. In other words, seven out of every ten non-regular workers are "low wage earners", while one fifth of regular workers belong to the OECD low wage group. In accordance with the statutory minimum wage, which was set at 2,275 won per hour in 2002, the number of workers who are below the minimum wage is 774,000 in total. In specific, the number of non-regular workers below the minimum wage is 736,000 won, nearly 19.5 times the number of regular workers in the same condition. And, one of every ten non-regular workers is not protected by the statutory minimum wage. It should be noted that even this number, based on the Economically Active Population Survey, is somehow underestimated, since the EPS data is indicative of the gross wage amount, differently from the statutory minimum wage to be estimated by the basic wage.

Table 6: Workers of Low Wage Earnings by Employment Status, in Thousands

	Low Wage Workers, 2001		Low Wage Workers, 2002		Below Minimum Wage, 2001		Below Minimum Wage, 2002	
	Total	Share	Total	Share	Total	Share	Total	Share
Regular Worker	1,387	23.7 %	1,217	20.6 %	22	0.4 %	38	0.6 %
Non-regular Worker	5,504	74.7 %	5,408	70.0 %	616	8.0 %	736	9.5 %

Source: The 2001-2002 Economically Active Population Survey – Additional Survey.

The proliferation of cheaper non-regular labor is accompanied by the deepening inequality of wage earnings among the workforce. As demonstrated in figure 5, Gini coefficients and the ratio of wage earnings dispersion[3], both of which are indicative of wage inequity, abruptly soared in 1998 to the highest level during the past 15 years, and have since remained at that level. Interestingly, the trend of wage earnings inequity appears to match that of non-regular employment to a large extent. Therefore, the segmented quality of working life between the regular and non-regular workforce has resulted in the increase of income inequity and social disintegration in the country.

Moreover, the vast majority of non-regular workers are excluded from social welfare and statutory working conditions. As shown in table 7, although the entire wage labor force is entitled to social welfare, less than a quarter of non-regular workers have access to such public benefit programs as national pension (21.6 %), medical insurance (24.9 %), and employment insurance (23.2 %). This is quite contrasting to the regular worker group, whose coverage of social welfare plans ranges from 79.1 % to 94.6 %. The case of statutory working conditions, like severance pay (a legal payment given to employees, when quitting after one year service) and extra work allowances (a legal premium payment for overtime (50 %) and holiday (100 %) work), is even worse.

Figure 5: Trends of Earnings Inequity , 1989-2002

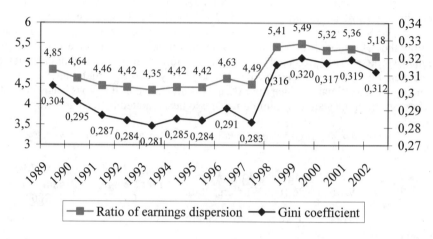

Source: KLI (2003).

Severance pay and extra work allowances are respectively provided to 13.9 % and 10.1 % of the non-regular workforce, whereas these legal payments are given to 93.2 % and 76.8 % of regular workers. Bonuses, which are not legal payments are paid to only 14.0 % of non-regular employees, although, in many instances, they work together with regular workers and contribute to their affiliated firms' business performance. Besides, according to Lee and his colleagues (2002), while a very luxurious list of corporate-level infringe benefit plans are offered to regular workers, non-regular workers have very limited access to or are totally excluded from the use of the corporate welfare programs. As such, non-regular workers have suffered from social exclusion of statutory and corporate welfare as well as wage inequity.

Table 7: Beneficiary Rate of Social Welfare & Statutory Working Condition in 2002, in %.

	National Pension	Medical Insurance	Employment Insurance	Severance Pay	Extra Work Allowances	Bonuses
Regular Worker	92.3	94.6	79.1	93.2	76.8	92.5
Non-Regular Worker	21.6	24.9	23.2	13.9	10.1	14.0

Source: The 2002 Economically Active Population Survey – Additional Survey.

FACTORS INFLUENCING THE POLARIZED
QUALITY OF WORKING LIFE

The segmentized quality of working life can be explored with the following two questions: why the disadvantaged worker group of non-regular employment has grown, and why those non-regular workers suffer from the discriminatory employment condition. As for the first question, we can point out three actor-oriented factors influencing the sharp increase of non-regular labor. The first and most important factor is employers' market-driven HRM strategy on the labor demand side. During the 1990s, employers have pursued the externalization of employment relations, including downsizing, outsourcing, spin-offs, and the utilization of non-regular labor. In particular, employers carried out massive downsizing of regular employees during the economic crisis, and re-filled those regular jobs with non-regular workers during the period of economic recovery (since 2000). The growing use of 'external' non-regular labor by firms has been a main part of their strategic effort to gain the reduction of labor cost and numerical labor flexibility, tailored to market demand. According to the KLI workplace panel survey, which was conducted in 2002, 32.1 % of surveyed establishments (N=832) use non-regular employment to save labor cost, while 30.3 % employ disposable labor to be easily adjustable to changing business situations (Ahn et al., 2003).[4] An additional hidden reason for the use of non-regular labor may be employers' intention to avoid unionization, in that those marginal workers can be hardly integrated into the current enterprise-based union structure.

The second factor is the government's policy to promote labor market flexibility. Since the early 1990s and particularly during the economic crisis, the government stressed the flexibilization of labor markets as a key means to enhance the competitiveness of the national economy in the context of globalization and a liberalized domestic market, and attempted to reform labor laws for permitting employers' massive lay-offs and their use of dispatched labor in the face of labor unions' strong opposition. (Lee, 2003a) The government's neo-liberalistic policy for labor market flexibilization has provided a favorable condition which indirectly promotes employers' increasing utilization of non-regular labor. Moreover, the government has expanded its use of non-regular labor, since it was obliged to employ a number of those cheaper workers due to budget constraints, following massive downsizing of the public sector during the economic crisis. In fact, the increasing use of non-regular labor in the public sector (i.e. schools, hospitals, post office, and many public enterprises) offers a good reference to justify the employment practices of those flexible workers in the private sector.

The third and last factor is the weakening of union power regulating employers' use of non-regular labor. This is represented by a sharp decline of union density. The union density peaked at 18.6 % in 1989, following the political democratization in the mid of 1987, and has since fallen down to the level of 11 % in 1997 and thereafter. Although the union movement in Korea has been very militant, the unions have not been able to effectively constrain employers from using non-regular labor and pressure the government to protect those powerless workers, due to their shrunken organizational base. The results of Kim's (2003) empirical analysis confirm that the three actor-related factors have had significant influence on the increase of non-regular labor.[5] He adds that other factors, such as labor supply, industrial changes, economic environments, are not significantly related to the growth of atypical employment in Korea.

Now, we turn to the second question of why the discriminatory treatment of non-regular labor has been persistent (or increasing) over the recent years, by shedding light on institutional aspects. Above all, the existing labor laws were enacted to protect permanent and full-time employment (regular workers) over 50 years ago, and, therefore, they do not reflect the recent changes of labor markets, particularly the proliferation of non-regular labor. As a result, the labor laws are very limited in protecting the "flexible" workforce. For instance, the Labor Standards Act, which regulates the minimum working conditions, stipulates the prohibition of discriminatory treatment by gender, religion, and nationality, yet does not deal with the discrimination against non-regular labor. Similarly, this labor law does not regulate employers' use of non-regular labor (i.e. legal qualifications for the use of non regular labor, the renewal of non-regular employment contract, and the transferability of non-regular employees into regular status) in a proper way, nor does it provide any statutory vehicle to represent those peripheral workers' interests. Another example is the Minimum Wage Act, which excludes such non-regular employment patterns as home workers and discretely-employed workers from its protection. The limited statutory protection of non-regular labor enables employers to use these atypical workers at a cheaper price and impose inferior working conditions on them. To make matters worse, employers in Korea often ignore and violate even the existing legal clauses to protect non-regular workers by taking advantage of their vulnerable status, as illustrated by Lee (2003b). For instance, employers do not provide the statutory welfare and working conditions, including extra work allowances, severance pay, and paid vacations, to non-regular workers, in order to save labor cost in an illegal way. Although labor unions and civil activists have demanded the reform of labor laws to protect non-regular workers, the government has not yet taken any active policy move in the face of employers' strong opposition. As such, the lack of proper statutory protection and legal enforcement places non-regular workers into a very disadvantaged position.

The other factor to influence the discrimination against non-regular workers is the existing enterprise-based union structure in Korea. Given the decentralized organizational and bargaining structure, labor unions are basically obliged to focus on the protection of affiliated regular workers, particularly at large firms. In 2001, when the nation-wide union density was 11.6 %, labor unions organized only 1.2 % of the contingent workforce, while representing respectively 41.5 % and 26.5 % of the regular workforce, employed by large firms with the employment size of 500-999 and 1000+, according to the 2001 KLI labor panel survey (Kim 2002). Although labor unions, which are concerned with the rapid growth of non-regular labor, have launched various campaigns to demand labor reforms for protecting non-regular workers and organize those marginal workers, their efforts have taken little effect, due to not only the government's inactive stance and employers' persistent opposition, but also their own decentralized structure. As a consequence, the current union structure leads, to a large extent, to the segmentation of working life between organized regular and unorganized non-regular workers, by focusing on the enhancement of the former group's employment conditions and excluding the interest representation of the latter group.[6]

CONCLUSION: POLICY IMPLICATIONS

Now, Korea is confronted with a grave social problem of polarized working life, mainly derived from the proliferation of the non-regular workforce and their discriminating employment conditions. The fact that non-regular workers have experienced various forms of social exclusion to differentiate their working life from regular workers' creates social disintegration among working people and, as a result, draws a focal attention from labor unions (and the government). In order to tackle this problem, we can make several policy suggestions, based on the above analysis of factors influencing the polarized QWL between regular and non-regular workers. First, the government, which pursued the neo-liberalistic restructuring of labor markets over the past decade, needs to re-align its labor policy to harmonize economic efficiency and social equity from the long-term perspective, in that the market-driven policy is likely to produce the polarization of QWL in the working population and the resulting social division and tensions. In other words, the government is required to constrain employers' excessive use of non-regular labor, damaging social integration to a large extent.

Secondly and as noted above, the reform of labor laws to protect non-regular labor is a matter of utmost urgency. In fact, a tripartite dialogue on the labor law reform to tackle the issue of non-regular labor has been underway for the past two years, yet there has been little progress owing to employers' strong concern that the protection of non-regular workers would severely weaken business competitiveness under the over-protection of regular employees. Thus, when attempting to reform the existing labor laws, we have to balance the interest of organized labor and employers. On the one hand, the revised labor law should include protective provisions to reduce the gap of employment conditions between regular and non-regular workers. On the other hand, the functional flexibility of the regular workforce needs to be promoted in order to ease employers' burden of rigid and expensive utilization of internalized labor, which is likely to result in their expanded use of non-regular employment. Furthermore, legal regulation should be strictly enforced employers' infringement of non-regular workers' labor rights, and a policy plan to enable labor unions and NGOs to supervise employers' illegal use of non-regular labor can be implemented in the light of the shortage of governmental resources.

Lastly, labor unions are required to transform their bargaining and organizational structure from the current enterprise-based model to a more centralized one in order to represent the interests of non-regular labor effectively.. This is affirmed by research findings in Lee & Kim (2003) and Kim (2003), arguing that the centralized bargaining structure is likely to limit employers' use of non-regular labor. In this context, the government needs to be supportive of labor unions' strategic move towards centralized bargaining as an indirect means to regulate employers' excessive reliance on non-regular labor.

NOTES

1   The total number of non-regular workers in the EPS-additional survey, which began being conducted in 2000, is higher than the figure in the EPS, in that the former includes on-call, dispatched, contract, home workers and independent contractors, in addition to the latter's temporary and part-time employees.

2   In a similar vein Ahn et al. (2002) indicate that the segmentation of labor markets between the two worker groups is a structurized problem, rather than a temporal phenomenon.

3   The ratio of earnings dispersion is calculated by the sum of top 20 % workers' wage earnings divided by that of bottom 20 % workers' wage earnings.

4   This survey result adds that 18.5 % and 13.9 % of the respondent establishments use non-regular labor respectively for unskilled simple jobs and short-term job assignments.

5   Kim (2003) shows in his time-series analysis that union density has a significantly negative impact on the use of non-regular labor. In addition, he also addresses that unemployment rate influence the use of non-regular labor in the negative direction.

6   In a similar vein, OECD (1997) shows that the centralization of collective bargaining (and union density) has a significantly negative effect on earnings inequality.

REFERENCES

Ahn, J., Y. Noh, W. Park, C. Park, J. Lee & J. Hur (2001): Situation of Non-regular Labor and Policy Issues (I), Seoul: Korea Labor Institute (in Korean).

Ahn, J., J. Cho & J. Nam (2002): Situation of Non-regular Labor and Policy Issues (II): Seoul: Korea Labor Institute (in Korean).

Ahn, J., D. Kim & S. Lee (2003): Situation of Non-regular Labor and Policy Issues (III), Seoul: Korea Labor Institute (in Korean).

Doeringer, P. & M. Piore (1971): Internal Labor Markets and Manpower Analysis, Lexington: D.C. Heath.

KLI (2003): 2003 KLI Labor Statistics, Seoul: Korea Labor Institute (in Korean).

Kim, Y. (2003): The Forces Propelling the Growth of the Nonstandard Workforce in the Korean Labor Market: Cross-section and Time-series Analyses, Ph.D. Dissertation of Economics Dept., Korea University (in Korean).

Kim, Y. (2002): Determinants of Union Affiliation. Korean Journal of Labor Economics 25 (1), 23-45 (in Korean).

Kim, Y. (1999): Policy Issues for the Protection and Organizing of Part-time Workers, Seoul: Korea Labor and Society Institute (in Korean).

Korea Contingent Workers Center (2002): Statistics of Korean Non-regular Workers, Seoul: KCWC (in Korean).

Korea Metal Workers Federation (2003): A Study on the Situation of Contract Workers in the Metal Industry, Seoul: Korea Contingent Workers Center (in Korean).

Kwon, H. (1996): Situation of Non-regular Workers and Labor Movement, Seoul: FKTU Research Center (in Korean).

Lee, B. (2003a): Globalization and Industrial Relations in Korea. Korea Journal 43 (1), 261-88.

Lee, B. (2003b): Case Study on the Infringement of Non-regular Workers' Labor Rights. FKTU Research Center (ed.): Problems of Non-regular Labor and Unions, 21-70 (in Korean).

Lee, B. & S. Frenkel (forthcoming): Divided Workers: Social Relations between Contract and Regular Workers in a Korean Auto Company. Work, Employment and Society.

Lee, B. & D. Kim (2003): Union Effect on the Externalization of Employment Relations. Paper presented to the 11th annual conference of the IERA, held in Greenwich University, London, July, 8-11.

Lee, B., Y. Kim, M. Ryu & S. In (2002): A Study on Labor Policy to Promote Corporate Infringe Benefits. Working Paper presented the Ministry of Labor (in Korean).

Nam, J. & T. Kim (2000): Non-regular Labor, Bridge or Trap? Korean Journal of Labor Economic 23 (2), 85-105 (in Korean).

OECD (1997,1998): OECD Employment Outlook, Paris: OECD.

Peetz, D. & N. Ollett (forthcoming): Union Growth and Reversal in Newly Industrialized Countries: The Case of South Korea and Peripheral Workers. G. Wood & M. Harcourt (eds.): Trade Unions and the Crisis of Democracy: Strategies and Perspectives, Manchester: University Press.

Ryu, K. (2001): Situation of Nonstandard Workers: Analysis of Workforce Survey. Paper presented to the 2001 KLEA conference (in Korean).

Tsui, A., H. Pearce, L. Porter & J. Hite (1995): Choice of Employee-Organization Relationship: Influence of External and Internal Organizational Factors. Research in Personnel and Human Resources Management 13, 117-51.

Way, P. (1992): Staffing Strategies: Organizational Differences in the Use of Temporary Employment. Industrial Relations Research Association 44th Annual Proceedings, 332-39.

13. DOES HAPPINESS PAY?

An Exploration Based on Panel Data from Russia

Carol Graham, Andrew Eggers, and Sandip Sukhtankar
The Brookings Institution, Washington DC, USA

ABSTRACT

This paper uses panel data from Russia to identify "residual" happiness levels that are not explained by the usual demographic and socioeconomic determinants of happiness. We then test whether our residual happiness variable has causal properties in addition to those of the observed demographic and socioeconomic variables on future income. We find that both residual happiness and positive expectations for the future in the initial period are positively correlated with higher income in future periods. People with negative perceptions of their own progress and with higher fear of unemployment increase their incomes less, on average. Psychologists attribute stability in happiness levels over time – analogous to the "residual" happiness levels that we identify – to positive cognitive bias, such as self-esteem, control, and optimism. The same factors may enhance individuals' performance in the labor market.

INTRODUCTION[1]

The study of happiness, or subjective well-being, and its implications for economic behavior is a fairly new area for economists, although psychologists have been studying it for years. The findings of this research highlight the non-income determinants of economic behavior. For example, cross-country studies of happiness consistently demonstrate that after certain minimum levels of per capita income, average happiness levels do not increase as countries grow wealthier.[2] Within societies, most studies find that wealthier individuals are on average happier than poor ones, but after a minimum level of income, more money does not make people much happier.[3] Because income plays such an important role in standard definitions and measures of well being, these findings have theoretical, empirical, and policy implications.

Some of the earliest economists – such as Jeremy Bentham – were concerned with the pursuit of individual happiness. As the field became more rigorous and quantitative, however, much narrower definitions of individual welfare, or utility, became the norm, even though economics was still concerned with public welfare in the broader sense. In addition, economists have traditionally shied away from the use of survey data because of justifiable concerns that answers to surveys of individual preferences – and reported well being – are subject to bias from factors such as respondents' mood at the time of the survey and minor changes in the phrasing of

179

Wolfgang Glatzer, Susanne von Below, Matthias Stoffregen (eds.), Challenges for Quality of Life in the Contemporary World, 179-204.

survey questions, which can produce large skews in results.[4] Thus traditional economic analysis focuses on actual behavior, such as revealed preferences in consumption, savings, and labor market participation, under the assumption that individuals rationally process all the information at their disposal to maximize their utility.[5] More recently, behavioral economics has begun to have influence at the margin, as an increasing number of economists supplement the methods and research questions more common to economists with those more common to psychologists.[6]

In this same vein, the research on subjective well being relies heavily but not exclusively on surveys, and combines methods from both professions. Typically, the questions are very simple ones about how happy or satisfied respondents are with their lives, with responses ranging from not very or not at all to very or fully satisfied.[7] While there are justified criticisms of how accurate such questions are in assessing life satisfaction at the individual level, there is remarkable consistency in the patterns generated by the answers to these questions aggregated across populations and over time. In addition, a number of psychologists have been able to "validate" the use of these questions through other measures, for example by showing that individuals who answer happiness questions positively also demonstrate other measures of positive affect, such as smiling more frequently.[8]

Some of the most recent work on subjective well being has resulted in a new collaboration between economists and psychologists, and contributes to our understanding of seemingly non-rational economic behavior. Examples of such behavior are the remarkable contrast between predicted and experienced utility, such as individuals valuing economic losses disproportionately more than gains; conspicuous consumption to demonstrate wealth at the margin; and/or the contrast between observed time preferences and the standard economic analyses of discounting.[9] Better understanding of such behavior helps explain unusual patterns in consumption and savings; in voting; in the structure of redistributive policies; in attitudes about insecurity and social insurance; and in support for market policies and democracy, among others.

Another of the many important insights from the happiness research, which has been written about extensively in the sociological and economics literature, is the important role of adaptation and rising expectations. As individuals – and those in their reference group – earn more income, their expectations also rise or adapt.[10] Thus higher levels of income are needed to achieve the same levels of well being.[11] Adaptations can also adjust downwards. A good example is in the case of health and aging. Several studies show that individuals adapt to changes in health status – such as the onset of a serious disease – by changing their reference point for "good" health, and, after a temporary drop, continue to evaluate their well being at the same or similar levels as before.[12]

An important unanswered question in much of this research is the direction of causality. In other words, it is difficult to establish cause and effect with many of the variables that are at play, and in many cases they may interact. For example, are married people happier, or are happier people more likely to get married? Are wealthier people happier, or are happier people more likely to be successful and earn more income over time? Similar questions can be posed in a number of areas, including the positive relationship between health and happiness, between happiness and support for market policies and democracy, and happiness and tolerance for inequality. A better understanding of the direction of causality question will help determine the extent to which the findings from this research should be incorporated into policy analysis.

One of the primary difficulties in establishing this direction of causality is the lack of adequate data. Most of the happiness research is based on cross-section data, while to answer these questions, we need panel data – i.e. surveys that follow the same people over time. Such data are particularly rare for developing countries. A few isolated studies by psychologists in the United States and Australia shed some light, and establish that happier people earn more income in later periods than do their less happy cohorts.[13] Yet for the most part, research on subjective well being has not addressed these questions.

Table 1: Variable Means, Standard Deviations (in Parentheses) and Definitions

Variable	1995	2000
Happiness: "To what extent are you satisfied with your life in general at the present time?" (1=not at all; 5=fully)	2.209 (1.06)	2.355
Age	40.673 (19.17)	45.677 (19.17)
Age, squared	2104.208 (1674.04)	2453.682 (1822.74)
Log equivalence income (real household income in 1992 rubles/square root of the number of people in household)	7,873 (.86)	7,826 (.81)
Education level (school grade level completed, 0-12)	8.684 (2.17)	8.741 (2.15)
Gender (1=male)	0.422 (.49)	0.422 (.49)
Minority (1=minority, i.e. non-Russian)	0.164 (.37)	0.164 (.37)
Married (1=married)	0.559 (.49)	0.542 (.50)
Student (1=student)[14]	0.169 (.37)	0.116 (.32)
Retired (1=retired)	0.236 (.42)	0.305 (.46)
Housewife (1=housewife)	0.043 (.20)	0.033 (.18)
Unemployed (1=unemployed)	0.064 (.24)	0.085 (.28)
Self-employed (1=self-employed)	0.011 (.11)	0.012 (.11)
Health index (Index for 3 equally weighted questions about recent health problems, missed work or study, and hospital stays. 1=yes for all three)	0.838 (.22)	0.820 (.22)
Observations	5,269	5,269

Source: RLMS Round 6 and 9; authors' calculations (Graham and Pettinato, 2002). In a paired t-test, the difference between the 1995 and 2000 means was significant for all variables except male and minority (unchanging), self-employment, education level, and amount of drinking.

In this paper, we take advantage of a large panel for Russia, the Russia Longitudinal Monitoring Survey (RLMS), which covers an average of almost 13,000 Russians per year from 1992 to 2001, and from which we create a panel data set containing data in 1995 and 2000[15] (summary statistics are in table 1). Among many other questions, there is a standard happiness question in the RLMS, which asks "to what extent are you satisfied with your life at the present time", with possible answers being "not at all satisfied", "less than satisfied", "both yes and no", "rather satisfied", and "fully satisfied".[16]

A very clear drawback of this dataset is that it covers a time period of tremendous economic and structural change, with far reaching changes for many people's livelihood and economic well being, which limits the extent to which we can draw broader generalizations. On the other hand, data containing observations on both happiness and income for the same respondents at more than one point in time is extremely rare. In addition, the instability in economic conditions provides us with a better than average reference point for stability in subjective well being despite extensive contextual change.

We depart in this study from earlier analysis by Graham and Pettinato which compares happiness in Latin America and Russia. In contrast, we analyze happiness data on the same individuals for two points in time and examine a number of questions in which the direction of causality is not clear from cross section data alone.[17] Our central goal is to test whether people who reported higher happiness in 1995 than would be expected based on their socioeconomic and demographic characteristics fared differently in 2000 than others. Presumably, these differences are due to psychological or other non-economic or demographic factors. The purpose of this exercise is to determine whether these differences, appearing in people's reported happiness levels in the first period, have effects on outcomes such as income, marriage status, and employment in the second.

Psychologists find that there is a remarkable degree of consistency in people's level of well-being over time. They attribute this stability in happiness levels to homeostasis, in which happiness levels are not only under the influence of experience, but also controlled by positive cognitive bias, such as self-esteem, control, and optimism.[18] We use our panel data to create a "residual" or unexplained happiness variable, which is an attempt to capture or proxy this psychological element of happiness. We can then test whether it has causal properties in addition to the observed demographic and socioeconomic variables on future income. Of course, some of what is captured by our residual term could well be other unobservable socioeconomic, demographic, or stochastic characteristics that are unrelated to cognitive bias. It remains to be seen to what extent the causal properties of unexplained happiness depend on cognitive bias as opposed to other unobserved factors.

Our analysis is a first attempt to examine these questions in detail with this kind of data, and has an exploratory element. We first use the standard variables to explain as much as we can about happiness levels at a given point in time. We take advantage of having two observations on the same people to see if there are any changes in the relative weights of these variables over time. We then correct for the effects of individual traits or characteristics that could be driving the results (for example, happier people may be more likely to get married rather than marriage enhancing happiness) by using panel fixed effects to see if changes in individual status make a difference to the results. We then turn to the effects of unexplained or residual happiness on our key variables, such as income, health, and marital status. Finally, we examines the effects of changes in these variables that are not explained by our residual happiness variable – such as quitting smoking and getting divorced – on happiness.

RUSSIA IN THE 1990S

Any attempts to generalize from analysis based on Russia in the 1990s must take into account the far reaching nature of the changes in that country's economy and polity over the course of the decade. During that period, Russia underwent a transition from a centrally planned economy and communist government to a free market, presidential-parliamentary democracy.[19] At the same time, much of its large federation – which was part and parcel of its status as a superpower – was parceled into a number of newly independent states.

The transition had high social costs, with some of the worst losers being pensioners and others on fixed incomes. Poverty and inequality increased markedly. Depending on the data sources, the prevalence of poverty in Russia was between 22 and 33 % in 2001, while the Gini coefficient increased from .29 to .40 between 1992 and 1998, with some estimates as high as .48, a level which is comparable to some of the most unequal countries in Latin America.[20] An additional shock, particularly to those on fixed incomes, came from a financial crisis and sharp devaluation of the ruble in August 1998. The devaluation, in which the ruble fell to 25 % of its previous rate against the US dollar, was accompanied by fiscal austerity.[21]

Since the crisis and devaluation, Russia's economy has experienced positive growth rates for several years in a row. Yet a large part of Russia's economy remains "virtual" – outside the monetary, market economy. Numerous city-sized factories throughout Russia conduct a large share of their transactions on a non-monetary basis. Their workers in turn receive their wages and benefits in kind. To survive, Russians engage in extensive self-subsistence activity, beginning with food production. Russians – and this includes not only rural residents but also middle-class urban professionals such as scientists, doctors, and military officers – produce an astounding 50 % of the nation's meat supply and 80 % of all vegetables and fruits on their family garden plots.[22] Russia's "virtual" economy acts as a de facto safety net, limiting the impact of devaluation-induced price changes on the average consumer at the time of devaluation, for example.

There is considerable debate over the extent to which Russia's transition to the market has been a success or a failure, and whether the pace and sequencing of reform was appropriate. This is a debate that is well beyond the scope of this paper.[23] Yet it is important to recognize that our panel data cover a period of extensive economic and political change, and the effects of those changes have not been even across individuals and across economic sectors. This, in turn, could affect the relationship between income and well being.

There are some peculiarities in the data that seem to reflect the reality of the Russian situation – both in terms of a large black market and a large barter or virtual economy.[24] For example, we had 54 observations from respondents that reported zero household income. Yet the results of our econometric analysis including these respondents produced results which were quite counter-intuitive, such as a consistently positive and significant sign on the zero income dummies in relation to both future happiness and future income. About half of the zero income respondents reported that they were employed. It is quite plausible that they are earning substantial income on the black market, which they are reluctant to report, and/or have earnings in kind. These earnings still have effects on their well being, but do not show up as reported income.[25]

Another caveat is that all panel data suffer from attrition bias. Those on the extreme tails of the distribution are the most likely to drop out of the panel, as the wealthiest may move to better neighborhoods and the poorest who "don't make it" may move in with other family members or opt for other kinds of coping strategies. Thus panels can be biased in their representation of all income groups. In the case of Russia, with extreme levels of economic and political turmoil, it is plausible that this attrition occurs more than it would under more stable circumstances. Our analysis of the data, however, finds no difference between the characteristics of those respondents in the panel and the entire group of respondents in the original 1995 survey, at least as measured by age, education, income, gender, marital status, and happiness.[26]

A second problem, measurement error, involves possible error stemming from the difficulty of accurately measuring the incomes of those individuals who work in the informal economy or in the agricultural sector. As noted above, this informal sector is disproportionately large in Russia.[27]

There are also concerns that because of Russia's political legacy, respondents might view survey questions with suspicion and answer them less honestly then they would in other contexts. Thus the unusually low levels of happiness in Russia could be due to such suspicions, or to unfavorable comparisons with the West, and/or to a culture of negativism. However, research by Veenhoven (2001) finds that the unusually low levels of happiness in Russia have more to do with the troublesome transitions than with Russian national character or other biases in responses. Finally, despite these many caveats, the relatively large sample size and the intuitive nature of many of our results make us cautiously optimistic about their broader applicability.

MEASURABLE AND UNEXPLAINED DETERMINANTS OF HAPPINESS

A fairly wide body of literature has found consistent links between a number of demographic and socioeconomic variables and reported happiness. These include income, health, marital status, gender, race, and life cycle effects. In this section, our objective is to explain happiness in Russia as accurately as possible based on these standard measures. Our first step was to examine the effects of the usual socioeconomic and demographic determinants of happiness, such as age, education, income, gender, and marriage, on happiness levels in Russia.

These variables have fairly consistent effects on happiness across societies and across time – in both the developed and developing economies for which there is data.[28] Yet there are a number of plausible reasons why these effects might not hold in Russia. These include the dramatic nature of economic and political change in Russia during the period under study, as well as cultural differences in answering this kind of survey question.[29]

We ran standard happiness regressions for both 1995 and 2000, and then conducted a T-test for equivalence to see if there was any significant difference in the results between the two years. As in many other countries, there is a quadratic relationship between age and happiness, a U-shaped curve with the lowest point on the curve being 47 years of age (this is slightly older than the turning point for most OECD countries and the United States, which is typically in the early forties). Men were happier than women in Russia, both in 1995 and in 2000 (table 2). Higher levels of education are correlated with higher levels of happiness in Russia, as they are in most countries.[30] Retirees are less happy than others, which reflects the oft-described plight of pensioners in Russia.

Table 2: The Correlates of Happiness, 1995 and 2000

Independent Variables	1995 coef	z	2000 coef	z	T-stat for Equivalence
Age	-0.0742	-6.27	-0.0668	-7.42	0.498
Age squared	-0.0008	6.35	0.0007	7.15	-0.498
Male	0.1419	2.41	0.1521	2.80	0.128
Married	0.1490	2.15	0.0875	1.40	-0.659
Log equivalent income	0.4777	13.97	0.3892	11.48	-1.839
Education level	0.0305	1.87	0.0150	0.96	-0.688
Minority	0.3835	5.21	0.1721	2.46	-2.082
Student	0.4561	2.91	0.1991	1.59	-1.281
Retired	-0.3029	-3.05	-0.3783	-3.97	-0.548
Housewife	0.1814	1.34	0.0490	0.33	-0.661
Unemployed	-0.2434	-2.19	-0.6568	-6.51	-2.756
Self-employed	0.7676	3.00	0.5375	2.23	-0.654
Health index	0.2744	2.22	0.4462	3.82	1.010
Observations	4,524		5,134		
Pseudo R^2	0.0330		0.0331		

Dependent Variable: Happiness (Ordered Logit Regression)

Source: RLMS Round 6 and 9 data; authors' calculations (cf. Graham and Pettinato, 2002).

Minorities in Russia are, on average, happier than other respondents (16 % are in the former group, 84 % identify as Russian). This is distinct from trends in many other countries, where minorities tend to be less happy than other groups. In the U.S., blacks are, on average, less happy than other groups, and in Latin America, those who identify first as a minority rather than as the nationality of their country are less happy than other groups.[31] There are many plausible reasons for this, including the dramatic changes in Russia's status as a superpower and its effects on national morale, as well as longer term cultural traits. Similarly, in a related but separate question, those that identify themselves as Muslim – 8 % of the sample – were, on average, happier than others in 2000, although the coefficient was just short of significant at the 5 % level. More generally, having faith or a religious affiliation is positively associated with happiness in most countries.[32]

Happiness research finds general patterns in the relationship between socioeconomic variables and happiness across countries and across time, but with subtle variations. Given the extent of economic change and mobility in Russia during the period under study, we expected there to be more than the usual variation across time. The 1990's crisis hit retirees, the unemployed, and lenders in particular very hard. Rather remarkably, there was very little change in the relationship among the standard variables and happiness during this time period. When we tested the difference between the two years' results, however, the only two coefficients in our basic happiness model that experienced a significant change in value were being a minority and being unemployed; even then there was not a change in direction in the sign of either coefficient (table 2 – column 3).

In 2000, while minorities were still, on average, happier than other respondents, they were far less happy than they were in 1995. The war in Chechnya, which started at about the time the first survey was conducted, has changed the image of Muslims and minorities in general in Russia, and a number of surveys find that the majority of Russians support the efforts of their military against a mainly Islamic population.[33] Thus respondents who are Muslim or minorities have, on average, higher happiness levels than Russians, but have experienced a transitory (hopefully) decline in happiness due to the change in the status of Muslims related to the war.

The second coefficient that experienced a change in value was being unemployed. While unemployed people were less happy on average than others in both years, the negative effects of being unemployed were significantly greater in 2000 than they were in 1995 (table 2, column 3). This probably reflects the effects of the financial crisis and the devaluation on the fixed and/or very meager incomes of the unemployed.

If our simple cross-sectional model completely captured the determinants of happiness, then conducting a panel fixed effects regression – essentially, measuring the effect of *changes* in the determinants on *changes* in happiness – would produce identical coefficient results. However, we have good reason to believe that the fixed effects regression will yield different and better estimates.

Most importantly, panel fixed effects analysis corrects some of the bias associated with unobserved characteristics of the survey respondents in cross-sectional analysis. Although we observe a great many characteristics of each respondent, these factors leave much of the variation in happiness unexplained (the R-squared in our happiness models is in the neighborhood of .03, suggesting that about 97 % of the variation in happiness responses is due to factors we do not observe). For example, a person's disposition or personality is assuredly one of the determinants of his/her level of reported happiness, so we would expect a person with a generally sunnier disposition to report a higher level of happiness than a person who is identical in every other respect but has a gloomier outlook. Disposition, of course, is not captured in survey data.

Table 3: First Difference Regression

Dependent Variable: Change in Happiness, 1995-2000 (ordered logit regression)			
		coef	z
Static Variables	Age	-0.0400	-1.70
	Age^2	0.0004	1.54
	Male	0.0390	0.35
	Minority	-0.0632	-0.51
Changes in Continuous Variables	Change in log Equivalence Income	0.1875	4.21
	Change in Education Level	0.0312	0.62
	Change in Health Index	0.0757	0.47
Changes in Status Variables			
Marriage (Omitted Group: Remained Single)	Got Married	-0.03802	-1.20
	Got Divorced	-0.5681	-3.20
	Stayed Married	-0.1905	-1.57
Employment (Omitted Group: Remained Un-employed)	Got Employed	0.0608	0.19
	Got Unemployed	-0.2054	-0.65
	Stayed Employed	0.3554	1.35
Smoking (Omitted Group: Remained a Non-smoker)	Quit Smoking	0.1451	0.58
	Started Smoking	0.2488	1.19
	Kept Smoking	-0.0356	-0.31
Schooling (Omitted Group: Remained a Non-student)	Entered School	*	*
	Left School	-0.8415	-2.38
	Stayed in School	-0.7139	-1.29
Retirement (Omitted Group: Remained a Non-retired)	Became Retired	-0.0699	-0.38
	Came out of Retirement	0.2638	0.55
	Stayed Retired	-0.0731	-0.35
	Observations	1,673	
	Pseudo R^2	0.0089	

Source: Own calculations. *=dropped because of multicollinearity.

These unobserved determinants of happiness will bias our coefficient estimates in cross-sectional analysis if they are correlated with the observed determinants. For example, if a person's disposition affects both his income and his happiness results in the same way, then our estimate of the effect of income on happiness will be biased upwards, since disposition is unobserved. Using panel data allows us to filter out the set of unobserved determinants of happiness that are unchanging over time, which should remove this bias and improve upon our coefficient estimates from cross-sectional analysis.

On the other hand, the volatility in late-90s Russia can be seen as a unique opportunity for analysis. Panel studies rely on changes in the observed variables to detect causal effects, so panel studies on populations that change very little tend to be unrevealing. Yet in this instance, most likely due to the extensive economic changes in Russia during the period, the data reveal a high degree of mobility. There was significantly more movement among income quintiles in the second half of the 1990s (1995-2000) in Russia than there was during the entire 1980s in the United States, for example. Happiness levels also fluctuated a great deal during the period, with downward shifts more common than upward ones. While this is certainly an exceptional period in Russia, which suggests that caution is necessary in drawing some conclusions, there are also some very clear analytical advantages to the extent of change in the key variables.

The results are reported in table 3. We find that the only variables that have significant effects on changes in happiness are changes in income, which has positive effects; getting divorced, which has negative effects; and leaving school, which also has negative effects. The effects of income and divorce are both unsurprising, and would probably hold in any context. The effects of leaving school, which may or may not hold in other contexts, are intuitive in the Russian context, where the labor market is very precarious, and highly educated people are often unable to find satisfactory jobs.

Finally, it is quite interesting that while both unemployment and retirement are negatively correlated with happiness in our standard regression, neither retiring nor becoming unemployed had significant effects in the panel regression. This may reflect the rather mixed fate of pensioners and the unemployed in Russia. Recent retirees are probably much better prepared to cope with the current economic environment than are those who retired many years ago on fixed incomes.[34] And many jobs in Russia pay unstable if any wages, while many highly educated workers are often over-qualified for what they are doing, which may mitigate the usual effects of becoming unemployed on happiness.

HOW INCOME AFFECTS HAPPINESS AND VICE VERSA

One issue that we have still not resolved is the direction of causality. In other words, do happier people earn more money, or does earning money make them happier? Are happier people more likely to get married, or does marriage make them happier? We turn to these questions in the following sections. While we attempted to correct for the unobserved or unexplained differences in happiness among our respondents in the above estimations, we will now use this unexplained happiness to see how happiness affects behavior pertaining to earnings activities, health, and social relations.

Table 4: The Effects of Happiness on Income

Dependent Variable: Log Equivalence Income, 2000 (OLS)					
Independent Variables (2000, exc. noted otherw.)	a		b		c
	coef	t	coef	t	coef	t
Age	-0.0133	-3.00	-0.0132	-2.97	-0.0146	-3.25
Age^2	0.0001	3.18	0.0001	3.15	0.0002	3.52
Male	0.0102	0.42	0.0102	0.42	-0.0004	-0.02
Married	0.2053	7.84	0.2054	7.84	0.2050	7.84
Education Level	0.0301	4.51	0.0301	4.51	0.0296	4.44
Minority	0.1213	3.98	0.1227	4.03	0.1216	4.00
Student	-0.0336	-0.34	-0.0301	-0.31	-0.0367	-0.38
Retired	-0.1906	-4.85	-0.1899	-4.83	-0.1659	-4.18
Housewife	0.2488	-3.90	-0.2492	-3.90	-0.2388	-3.73
Unemployed	-0.3450	-8.16	-0.3435	-8.12	-0.3426	-8.07
Self-employed	0.1415	1.46	0.1411	1.46	0.1284	1.33
Health Index	0.0601	1.11	0.0588	1.09	0.0559	1.04
Log Equiv. Income 1995	0.2420	18.11	0.2429	18.12	0.2244	15.69
Log Equivalence Income 1995, poor	*	*	*	*	0.0094	2.60
Log Equivalence Income 1995, rich	*	*	*	*	0.0180	4.36
Unexplained Happiness, 1995	0.02298	2.64	0.0634	2.32	0.0269	2.38
Unexpl. Happiness 1995, 2nd quintile	*	*	-0.0436	-1.14	*	*
Unexpl. Happiness 1995, 3rd quintile	*	*	-0.0361	-0.95	*	*
Unexpl. Happiness 1995, 4th quintile	*	*	-0.0626	-1.71	*	*
Unexpl. Happiness, 1995 5th quintile	*	*	-0.0229	-0.65	*	*
Constant	5.88325	36.35	5.8234	36.19	5.9365	34.62
Number of Observations	4,457		4,457		4,457	
R^2_{adj}	0.1335		0.1333		0.1518	

Source: Own calculations. Regression a: no income quintile distinctions; regression b: testing for a difference in the effect of unexplained happiness on 2000 income, by 1995 quintile; regression c: testing for a difference in the effect of 1995 income on 2000 income, by 1995 income quintile.*=omitted. "Unexplained Happiness" is the residual of basic happiness regression (table 2). "Poor" is defined as bottom 40 % of the income distribution; "rich" is the top 20 % of the income distribution.

Only part of what we are able to observe and measure as "happiness" can be explained by the demographic and socioeconomic variables available to us. There are clearly psychological traits that seem to account for consistency in happiness levels, which persist regardless of variations in demographic and socioeconomic variables. We took advantage of having over-time observations on happiness in the Russia data to attempt to capture this unmeasured or psychological component of happiness. We began with the standard regressions estimating the effect of the standard socioeconomic variables on happiness in Russia. Based on the residual from this regression we created a variable for each respondent's unexplained happiness. We then test whether this element of happiness has any additional causal properties.

What do we know about residual happiness? We know that it is very close in value to happiness itself, since the pseudo R-squared statistics on our standard happiness regressions are quite low (in the neighborhood of .03). In other words, a great deal of happiness is "unexplained happiness". We also know that while unexplained happiness is not correlated (by definition) with the observable socioeconomic variables that we believe affect happiness, it is positively correlated across time for individuals: People with high unexplained happiness in 1995 were likely to have high unexplained happiness in 2000. The simple correlation between the two is .2198. This result is consistent with the view that unexplained happiness includes stable factors which affect happiness and which might include cognitive bias.

The research on subjective well being has focused a great deal on the relationship between income and happiness. Here we focus on the classic direction of causality question. While we know that, on average wealthier people are happier, the reverse may also be true: that happier people, on average, earn more income. We attempt to shed some light on these questions in this section.

We began by exploring whether happier people earn more income than less happy people. In order to do this, we first calculated the residual or unexplained happiness levels for each respondent from our standard happiness regression. We then regressed log equivalence income in 2000 on unexplained happiness in 1995, log equivalence income in 1995, and the usual socio-demographic variables.[35] We find that unexplained or residual happiness has positive and significant effects on second period income (table 4). To date most analysis has focused on the effects on the effects of income on happiness. This result establishes that there is an additional causal effect of happiness on income.

We also separated the unexplained happiness residual variable by income quintiles, to see if the effects of happiness varied according to respondents' position in the income distribution. In comparison to those respondents in the lowest quintile, happiness matters less to those in wealthier quintiles, although the difference is just short of significant. In other words, happiness matters more to future income to those at lower levels of income (table 4).

Having established that happiness has effects on income, we wanted to make sure that the usual effects of income on income still hold. We regressed second period income (log equivalence income) on initial period income and unexplained happiness, using dummies for the poorest (40 %) and wealthiest (20 %) of the respondents in the sample.[36] We found that the effects of unexplained happiness were still positive and significant on second period income. In addition, initial income was more important (significant) to second period income for the poor and the rich compared to the omitted, middle income category, with the effect being strongest for the rich. Initial period income seems to matter most for those at higher levels of income. It also matters more for the poor compared to those in the middle (table 4).

This suggests that initial period income provides advantages in earning even more income in the future for the wealthy, who can use their income as an asset in addition to consumption. Initial period income also matters more for the poor than for those in the middle, suggesting that some minimal amount of income (basic needs?) is necessary for people to increase their income in the future. Meanwhile happiness seems to matter to future incomes across the board, but more for those at lower levels of income. In other words, in the absence of income, a good attitude can make a difference to one's future earnings.

Table 5: The Effects of Income on Happiness

Dependent Variable: Happiness, 2000 (Ordered Logit)				
Independent Variables (2000, except noted otherwise)	ab		b	
	coef	z	coef	z
Age	-0.0781	-7.06	-0.0830	-7.41
Age^2	0.0008	6.97	0.0008	7.20
Male	0.1572	2.65	0.1430	2.39
Married	0.0698	1.08	0.0717	1.11
Education Level	0.0211	1.27	0.0175	1.05
Minority	0.2088	2.80	0.2195	2.94
Student	-0.3473	-1.48	-0.2912	-1.24
Retired	-0.3972	-4.08	-0.3694	-3.75
Housewife	-0.0803	-0.53	-0.0446	-0.29
Unemployed	-0.6742	-6.34	-0.6434	-6.02
Self-employed	0.4541	1.89	0.4439	1.84
Health Index	0.4000	3.05	0.3966	3.02
Log Equivalence Income 2000	0.2438	7.21	0.3176	8.38
Log Equivalence Income 1995	0.3199	8.46	0.2128	5.94
Log Equivalence Income 1995, rich	*	*	0.0163	1.62
Log Equivalence Income 1995, poor	*	*	-0.0146	1.65
Unexplained Happiness, 1995	0.4158	14.50	0.4096	14.24
Number of Observations	4,414		4,414	
Pseudo R^2	0.0474		0.0481	

Source: Own calculations. Regression a: No Income Quintile Distinctions; regression b: testing for a difference in the effect of 1995 income on 2000 income by 1995 quintile.*=omitted. "Unexplained Happiness" is the residual of basic happiness regression (table 2). "Poor" is defined as bottom 40 % of the income distribution; "rich" is the top 20 % of the income distribution.

Given that happiness has positive effects on income in Russia, does income still lead to happiness? We examined the effects of initial period income – controlling for residual happiness in 1995, and the usual socio-economic and demographic variables, on happiness in 2000. We included income in both periods in order to control for the effects of income in 2000 on happiness in 2000. We found that income was indeed positively and significantly correlated with happiness, in addition to the positive and significant effects of unexplained happiness. Thus income clearly does matter to happiness, even for happy people (table 5).

We broke this down by income levels, using our dummies for poor and rich categories as the independent income variables and controlling for initial period happiness. We found again that income matters for happiness, and evidence to suggest that the effect increases as people's income levels increase. The result is significant at the 10 % level (table 5).[37] Thus initial period income seems to matter more for happiness for those at the top of the distribution.

It seems that income needs to be sufficiently above a minimum level to have effects on happiness – a sort of "greed" effect, where additional income increases happiness more for the very wealthy than for others. Some of the findings in the literature on happiness suggest that the relative importance of income as both a motivating force for behavior and in determining well being is greater at very low levels of income, where basic needs are not yet met, while at higher levels of income, other variables have more importance.[38] In contrast, our findings suggest that when people reach a certain high level of income, money begins to matter more to them.

These findings are complementary to our findings for the effects of happiness on income, where residual happiness matters more for second period income for those at the lower end of the income ladder, while income matters most for second period income for those at the higher end of the income ladder. These findings suggest that income matters more for happiness to wealthy people. They may also reflect the peculiarities of the Russian situation, in which large numbers of people operate in the non-monetary economy, and therefore reported income plays much less of a role in evaluating their well being than it might in other contexts.

We also tried to capture the effects of changes in income on happiness to determine if income mobility itself has additional effects. When we use percentage change in equivalence income (1995 to 2000), controlling for initial (1995) levels of income, we find a positive and significant effect on happiness. In other words, when one compares people that start out at the same level of income, a higher percentage change in income has positive effects on happiness (table 6).

In sum, unexplained happiness levels had positive and significant effects on future earnings.[39] This analysis supports the evidence from the psychology literature that happier people earn more income or, more broadly speaking, perform better economically. It is certainly plausible that the same positive cognitive biases that affect normal happiness levels – such as self-esteem, control, and optimism – may also have positive effects on people's performance in the labor market. An additional finding is that the effects of unexplained happiness on future income and on future happiness seem to be more consistent across all income groups than are the effects of income on future income and future happiness. The effects of initial period income seem most important for those at higher levels of income, at least in the Russian context.

Table 6: The Effect of Changes in Income on Happiness

Dependent Variable: Happiness, 2000 (Ordered Logit)		
Independent Variables (2000, except noted otherwise)	coef	z
Age	-0.0781	-7.06
Age^2	0.0008	6.97
Male	0.1572	2.65
Married	0.0698	1.08
Education Level	0.0211	1.27
Minority	0.2088	2.80
Student	-0.3473	-1.48
Retired	-0.3972	-4.08
Housewife	-0.0803	-0.53
Unemployed	-0.6742	-6.34
Self-employed	0.4541	1.89
Health Index	0.4000	3.05
Unexplained Happiness, 1995	0.4158	14.50
Log Equivalence Income, 1995	0.5637	12.83
Change in Log Income, 1995-2000	0.3199	8.46
Number of Observations	4,414	
Pseudo R^2	0.0474	

Source: Own calculations. "Unexplained Happiness" is the residual of basic happiness regression (table 2).

PERCEPTIONS, EXPECTATIONS, HAPPINESS, AND INCOME

Aspirations and expectations also affect both subjective well being and actual economic behavior. A wide body of political economy literature, for example, documents the effects of individuals' perceived prospects of upward mobility on their savings and investment behavior, on their voting behavior and views about redistribution, and on their attitudes about market policies.[40] Psychologists, meanwhile, have explored the links between aspirations and well being fairly extensively, and find that aspirations temper the effects of other variables, such as increases in incomes, on well being.[41]

Graham and Pettinato find that happiness is correlated with more positive perceptions about a whole set of economic and political variables.[42] These include perceived prospects of upward mobility, perceived past progress, satisfaction with current financial situation, satisfaction with democracy, support for free market policies, support for redistribution (it is negatively correlated with happiness in both Latin America and the United States); and position on a notional societal economic ladder – the Economic Ladder Question (ELQ). Controlling for income, they find that happier people tend to place themselves higher on the notional ladder.

While these findings are interesting, two questions remain. The first is the usual problem of direction of causality. It is quite plausible that happier people perceive all sorts of things more positively than less happy people, and therefore they will be more satisfied with whatever policy regime they live in, as well as with the existing distribution of resources, no matter how equal or unequal.

Table 7: Correlation of Perceptions Variables with Happiness

Dependent Variable: Happiness, 2000 (Ordered Logit Regression)				
Independent Variables	a		b	
	coef	z	coef	z
Age	-0.0742	-6.27	-0.0707	-2.90
Age^2	0.0008	6.35	0.0009	3.00
Male	0.1419	2.41	0.2061	2.35
Married	0.1490	2.15	0.0246	0.24
Log Equivalence Income	0.4777	13.97	0.2361	4.08
Education Level	0.0305	1.87	-0.0198	-0.53
Minority	0.3835	5.21	-0.1504	-1.23
Student	0.4561	2.91	-0.7337	-0.97
Retired	-0.3029	-3.05	**	**
Housewife	0.1814	1.34	0.1277	0.36
Unemployed	-0.2434	-2.19	**	**
Self-employed	0.7676	3.00	0.0032	0.01
Health Index	0.2744	2.22	0.0140	0.08
Fear of Unemployment	*	*	-0.1221	-4.05
Economic Ladder Question	*	*	0.4789	15.14
Perceived Past Mobility	*	*	0.2203	5.34
Pro-Democracy	*	*	0.2462	5.43
Observations	4,524		1,969	
Pseudo R^2	0.0330		0.0906	

Source: Own calculations. Regression a: No perceptions variables included; regression b: perceptions variables included.*=omitted. **=dropped due to multicollinearity.

Alternatively, it may well be that many of these variables – such as having high expectations for future progress and/or positive assessments of one's past progress;

living in a democracy and with free markets; and believing that one is relatively high on a notional economic ladder – have positive effects on happiness. Causality may run in both directions, and it is extremely difficult to definitively assess which is more important.

The second unanswered question is the effects of these perceptions on future economic and political behavior. In other words, even if we establish that happiness and positive perceptions about individual economic situations and about desirable policy regimes are positively correlated, does it matter for policy? If we can establish that happier people who have higher expectations for the future also work harder, save more, invest more in their children, and support democracy, then certainly it does matter. Similarly, if we find that frustrated or less happy respondents, who assess their situations and future prospects negatively (even if they are relatively well off), spend conspicuously to keep up with the Jones rather than saving, and vote for anti-market policies, then that is of concern for policy.[43]

While we cannot fully answer these questions, our analysis sheds light on them. As a benchmark, we checked to see if the usual positive correlation between perceptions and happiness levels held for our panel. When we include the perceptions variables in the happiness regression, the explanatory power of the regression rises markedly. And all of our perceptions variables: Perceived past mobility, prospects of upward mobility, ELQ, and pro-democracy (preferring democracy to pre-perestroika times) were positively correlated with happiness. Fear of unemployment was, not surprisingly, negatively correlated with happiness (table 7).[44]

At the same time, many of the variables that were previously significant, such as marriage, minority and student status, and self employment, lose significance. This suggests that the difference in happiness between married and unmarried people, between minorities and non-minorities, and between the self-employed and others, are explained by differences in attitudes among them rather than by some other characteristics. It may be that happier people or those with more positive attitudes are more likely to get married; that minorities are happier because they have different attitudes or beliefs; and that the self-employed are both self-employed and happier because of their attitudes.

What are the implications of perceptions for economic behavior and outcomes? We examined the effects of perceptions scores in 1995 on income in 2000. In separate regressions, we find that having positive prospects of upward mobility and higher responses on the economic ladder question in the initial period has significant and positive effects on income in the second period, controlling for residual happiness. Indeed, we find that including the perceptions variables in the equation renders the effects of residual happiness insignificant (table 8). It is likely that our perceptions variables and our residual happiness variable are capturing similar traits, which is the element of happiness or optimism that is not captured by the standard demographic variables.[45] This supports our earlier findings that this element of happiness or well being has positive effects on peoples' performance in the labor market.

Table 8: Effect of Perceptions Variables on Future Income

Dependent Variable: Log Equivalent Income, 2000 (Ordered Logit Regression)				
Independent Variables (2000, except noted otherwise)	a		b	
	coef	t	coef	t
Age	-0.0133	-3.00	-0.0087	-0.78
Age^2	0.0001	3.18	0.0001	1.24
Male	0.0102	0.42	-0.0081	-0.23
Married	0.2053	7.84	0.2410	6.15
Education Level	0.0301	4.51	0.0325	2.44
Minority	0.1213	3.98	0.0806	1.80
Student	-0.0336	-0.34	0.4268	1.07
Retired	-0.1906	-4.85	-0.2726	-4.60
Housewife	-0.2488	-3.90	-0.1659	-1.60
Unemployed	-0.3450	-8.16	-0.3726	-5.82
Self-employed	0.1415	1.46	0.0936	0.72
Health Index	0.0601	1.11	0.0609	0.84
Log Equivalent Income, 1995	0.2420	18.11	0.2299	11.55
Unexplained Happiness, 1995	0.0298	2.64	-0.0020	-0.11
Fear of Unemployment, 1995	*	*	-0.0143	-1.22
Prospects of Upward Mobility, 1995	*	*	0.0411	2.27
Economic Ladder Question, 1995	*	*	0.0274	2.17
Constant	5.8325	36.35	5.5325	17.49
Observations	4,457		2,296	
R$^2_{adj}$	0.1335		0.1262	

Source: Own calculations. Regression a: no perceptions variables; regression b: perceptions variables included.*=omitted. "Unexplained Happiness" is the residual of basic happiness regression (table 2). Not surprisingly, the effect of unexplained happiness 1995 on income 2000 also disappears when we calculate unexplained happiness using these perceptions variables as explanatory variables (results available from authors on request).

Our findings on fear of unemployment, our negative perceptions variable, also support this intuition. We find a negative (though insignificant) correlation between fear of unemployment in the initial period and income in the second period, and again the residual happiness variable is insignificant. This time the effect of negative perceptions is working in the reverse direction of residual happiness (table 8).[46]

Perceptions – both positive and negative – seem to have effects on future economic behavior and outcomes, although at this point we do not know if the outcomes are due to greater effort or to other variables such as better social skills, given that we control for initial income, education, and age. While wealthier people and those with positive expectations are happier, we also find that being happier and having higher expectations affects future economic performance. The effects of perceptions seem to be stronger than those of our residual happiness variable, although they run in the same direction.

MARRIAGE, EMPLOYMENT, AND HEALTH

One of our most important findings is that unexplained or residual happiness has positive effects on future income. An additional question, which we explore in this section, is if unexplained happiness also has effects on other socioeconomic variables, such as on the probability of getting married or divorced, of being healthy, of being unemployed, and on behaviors such as smoking and drinking.

As expected, married people are, on average, happier than non-married people in Russia in 2000.[47] We created dummy variables for changes in marital status during the 1995-2000 period. 45 % of the sample – 2,935 respondents – stayed married, while others experienced a change in status: 226 respondents or 3 % of the sample got married and 529 respondents, or 8 % of the sample got divorced. Our first set of regressions explored whether residual or unexplained happiness was a predictor of change in marital status. Rather surprisingly, given the strong relationship between marriage and happiness, there was no significant relationship between residual happiness and getting married. In other words, happier people are not more likely than others to get married (table 9).

Divorce is a marital status variable that has notable effects on happiness in most studies: Divorced individuals are, on average, less happy than others. This is also the case in our Russia data set. Becoming divorced had negative and significant effects on both happiness levels in 2000 and changes in happiness levels from 1995 to 2000 in Russia. Yet we found that residual happiness – or more accurately put unhappiness – had no significant effect on the probability of getting divorced (table 9).[48] Thus while unhappiness does not cause divorce, divorce clearly causes unhappiness. In contrast, when we looked at the effects of getting married on happiness and HAPPYCHANGE, the sign on the coefficient was positive, but it was – rather surprisingly – insignificant for both happiness levels and for changes in happiness (table 3).

Not surprisingly given the consistent negative effects of unemployment on happiness across countries and time, those that became unemployed in our sample were significantly less happy than other respondents (table 2). Unexplained happiness, however, had no effects on the probability of being employed. While the sign on the coefficient is negative, it is short of significant (table 9). Interestingly enough, education levels also had no effects on the probability of being employed.[49] This most likely reflects the dramatic nature of the economic transition in Russia, and the fact that many highly educated people are either overqualified for what they are doing and/or are unable to find jobs.[50]

Health is one of the most important variables affecting subjective well being. In our first exploration on the determinants of happiness discussed above, we find that health – as measured by a neutral index based on a number of questions about days missed due to illness, hospitalization, etc. – is positively and significantly correlated

Table 9: The Effects of Happiness an Marriage Status, Employment, and Health

Dep. Variables	Divorce by 2000		Married by 2000		Unemployed by 2000		2000 Health Index	
Condition:	(Given Married 1995)		(Given Unmarried 1995)					
Regression:	Logit		Logit		Logit		OLS	
	a		b		c		d	
Ind. Variables	coef	z	coef	z	coef	z	coef	t
Age	-0.01061	-4.00	0.1023	2.12	0.1609	3.86	-0.0023	-1.89
Age^2	0.0012	4.57	-0.0017	-2.71	-0.0023	-4.62	0.0000	0.97
Male	-0.8974	-7.50	0.1331	0.62	0.8566	6.85	0.0319	4.76
Married	*	*	*	*	-0.3410	-2.55	0.0109	1.51
Educ. Level	-0.0134	-0.43	-0.0171	-0.21	0.0356	0.71	-0.0001	-0.04
Minority	-0.2832	-1.77	-0.1190	-0.44	0.4020	2.94	0.0129	1.54
Student	**	**	-1.1540	-2.08	0.8497***	3.08	-0.0638	-2.38
Retired	0.1634	0.84	-0.7226	-1.39	-0.9747***	-2.15	-0.0507	-4.69
Housewife	*	*	*	*	0.8314***	3.59	0.0345	1.96
Unempl.	0.5603	2.79	0.1352	0.50	1.7353***	11.69	0.0332	2.84
Self-empl.	0.1159	0.24	**	**	0.4387***	1.10	0.0014	0.05
Log Equiv. Income	-0.3646	-5.45	0.4490	3.40	-0.2341	-3.96	0.0040	1.00
Health Index	-0.7259	-2.88	-0.2853	-0.65	0.7837****	2.70	0.1524***	10.68
Unexpl. Happiness, '95	-0.0365	-0.65	-0.0044	-0.04	-0.0886	-1.56	0.0127	4.09
Constant	4.0965	4.75	-6.2979	-3.78	-4.4105	-4.06	0.7368	16.09
Observ.	3,050		1,397		4,491		4,457	
Ps. R^2	0.0759		0.1541		0.2077		0.0930	

Source: Own calculations. *=omitted. **=dropped: perfect predictor. ***=1995 values employed. ****=The unexpected sign here is a spurious artifact of one of the three questions underlying the health index: "In the last 30 days did you miss any work or study days due to illness?" We obtain the expected negative relationship between good health and unemployment when we use other measures of health.

with happiness (table 2) (The three questions that made up the index were: In the last 30 days did you miss any work or study days due to illness? Have you been in the hospital in the last 3 months? Have you in the last 30 days had any health problems?).

We then examined the effects of residual or unexplained happiness on our health index. We found that residual happiness had positive and significant effects on health (table 9). Thus not only does good health make people happier, but our findings suggest that happiness may have additional positive effects on health, something which is often alluded to in the literature but is more difficult to prove empirically with most data. The same cognitive bias or other attitudinal traits that seem to have positive effects on individuals' labor market performance may also influence the manner in which they take care of their health.

CONCLUSIONS

Studies by psychologists find that most individuals have fairly stable levels of happiness or subjective well being, but that those levels are also subject to short-term fluctuations. Our findings support the idea that there are different elements of well being, some of which are behaviorally driven, and others that are determined by socio-economic and demographic variables. The latter are much more vulnerable to day to day events, such as changes in employment and marital status, and fluctuations in income.

Our study used panel data from Russia to identify "residual" happiness levels that are not explained by the usual demographic and socioeconomic determinants of happiness. We then tested whether our residual happiness variable had causal properties on future income and other variables. In other words, while we know that more income (up to a certain level) and stable marital status and more education make people happier, does happiness matter to future outcomes? Does happiness pay? Are happier people healthier and/or more likely to get married? Related to this, do positive expectations and perceptions also have an effect on economic behavior?

We find that residual happiness is associated with higher levels of income in future periods, controlling for income, education, and other socio-demographic variables. Thus people with higher levels of happiness are more likely to increase their own income in the future. When we divided the sample by income level, we found that happiness matters more to future income to those at lower levels of income. In contrast, the effects of initial period income on both future income and future happiness seem more important for those at higher levels of income. Thus, at least in the Russian context, happiness matters more to future income for those with less income, while income matters more to both happiness and income to those with more income.

We also found that residual happiness had positive effects on health. Divorce made people significantly less happy, although unhappier people were not more likely to get divorced. In short, happiness seems to have effects on people's outcomes in the labor market and at the doctor's office. In contrast, divorce affected people's happiness but unhappiness did not cause divorce.

Psychologists attribute stability in happiness levels over time – analogous to the "residual" happiness levels that we identify – to positive cognitive bias, such as self-esteem, control, and optimism. The strong correlation between happiness and our perceptions variables suggest that these same factors may be at play and that, in turn, they affect peoples' performance in their earnings activities. Those respondents with positive expectations for their own upward mobility were more likely to increase their income in the future. Along the same vein, people with more negative perceptions – about their own past progress – and those that have higher fears of being unemployed in the future – increase their incomes less, on average, in future periods.

In conclusion, our findings about the effects of well being on future economic performance – in particular that both happiness and high expectations seem to have positive effects on income in future periods and not only the other way around – suggest that better understanding of subjective well-being can contribute to policy questions, such as about labor market performance and about health. The results are tempered, however, by the exceptional nature of the time period and country from which they come. An important next stage is to test the broader relevance of these results against those from similar data – to the extent it exists – from other countries.[51]

NOTES

1 We would like to thank Bill Dickens, Gary Burtless, Robert Cummins, Clifford Gaddy, Michael Kremer, Andrew Oswald, and Stefano Pettinato for helpful comments on an earlier version, as well as the participants of the MacArthur Network on social interactions and inequality and at a Brookings work in progress seminar for comments. We also thank two anonymous reviewers for extremely helpful comments. The authors acknowledge the generous support of the Tinker Foundation for this research. Please direct all comments to cgraham@brookings.edu. A slightly different version of this paper is forthcoming in the *Journal of Economic Behavior and Organization*

2 Easterlin (1974).

3 See, among others, Blanchflower and Oswald (2000); Diener (1984); Frey and Stutzer (2002); and Graham and Pettinato (2002a). A contrasting view, in a study by psychologist Bob Cummins, starts from the assumption that subjective well being is held within a narrow range determined by personality, and that then is influenced by a number of environmental factors, including income. This study finds that there are significantly different levels of subjective well being for people who are rich, those who are of average Western incomes, and those who are poor. They also note that the effects of income are indirect, i.e. in terms of the other resources that income allows people to purchase, ranging from better health to nicer environments. See Cummins (2000), Personal Income and Subjective Well Being: A Review, Journal of Happiness Studies, Vol. 1, pp. 133-58.

4 For a critique of the use of survey data, see Bertrand & Mullainathan (2001).

5 Assumptions about how much information individuals have and how they process it have become much more sophisticated over time, including the concept of bounded rationality. With bounded rationality, individuals are assumed to have access to local or limited information, and to make decisions according to simple heuristic rules rather than complex optimization calculations. See Conlisk (1996) and Simon (1978).

6 A particularly important sign of support for this line of work was the granting of the 2002 Nobel Prize in economic science to Daniel Kahneman, a psychologist.

7 Most surveys use a four point scale, although more recently psychologists have begun to advocate the use of either seven or ten point scales as more accurate.

8 See, for example, Diener & Biswas-Diener (1999). More recently, Daniel Kahneman has been conducting studies to determine differences in the determinants of positive affect from those of life satisfaction at the Center for the Study of Well Being at Princeton. He presented preliminary findings at a Center on Social and Economic Dynamics seminar at Brookings, February 2002 (Kahneman et al., 2002). Psychologists tend to make a distinction between happiness and life satisfaction, while

economists tend to use the terms satisfaction and happiness interchangeably, as we do in this paper. The correlation between responses to life satisfaction and happiness questions, meanwhile, tends to be on the order of .95.

9   Kahneman & Tversky (2000); Thaler (2000).

10 This literature is summarized in Graham & Pettinato (2002a).

11 This has also been referred to as the "hedonic tread mill".

12 Groot (2000).

13 These effects seem to be more important for those at the higher end of the income ladder. Diener & Biswas-Diener (1999).

14 The drop in percentage of respondents who were students is a result of the aging of the respondent pool. Our dataset consists of 5,269 people who responded to the survey in both 1995 and 2000. Since our youngest respondents are 10 years old in 1995 and 15 by 2000, there is a greater student population in the first round of the survey.

15 The RLMS is a nationally representative panel study for Russia, carried out in collaboration with the University of North Carolina at Chapel Hill, and with funding from U.S. AID among others. More information on the survey can be found at www.cpc.unc.edu/projects/rlms/. Critics of the survey question its degree of representation. Accepting that some of these criticisms may have validity, we believe it is an extremely valuable data set.

16 Two possible problems with the question, however, which need to be taken into account, is that the question allows respondents to have a neutral option, which skews responses to the middle of the distribution, and the ordering of the question in the survey. Rather than asking the happiness question first in the survey, before respondents are given a chance to evaluate other aspects of their life, the RLMS happiness question is in the middle of the survey, after a series of questions about occupational and income status, which might skew the responses negatively.

17 The 2000 results were not available at the time of that analysis. See Graham & Pettinato (2002a). In addition, the Journal of Happiness Studies had a special issue on happiness in Russia (Vol. 2, No. 2, 2001) which was based on the analysis of a separate panel of households, the Russet panel, which ran from 1993 to 1995. The articles in that volume tracked changes in happiness over time, but did not attempt to evaluate the affects of happiness on other variables such as income (cf. Veenhoven, 2001).

18 See, for example, Cummins & Nistico (forthcoming).

19 This is Freedom House's classification of the government in Russia in 2002.

20 There is considerable debate over these figures, in part due to problems with accurate over-time data. These figures are from the World Bank (www.worldbank.org.ru). For a more detailed discussion, see, for example, Ferrer-I-Carbonell & Van Praag (2001); and Klugman & Braithwaite (1998).

21 See Gaddy & Graham (2002).

22 For detail on this, see Gaddy & Ickes (2002).

23 For a critical view, see, e.g., Stiglitz (2002). For a more optimistic view, see Aslund (1995).

24 For a description of Russia's "virtual economy", see Gaddy & Ickes (2002).

25 We initially attempted to include these respondents by adding 1 to each of the 54 observations that reported zero household income in order to take a log and include them. We also created a dummy variable for these respondents, in order to control for any effects that were specific to them and/or that result from our arbitrary specification of their income level (adding 1). We also substituted this specification with a Box-Cox income variable transformation, but found that it did not have a (statistically significant) better fit than did the zero-plus-one logarithmic specification with zero income dummies. Including them produces skewed results (for example, log income in 1995 was negatively correlated with log income in 2000). Since they comprise only 54 observations in a sample of over 5000 – we chose to drop them and to use a simple log equivalence specification throughout the analysis. Results of this econometric analysis are available from the authors on request.

26 Results available from the authors on request.

27 We attempted to deal with this error in our sample by creating dummy variables for the 54 respondents that report zero income. Rather ironically, at least half of these respondents display other traits that suggest they have substantial assets if not monetary income (discussed below). Because of this, including them often skewed our econometric results and thus we did not include them in most of our analysis.

28 For studies in the U.S. and Europe see, among others, Blanchflower & Oswald (2000); and Frey & Stutzer (2002). For happiness in Latin America, see Graham & Pettinato (2002a).

29 Veenhoven (2001), for example, notes that results from Russia could be distorted by translation as well as a culture of "negativism". His own analysis, however, based on a different panel for Russia – the Russet panel for 1993-95, finds that the results are not biased by these factors.
30 This is true for the developed economies and for Latin America. For the latter, see Graham & Sukhtankar (2002).
31 On the U.S., see Blanchflower & Oswald (2000), among others; for Latin America, see Graham (2002).
32 For empirical evidence on this for Latin America and the U.S., see Graham (2002).
33 See Gerber and Mendelson (2002).
34 This contrasts with findings for the United States, for example, where workers are least happy in anticipation of retirement, but then happier, on average, after they retire. See the chapter by Lowenstein et al in Aaron (1999).
35 Our basic measure – the log of equivalence household income – is real household income in 1992 Rubles divided by the square root of the number of people in the household. While there are a number of other household equivalence scales, this is the most commonly used at the international level. For detail, see Figini (1998).
36 In contrast to happiness, which probably varies almost as much within each income quintile as it does over the whole sample, partitioning income by income quintiles loses much of the variation that occurs within the quintiles, particularly the higher ones. Therefore we opted to split the sample in a way that better captured at least some of this variation. The omitted category – middle – is the middle 40 % of the distribution.
37 The coefficient on the top quintile is short of significance at the 10 % level but the point estimate suggests our result. When we include the quintiles without the income variable, the coefficient becomes significant.
38 The studies by psychologists that find that happiness has positive effects on future income also find that these effects are stronger at the higher end of the income scale. See Diener & Biswas-Diener (1999).
39 An alternative exploration would be to use a Kernel estimation of income. Unfortunately, we do not have a statistical package in house that is able to do so.
40 See, among others, Benabou & Ok (1998); Piketty (1995); and Graham & Pettinato (2002a).
41 Cummins & Nistico (forthcoming).
42 Graham & Pettinato (2002a).
43 The "frustrated achievers" found in Graham & Pettinato (2002a, 2002b) also tended to be more negative in their scores on all of the other perceptions variables, including in their support for markets and democracy.
44 We also tried to separate the effects of perceptions from those specific to individuals by using person fixed effects and again dropping time invariant traits such as race, housewife, retired, and so forth. In a third best approximation, in which we had to use OLS rather than ordered logits to include person fixed effects, we still find that perceptions (POUM and ELQ) have positive and significant effects on happiness, while fear of unemployment has negative and significant effects. While using OLS on a categorical variable is not technically correct, we have found that OLS and the ordered logits yield very similar results on happiness regressions. Results available from the authors.
45 Not surprisingly we also find that residual happiness levels are positively correlated with more positive attitudes about democracy, more positive economic self assessments, and more positive prospects for upward mobility. Results are available from the authors.
46 As in the case of happiness, the log-log specification (with and without zero income dummies included) renders the perception variable insignificant.
47 One interesting finding is that in 1995, married people were not significantly happier than others, a finding that supports our intuition that overall happiness levels increased from 1995 to 2000 (for happiness in 1995, see Graham & Pettinato, 2002a). This is supported by the fact that 35 % of the sample had positive changes in happiness levels, while 28 % had decreases, plus the general improvements on the economic and governance fronts in Russia during the period.
48 The reverse of this was also true: Residual happiness had no significant effects on the probability of staying married.
49 In order to make sure that this result was not driven by selection bias – say by the few people not eligible for employment in the sample – we re-ran this same regression with only those employed in 1995, omitting students, retired, and the unemployed in 1995 – and got the same results on education.

50 Another rather interesting result on unemployment is that the health index was positively and significantly correlated with being unemployed in 2000. This may well be the result of spurious correlation,
as one question on the index asks "how days of work did you miss due to illness?", and obviously
unemployed people would answer zero.
51 One author, Graham, is currently in the process of compiling second period observations on happiness and other variables with a research team in Peru.

REFERENCES

Aslund, A. (1995): How Russia Became a Market Economy. The Brookings Institution Press. Washing-
ton, D.C.
Benabou, R. & E. Ok (1998): Social Mobility and the Demand for Redistribution: The POUM Hypothe-
sis. NBER Working Paper No. 6795.
Bertrand, M. & S. Mullainathan (2001): Do People Mean What They Say? Implications for Subjective
Survey Data. American Economic Review 91, 67-72.
Blanchflower, D. G. & A. J. Oswald (2000): Well Being Over Time in Britain and the USA. NBER
Working Papers 7487, National Bureau of Economic Research, Inc.
Conlisk, J. (1996): Why Bounded Rationality? Journal of Economic Literature 34, 669-700.
Cummins, R. & H. Nistico, H. (forthcoming): Maintaining Life Satisfaction: The Role of Positive Cogni-
tive Bias. Journal of Happiness Studies.
Diener, E. & R. Biswas-Diener (1999): Income and Subjective Well-Being: Will Money Make Us
Happy? Mimeo, Department of Psychology, University of Illinois.
Diener, E. (1984): Subjective Well Being. Psychological Bulletin 95, 542-75.
Easterlin, R. A. (1974): Does Economic Growth Improve the Human Lot? P. A. David & M. W. Reder
(eds.): Nations and Households in Economic Growth, New York: Academic Press, 89-125.
Ferrer-I-Carbonell, A. & B. van Praag (2001): Poverty in Russia. Journal of Happiness Studies 2, 147-72.
Figini, P. (1998): Inequality Measures, Equivalence Scales, and Adjustment for Household Size and
Composition. LIS Working Paper No. 185.
Frey, B. & A. Stutzer (2002): Happiness and Economics. Princeton, NJ.: Princeton University Press.
Gaddy, C. & C. Graham (2002): Why Argentina '02 is not Russia '98. The Globalist. February 11.
Gaddy, C. & B. Ickes (2002): Russia's Virtual Economy. Washington, DC.: The Brookings Institution
Press.
Gerber, T. P & S. E. Mendelson (2002a): How Russians Think about Chechnya. PONARS Policy Memo
No.243, CSIS, Washington, D.C.
Gerber, T. P & S. E. Mendelson (2002b): The Disconnect in How Russians Think about Human Rights
and Chechnya: A Consequence of Media Manipulation. PONARS Policy Memo No.244, CSIS,
Washington, D.C.
Graham, C. (2002): Crafting Sustainable Social Contracts in Latin America: Political Economy, Public
Attitudes, and Social Policy. Paper prepared for the Inter-American Development Bank Meeting on
Social Policy, Santiago, Chile.
Graham, C. & S. Pettinato (2002a): Happiness and Hardship: Opportunity and Insecurity in New Market
Economies, Washington, DC.: The Brookings Institution Press.
Graham, C. & S. Pettinato (2002b): Frustrated Achievers: Winners, Losers, and Subjective Well Being in
New Market Economies. Journal of Development Studies 38, 100-40.
Graham, C. S. Sukhtankar (2002): Is Economic Crisis Reducing Support for Markets and Democracy in
Latin America? Some Evidence from the Economics of Happiness. Center on Social and Economic
Dynamics Working Papers, No. 28, The Brookings Institution, Washington, D.C.
Groot, W. (2000): Adaptation and Scale of Reference Bias in Self Assessments of Quality of Life. Journal
of Health Econometrics 19, 403-20.
Hirschman, A. O. (1973): Changing Tolerance for Income Inequality in the Course of Economic Devel-
opment. Quarterly Journal of Economics 87, 544-66.
Kahneman, D., A. Krueger, D. Schkade, N. Schwarz & A. Stone (2002): Measuring Objective Happiness.
Work in Progress, Princeton University Center for the Study of Well Being.
Kahneman, D. A. Tversky (2000): Choices, Values, and Frames, New York: Cambridge University Press.
Klugman, J. & J. Braithwaite (1998): Poverty In Russia During The Transition: An Overview. World
Bank Research Observer, February.

Lowenstein, G., D. Prelec & R. Weber (1999): What, Me Worry? A Psychological Perspective on the Economics of Retirement. H. J. Aaron (ed.): Behavioral Dimensions of Retirement, Brookings Institution and Russell Sage Foundation, Washington, DC.

Merton, R. K. (1957): Social Theory and Social Structure, Glencoe: The Free Press of Glencoe.

Piketty, T. (1995): Social Mobility and Redistributive Politics. Quarterly Journal of Economics 110, 551-84.

Simon, H. (1978): Rationality as a Process and Product of Thought. American Economic Review 68, 1-16.

Stiglitz, J. (2002): Globalization and its Discontents, New York: W.W. Norton and Company.

Thaler, R. (2000): From Homo Economicus to Homo Sapiens. Journal of Economic Perspectives 14, 133-41.

Veenhoven, R. (2001): Are Russians as Unhappy as They Say They Are? Journal of Happiness Studies 2, 111-36.

PART IV:
CULTURAL CHALLENGES
FOR QUALITY OF LIFE

14. HAPPINESS AS AN EXPRESSION OF FREEDOM AND SELF-DETERMINATION

A Comparative Multilevel Analysis

Max Haller and Markus Hadler
University of Graz, Austria

ABSTRACT

In this paper, subjective well-being, as measured by survey questions on life satisfaction and happiness, is investigated from a sociological-comparative point of view. The central thesis is that happiness will be greater the more freedom a person has in her/his life decisions. It is hypothesized, therefore, that happiness will be higher in all those social contexts (micro and macro) which provide a person with greater freedom. Hence, happiness should be higher among the employed, among persons in higher positions and with higher incomes, and happiness should also be higher in free market and democratic, and in less stratified societies. A comparative empirical analysis (multilevel regression) is carried out, using survey data on 41 nations from the *World Value Survey* 1995-97. The finding that happiness is related significantly to the degree of individual freedom is fully confirmed. It also has been proven that people who live in circumstances providing more freedom of personal choice are happier. However, macro-social conditions are not directly relevant for personal freedom and happiness; this happens only through their perception and through their expected change (improvement or stagnation) in the future.

INTRODUCTION

In recent decades, happiness has become a topic investigated intensively by social psychologists (Argyle, 1987; Michalos, 1991; Myers, 1993; Kahnemann & Diener, 1999), sociologists (Veenhoven, 1989; 1993; Bellebaum, 1992), political scientists (Lane, 2000) and economists (Frey & Stutzer, 2002). Already in the Sixties, large-scale empirical surveys on mental health and the subjective quality of life of the population have been carried out in the United States (Gurin et al., 1960; Bradburn, 1969); recently, in many advanced countries regular surveys on subjective quality of life have been established (Campbell, 1981; Glatzer & Zapf, 1984). The relevance of happiness from the personal, social-scientific and political-practical perspectives is evident (see also Veenhoven, 1994, pp. 102f.; Diener, 2000; Frey & Stutzer, 2002). To become and to remain happy is a fundamental goal and right of any human acknowledged not only by the political philosophy of utilitarianism. Thus, striving towards happiness has been embodied as a fundamental human right into the venerable constitution of the United States; today, many governments consider the advancement of happiness of their peoples at a primary political goal; the focus on

Wolfgang Glatzer, Susanne von Below, Matthias Stoffregen (eds.), Challenges for Quality of Life in the Contemporary World, 207-231.

economic growth is seen as the best means to achieve that goal (Eckersley, 2000, p. 4). Finally, empirical research has shown that happiness has positive consequences for other areas of human behavior, such as an increased openness and commitment of adolescents (Magen, 1996), increased chances of finding a job among unemployed (Verkley & Stolk, 1989) and the increase of life expectancy of middle- and older aged people (Deeg & van Zonneveld, 1989; Veenhoven, 1989).

In this paper, we take a sociological perspective which starts from the basic assumption that happiness must be seen as a concomitant and consequence of specific human action and their embedding into social structures. This perspective which may seem obvious at first sight, in fact has been considered only very seldom. Let us try to elaborate it in more detail and to deduce some testable hypotheses from it.

THEORETICAL CONSIDERATIONS

We do not assume that men are sluggish beings which must be "driven" to become active as theories of motivation usually do. Rather, we take it for granted that they – as all other creatures – are active by nature. Therefore, we must focus on the diversity and variability of action, and investigate the forms, preconditions and consequences of certain kinds of actions. This fundamental and simple idea which was central to the thinking of G. H. Mead, Max Weber and others (see Campbell, 1998; Haller, 2003) has far-reaching consequences.

First, it is a central element of human action – in contrast to pure "behavior" among animals – that it has a certain intent, a meaning. Through human action – which must be seen as a conscious and purposeful act – men try to realize some aim. Such an act requires a certain margin of decision, a certain degree of freedom. The broader this margin, the better the individual will be able to decide between the alternatives before him. In this perspective, the perennial, contested question of human sciences and philosophy, if men are free or not, is seen from a wholly new perspective. We take it as an axiological principle that an action must be free if it should be called „human" (see also Fromm, 1956; Boudon, 1999). This principle, however, is not a statement about every single human act. There exists also behavior which proceeds in a more or less automatic manner, such as everyday routine or traditional behavior (in Weber's terms) or behavior responding more or less automatically to internal or external stimuli (such as a pure affective behavior). Only if a certain act is carried out intentionally and with a specific aim, does freedom come in. Even such an action, however, can be enforced by others or circumstances to a certain degree. The basic assumption of our paper therefore is: If a human act has been carried out by free decision, and without external enforcement or constraint, it is gratifying per se because it deploys the essence of humans, the ability to act in a conscious, deliberate and reflexive manner.

If we see satisfaction with one's life as a whole as the highest form of happiness (Nozick, 1989), then it becomes also evident that freedom plays a decisive role. How could somebody really be happy with an over-directed life? This argument is in line with several socio-psychological findings. Doyle and Youn (2000, p. 207) report that a number of personality characteristics which influenced happiness are united by a freedom/control dimension. Mihaly Csikszentmihalyi (1990) has shown that the highest feelings of personal happiness and fulfillment (connected typically with absent-mindedness) result if a person is fully involved into a self-selected and demanding task or activity (see also Deci & Ryan, 1985). Our hypothesis is also in line with A. Sen's (1999) concept of "capabilities" which in essence means the degree of actual freedom of a person to lead a specific, self-chosen style of life (see also Sève, 1972).

From this simple and basic thesis, straightforward conclusions can be drawn about the significance of particular kinds of social behavior and action in different domains of life. The second general assumption of this paper, therefore, is that happiness should arise out of all those forms of actions, and in all those spheres of life, where the individual has at least some degree of freedom to decide. Free action is usually motivated intrinsically, by an inherent tendency to use knowledge and capacities to seek novelty and challenges (Ryan & Deci, 2000). It follows that the attainment of happiness will be easier in all those economic, social and political contexts and it will be facilitated by all those institutions which provide the individual with possibilities of participation, which give him the feeling that he has some personal influence and discretion on the events happening around him. Hannah Arendt (1958) has reminded us that in classical Greek philosophy political freedom was a precondition for the attainment of happiness (eudaimonia) which on its side was closely connected with health and prosperity. For the Greeks, freedom, a characteristic of the political sphere (as opposed to the private household), was closely related to equality between the citizens. This was a central point also in Alexis de Tocqueville's classical work on Democracy in America (Tocqueville, 1947). Thus, societal structures of opportunity and inequality play an important role in this regard.

As far as the personal and societal conditions for the exertion of free action are concerned, a twofold process will be at work. First, conditions and contexts will facilitate autonomous lines of action which will also increase individual happiness. From this point of view, an adequate job and income as well as good health will be important since they increase individuals' "capabilities" (Sen, 1999). Second, conditions and contexts which provide good opportunities in the future for those who find themselves in adverse situations will be conducive to happiness. Disadvantaged people then will have the feeling that they can look forward to and eventually move on into contexts providing better opportunities for personal freedom and advancement (Diener & Suh, 1997, p. 204). Thus, the future prospects of an individual might be as important or even more important than his/her present situation. Nobody would classify a student as "poor", even if his actual income falls below the statistical poverty line. Similarly, economic growth providing many new jobs and increasing the income of everybody, might have more positive effects than a high, but static level of wealth.

Based on these general considerations, four specific hypotheses are put forward:

(1) Happiness of individuals will be greater, the more they feel that they have a considerable degree of freedom of decision in their life and thus can control their destiny.

(2) Happiness will be higher in personal, social and macro-societal situations and contexts which accord individuals more opportunities for free decision. Here, we expect that gainful employment, a higher occupational position and higher income lead to more happiness, as well as a higher standard of living of a country as a whole. In all these regards we expect also that the subjective perception of present and future individual and societal conditions will be important.

(3) The variation of happiness between nations will reflect their economic, stratification and political order. In countries with a growing economy and positive socioeconomic prospects, with open and transparent stratification systems, and
with economic and political systems where citizens are free to express and put
forth their interests, happiness will be higher than in nations where political
suppression, rigid social hierarchies and non-transparent, clientelistic systems of
economic exchange and social advancement prevail. This will be so because in
the latter, wealth and privileges often must be attributed to external forces, unal-
terable by individual effort.

(4) Social class and status differences in happiness should be larger in more unequal societies and in countries with less open and free economic and political
systems .

EMPIRICAL RESULTS FROM THE WORLD VALUE SURVEY 1995-97

What we can present here, is only a partial test of the general theses developed in the
foregoing section. Since the focus of this paper is on happiness in the comparative
view, we must look primarily at international surveys. It was a felicitous circumstance that in the *World Value Survey* 1995-97 (WVS 95) questions on both dimensions – feeling of freedom and happiness – have been included which are relevant
from the theoretical perspective developed here.[1] A limitation arises from the fact
that this survey – as most others on "happiness" – has not been carried out within the
framework of the theory developed here. A direct test of our theory would require an
in-depth investigation of the actual processes of human action and a detailed grasp-
ing of the aims connected to certain lines of actions. It would also necessitate a differentiated coverage of the concept of "freedom" whose meaning might vary somewhat between different countries and cultures. Our indicators (questions) capturing
freedom and happiness, as well as socio-demographic variables, like sex, age or
marital status, are only approximations of the actual life circumstances of a respondent. We cannot expect, therefore, that the effect of these variables on happiness will
be very strong.

In the following subsection, the data set and items used are described; then, the
results of the analysis of feeling free are presented, followed by those of happiness
at the individual and the macro-social level.

a) Data Sets, Questions and Indicators, and Method of Analysis

The *World Value Survey* (WVS) is one of the few regular, large and international
comparative surveys. Beginning in the early 1980ies, it has already been carried out
three times in dozens of nations around the world (Inglehart et al., 2000). Its aim is
to provide an empirical base for the study of social and cultural change among the
populations of the different nations. The strengths of this project are obvious: It provides a unique and rich database for international comparisons of attitudes and values; it covers the whole range of basic social attitudes and its replication enables the
recording of value changes over time (Bréchon, 2002). However, there also exist
limitations of the WVS. One is the fact that – due to its coverage of a broad array of
social attitudes and values – specific dimensions often can be grasped only with a
single or a few questions.[2] Another one is the fact that for some large countries (e.g.

Russia, China, and others) only certain provinces were randomly sampled; these provinces tend to be the more urban and rich ones.[3]

The WVS 1995-97, which is used here, included about 70 different states, regions and cities around the world. After combining the sub-regions contained in the aggregated data set into one single country where necessary[4], 49 countries remained. Because of many missing values in important variables, several countries had to be excluded. Finally, 41 countries could be used for the multilevel regression analysis.

Our main dependent variables were captured by three questions. The following question (V66) grasps directly the dimension of subjective freedom of control:

> "Some people feel they have completely free choice and control over their lives, while other people feel that what they do has no real effect on what happens to them. Please use this scale where 1 means 'none at all' and 10 means 'a great deal' to indicate how much freedom of choice and control you feel you have over the way your life turns out:
>
> 1 ('Not at all') […] 10 ('A great deal')"

Two questions were asked about happiness and life satisfaction:

> "(V10) Taking all things together, would you say you are: very happy (1), quite happy (2), not very happy (3), not at all happy (4)";
>
> "(V65) All things considered, how satisfied are you with your life as a whole these days? Please use this card for your answer:
>
> 1 ('Dissatisfied') […] 10 ('Satisfied')"

Both these questions will be used as separate dependent variables in the following analysis, assuming that they – by and large – are measuring a similar dimension. Since they were asked at different places in the questionnaire the degree of correspondence in the results may be interpreted as an indicator of their validity.

We use the method of multilevel regression analysis in order to distinguish in a methodologically sound way between the effects of characteristics of the individuals (individual level) and the effects of characteristics of the countries as a whole (macro level). A multilevel analysis has several advantages over a simple regression analysis were no distinction between individual and macro-social characteristics is made (Goldstein, 1995, p. 3): First, it results in statistically efficient estimates of the regression coefficients; second, by using the context data (country characteristics), it produces correct standard errors, confidence intervals and significance tests, and these are usually more "conservative" than those obtained with an ordinary regression; third, by allowing the use of covariates measured at both levels, it enables one to explore interaction effects. Thus, one can investigate if the effects of an individual socioeconomic characteristic, such as income, on happiness are the same in all countries compared. For our statistical analysis, we used the program MlwiN (Rabash et al., 2000).

Three kinds of determinants of the dependent variable "freedom of decision" are distinguished here (see figure 1 and table 1):

Sociodemographic individual characteristics and behaviors: age and gender, education, employment participation and occupational status, income, marital status and presence of children; religious denomination and participation; membership in voluntary associations; these variables are related to the individual life situation of the respondents;

Attitudes and subjective evaluations; here, the following indicators were available: subjective social class placement, subjective health situation, satisfaction with financial situation, how often respondents think about the meaning of life, how the choices to escape poverty are perceived, altruistic orientation;

Macro-social indicators, that is, characteristics of the countries compared; By decomposing the global "black-box" variable "country" into a set of specific variables, it becomes possible to give a meaningful interpretation to differences between countries (Przeworski/Teune, 1970; Haller, 2002). Four macro-social characteristics of the countries were included: Level of economic development or wealth (GNP/head), economic growth during the Nineties (GDP/growth), income distribution (GINI coefficients) and degree of political freedom. The latter indicator was taken from a data set compiled by Freedom House, New York; it varies between 1 (fully free) to 8 (no freedom).[5] In this index, most Western-European and Anglo-Saxon countries have scores indicating high freedom (below 2); then follow Latin-American and post-communist countries (values 2-4); at the end we find China, Nigeria, Azerbaijan, Turkey, Belarus and Peru (over 5.0).[6]

Figure 1: The Multilevel Regression Models (Overview)

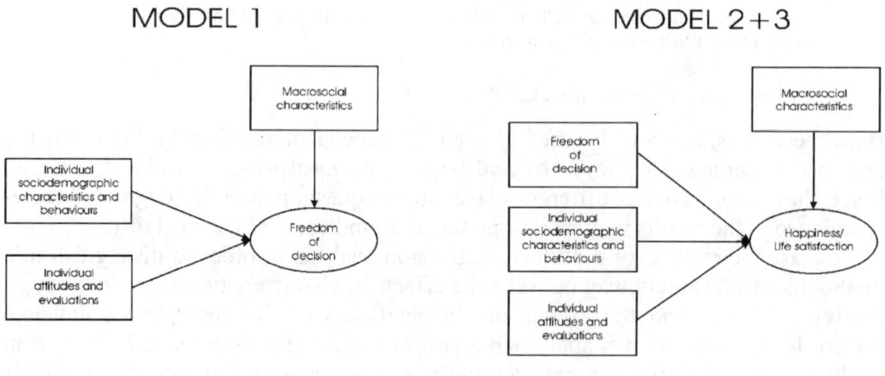

In the multilevel analysis, three models are estimated (see figure 1). In the first model, freedom of decision is taken as a dependent variable; in the second and third model life satisfaction and happiness, respectively, are the dependent variables.

b) Individual Social and Macro Structural Determinants of the Feeling of Freedom

In this section, we present the findings on the individual- and macro-level determinants of the feeling of being free in one's own life. First, let us look at the distribution of this variable in the 41 countries compared.

Figure 2: Freedom of Decision in 41 Countries (Mean Values)

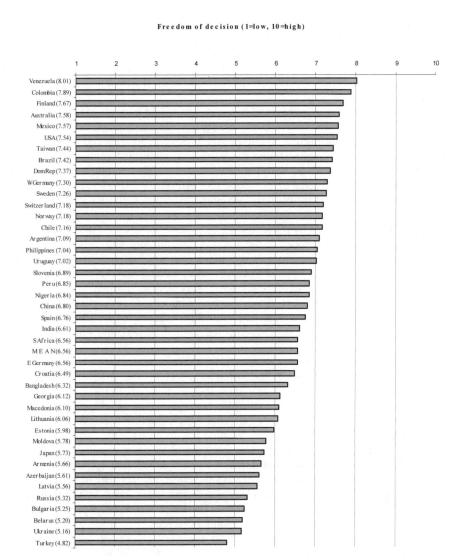

Source: World Value Survey 1995.

Figure 2 shows that there exist indeed significant international differences in this important dimension. The feeling of freedom was measured on a ten-point scale, 1 indicating none at all and 10 a high level of freedom. The mean value over the whole sample was 6.56, indicating an overall positive estimation. The international differences are considerable: On top, in Venezuela, the mean value is 8, but on bottom, in Turkey, it is only 4.82. Three groups of countries stand out with a very high level of subjectively felt freedom: Firstly, some advanced North Western European and Anglo-Saxon countries (Finland, Australia, and the United States); secondly – rather surprising – three Latin American countries; two of these – Venezuela and Colombia – are in fact on top of all; thirdly, Taiwan. In most of these countries, the mean value is above 7.30. The lowest values emerge in the post-communist Eastern European countries and in the successor states of the Soviet Union. Within this group, the higher developed nations, like Slovenia and Croatia, are about in the middle, and the lower developed ones, like Ukraine, Belarus, Russia and Bulgaria, on the bottom.

Two of these findings correspond to what one would expect: Market societies and democratic institutions have been established for the longest time and most firmly in North-Western Europe and in the Anglo-Saxon countries and these are also among the wealthiest nations around the world. In many post-communist Eastern European and Asian societies, however, free market and democratic institutions are of very recent origin and often do not work very effectively till today. Together with the dramatic worsening of the objective economic situation in those countries during the 1990ies (Haller & Hadler, 2002), this explains the very low level in the feeling of being in control of one's own life. Rather surprising, however, is the high level of the feeling of personal freedom in the Latin American countries, where socioeconomic inequality is often extremely large and democracy had a difficult fate in the last decades. One aspect correlated to this positive feeling may be that these countries experienced considerable economic growth as well as an opening and liberalization of their economic system in the Nineties. This could also explain the feeling of having a high degree of freedom and control in Asian countries like Taiwan (its value of 7.44 lies between Germany and the United States), the Philippines and China.

The multivariate multilevel regression gives more exact answers about the possible causes for these large international differences. Let us look, first, at the effects of individual sociodemographic characteristics, then at those of several subjective perceptions and attitudes and, finally, at the effects of the macro variables.

Table 1 shows that nearly all sociodemographic characteristics exert significant influence on the feeling of being free. Women feel to be less free then men; young people (below 29 years) feel to be more free than older ones; people with children feel more free than those without children; the unemployed, housewives and retired feel to be less free than those presently employed; managers feel to be more, the unskilled less free than the bulk of non-manual employees; those with high income feel more free than those with lower income. The latter two findings clearly support our hypotheses in this regard. The more pronounced feeling of freedom among men and among young people also corresponds to everyday experience. Somewhat contrary to our general assumption is the fact that people with children feel to be more free; we will see later, that close relationships to other people constitute an additional, independent source of happiness.

Table 1: Multilevel Regression Analysis of Freedom of Decision in 41 countries

	B	SE	Beta
Sociodemographic Characteristics			
Constant	6.26**	0.48	0
Women (Ref=Men)	-0.14**	0.02	-0.03
Age (-29)	0.14**	0.04	0.02
Age (30-39)	0.06	0.03	0.01
Age (40-49) (Ref)	-	-	-
Age (50-59)	-0.03	0.04	0
Age (60-69)	0.01	0.05	0
Age (70-)	0.1	0.06	0.01
Education (Low-High)	-0.01	0.01	0
Married (Ref)	-	-	-
Divorced, Separated, Widowed	0.05	0.03	0.01
Single	0.04	0.04	0.01
Children (No.s 1-4+)	0.03*	0.01	0.01
No Children or Missing Value	-0.04*	0.02	-0.01
Employment Status			
Employed (Ref)			
Retired	-0.19**	0.04	-0.02
Housewife	-0.11**	0.04	-0.01
Student	-0.07	0.05	-0.01
Unemployed	-0.08*	0.04	-0.01
Not Employed/Missing	-0.09	0.05	-0.01
Occupational Position			
Non Manual (Ref)	-	-	-
Manager	0.09*	0.04	0.01
Skilled Worker	-0.04	0.03	-0.01
Semi Skilled Worker	-0.12**	0.03	-0.02
Farmer	-0.04	0.06	0
Army	-0.19**	0.07	-0.01
Never Worked	-0.19**	0.04	-0.03
Income (Low-High)	0.02**	0.01	0.02

Table 1: Multilevel Regression Analysis of Freedom of Decision in 41 countries (continued)

Religious Denomination			
Catholic (Ref)	-	-	-
None	-0.08*	0.04	-0.01
Protestant	0.10**	0.04	0.01
Orthodox	0.04	0.04	0.01
Jew	-0.23**	0.09	-0.01
Muslim	-0.01	0.07	0
Other (Mainly Buddhist, Hindu, and other Asian Religions)	0.09	0.05	0.01
Interaction: Female-Muslim	-0.54**	0.07	-0.04
Individual Attitudes and Behavior			
Church Attendance (Often-Never)	0.02**	0.01	0.02
Voluntary Membership (No-Many)	0.04	0.03	0.01
Subjective Class (High-Low)	-0.12**	0.03	-0.04
Subjective Health (Bad-Good)	-0.25**	0.01	-0.1
Financial Satisfaction (Low-High)	0.23**	0	0.26
Think about Meaning of Life (Often-Never)	-0.11**	0.01	-0.04
Poverty Increased Last 10 Years (Not-Much)	-0.03	0.02	-0.01
Other/Own Preferences (Ref=other)	0.01	0.02	0
No Chance to Escape Poverty (Ref=Chance)	-0.19**	0.02	-0.04
Country Characteristics			
Political Freedom (High-Low)	-0.07	0.06	-0.06
GNP*1000 (Low-High)	0	0.01	-0.01
Gini-Index (Low-High)	0.01	0.01	0.06
Growth of GDP (Low-High)	0.04*	0.02	0.08
R^2_{makro}		0.678	
R^2_{total}		0.156	
N		64,605	

Source: World Value Survey 1995; own calculations. If an item was not asked in a country or not answered by a respondent, a dummy is included but not shown here.

Also religious affiliation and church attendance have significant effects. Catholics and Jews, as well as persons who often think about the meaning of life, feel to be less free in their decisions. The opposite is true for protestants and people who do not go to church. A very interesting and plausible interaction effect turned out in regard to gender and religion: Female Muslims feel significantly less frequent that they are free in their decisions.

Significant and often quite strong effects emanate from most of those items which concern the subjective perception of one's social position and life situation.

The feeling of being free is more widespread among those who assign themselves to higher social classes; among people who feel to be in good health; and among those who are satisfied with their financial situation.

A set of three additional individual attitudes in table 1 is related to social perceptions concerning our hypothesis 2, the stratification system of a society. Two questions were related to the perception of inequality and poverty in the immediate past and to the chances of poor people to improve their lot in the future (Items V171 and V173):

> "Would you say that today a larger share, about the same share, or a smaller share of the people of this country are living in poverty than were ten years ago?"

> "In your opinion, do most poor people in this country have a chance of escaping from poverty, or is there very little chance of escaping?"

Table 1 shows that the estimation of changes in the overall societal amount of poverty during the last ten years does not have any effect on the feeling of personal freedom. The estimation of the present chances of poor people to escape their lot, however, does have such effects. Persons who think that poor people in general have good chances to escape from poverty, feel that they themselves are in a better position to decide about important issues in their life.

Finally, let us look at the question of what determines freedom in the macro perspective. A lot of earlier research has shown that nations differ significantly in the mean level of happiness of their populations. We have shown that this is also true for the feeling of being free. It is a central tenet of our approach, however, to posit not only an overall "nationality" or "culture effect" on freedom and happiness (Inkeles, 1989; Inglehart & Rabier, 1986, p. 34ff.). Such an effect would be difficult to interpret. Rather, we decompose the variable nation into several specific, theoretically meaningful and measurable components (see Przeworski & Teune, 1970 and Haller, 2002 for this strategy). In our theoretical considerations we introduced three dimensions in this regard: wealth of a nation, economic inequality and political freedom.

Table 1 shows that the effects of these macro-social dimensions on the feeling of being free in one's own life are rather modest. Neither political freedom and the socioeconomic level of development (GNP per head), nor national income distribution (inequality) have significant effects on the feeling of being personally free in the daily decisions. Only growth of GDP over the last years has a significant (albeit only weak) positive effect on the feeling of personal freedom.

Summarizing these findings we may say that most of our hypotheses on the determinants of individual feelings of freedom have been supported. This was particularly true for the variables concerning employment and occupation; it was also true for the items on the subjective perception of one's status and life circumstances. Only a partial confirmation, however, was found for the hypotheses on the macro-social determinants of individual feelings of being free.

Two explanations might exist for this. First, the feeling of being in control of one's own daily life seems to be determined mainly by the immediate life situation of a person and his or her family. Second, the objective social structure and situation of a country seems to become relevant for the individual feeling of being free only through the subjective perception of the objective situation.

Now, let us go on to look at the factors which determine happiness and life satisfaction.

c) Personal and Social Circumstances Conducive to Happiness and Life Satisfaction

First, let us have a look at the distribution of life satisfaction over the 42 countries (see figure 3).

Figure 3: Life Satisfaction in 41 Countries (Mean Values)

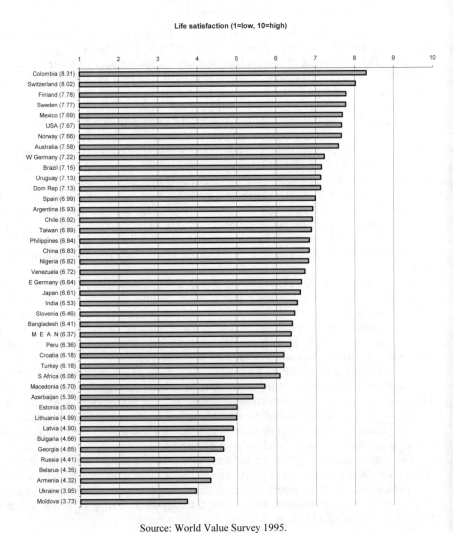

Source: World Value Survey 1995.

Here, we can see an even wider variation than in the case of freedom and self-control. The lowest value, found in Moldavia, is 3.73 (on the ten-point scale with 1 as the lowest, 10 as the highest value), the highest as much as 8.31 (found in Colombia). The general rank order of countries is rather similar to that in the degree of freedom, but not in all cases.

Again, a Latin American country, Colombia, lies on top with a mean satisfaction value of 8.31. This is indeed very high, 2 points above the overall mean (6.37). Next come two Scandinavian countries (Finland and Sweden), the USA and Australia. With some distance, West Germany and other Latin American countries follow. On the bottom of this scale, we find only the poorer post-communist countries: Moldova and the Ukraine show the lowest values (below 4) which indicate an overall rather negative evaluation of life (the median of the 10 point scale in life satisfaction is 5.5 points). If we compare the WVS-data of the mid-Nineties on happiness of nations with other data, the position of several single countries may be somewhat different. However, the main order of ranking does not differ: We always find the rich West-European and Anglo-Saxon countries on top, and the post-communist as well as very poor countries of the Third World on the bottom; the same is true for the conspicuously high position of the Latin-American countries (see Inglehart & Rabier, 1986; Veenhoven, 1993; Schyns, 1998; Diener, 2000; Frey & Stutzer, 2002; Vittersø et al., 2002). The rank order of the countries corresponds by and large with the objective life situation in these countries, albeit one clear exception exists. This is the very high level of life satisfaction in the Latin American countries whose level of development is rather modest and which are also characterized by high degrees of internal inequality, as well as many economic, social and political problems.

Let us now look at the central relationship, investigated in this paper. Figure 4 presents a scattergram of the relation between feeling of freedom and life satisfaction at the macro level.[7] We see a rather linear, strong association here; the Pearson correlation coefficient is .85. Thus, the first hypothesis of this paper is clearly confirmed also at this level of observation: In nations, where people feel to have a lot of freedom to decide about their own life, they are also happier. From this point of view, there seems to exist no contradiction between modernization, increase of freedom and individualism on the one, and happiness on the other hand (see also Veenhoven 1999; Boudon 1999).

A few countries deviate somewhat from the general pattern of a nearly linear relation between freedom and happiness: Especially in Turkey, but also in Japan, people feel to have relatively little freedom, compared to their life satisfaction; in Moldavia, Georgia, and Venezuela, people are less happy than one would expect based on their level of freedom of decision. We might note here that Turkey is the only Muslim society in our sample. As far as Japan is concerned, this finding corresponds to the fact that personal affiliation and dependence on authorities (the principle of "Amae") is a central characteristic of Japanese society (Doi, 1973).

Figure 4: Freedom of Decision and Life Satisfaction in 41 Countries

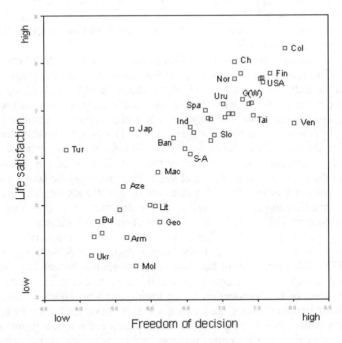

Source: World Value Survey 1995.

After this first, descriptive analysis we have to make sure that the central effects hold true even after controlling for other possible influences (see table 2). As far as the individual level variables are concerned, we describe and discuss only the effects of those variables which have been included in our hypotheses since they are also related to the feeling of individual freedom. These variables include employment participation and occupational status, income and a series of items related to subjective perception and evaluation of personal life circumstances.

Employment participation and occupational status: The deprivation of the unemployed and of unskilled workers. Work is one of the main bases for self-identity in modern society, and unemployment one of the most frequently occurring undesirable situations. In the foregoing section we found that all groups of the non-employed reported less freedom and self-control than the employed. The findings show also several significant effects of the employment situation on happiness. Housewives, students and the retired are happier, only the unemployed are less happy than employed persons. The findings for housewives and the retired are surprising since they are in the opposite direction as those on subjective freedom. Evidently, women who are not employed outside of the house have sources of satisfaction within the household and family which more than compensate for gainful work. A similar consideration may apply to retired people: While they certainly have less money, and less possibilities to participate in decisions, they have more time to spend with their relatives and hobbies, and, when they have reduced their material aspirations, they can lead a more quiet life.

Table 2: Multilevel Regression Analysis of Happiness and Life Satisfaction in 41 Countries

	Happiness (Low-High)			Life Satisfaction (Low-High)		
	B	SE	Beta	B	SE	Beta
Constant	-2.01**	0.13	0.00	3.62**	0.28	0.00
Employment Status						
Employed (Ref)	-	-	-	-	-	-
Retired	0.04**	0.01	0.02	0.09**	0.03	0.01
Housewife	0.06**	0.01	0.03	0.07**	0.03	0.01
Student	0.04**	0.01	0.01	0.11**	0.04	0.01
Unemployed	-0.04**	0.01	-0.01	-0.17**	0.03	-0.02
Not employed/ Missing	0.07**	0.01	0.02	0.16**	0,03	0.02
Occupational Position						
Non Manual (Ref)	-	-	-	-	-	-
Manager	0.01	0.01	0.00	-0.04	0.03	-0.00
Skilled Worker	0.02	0.01	0.01	0.02	0.03	0.00
Semi Skilled Worker	-0.02**	0.01	-0.01	-0.05**	0.02	-0.01
Farmer	-0.00	0.02	-0.00	-0.01	0.05	-0.00
Army	-0.00	0.02	-0.00	0.02	0.03	0.00
Never Worked	-0.01	0.01	-0.00	0.02	0.03	0.00
Income (Low-High)	0.00	0.00	0.01	-0.00	0.00	-0.00
Individual Attitudes and Behavior						
Subjective Class (High-Low)	-0.05**	0.00	-0.08	-0.1**	0.01	-0.05
Subjective Health (Bad-Good)	-0.21**	0.00	-0.28	-0.37**	0.01	-0.15
Financial Satisfaction (Low-High)	0.05**	0.00	0.20	0.44**	0.00	0.49
Decision Freedom (Low-High)	0.03**	0.00	0.11	0.18**	0.00	0.20
Poverty Increased Lat 10 Years (Not-Much)	-0.00	0.00	-0.00	0.00	0.01	0.00
No Chance to Escape Poverty (Ref=Chance)	-0.05**	0.01	-0.03	-0.13**	0.02	-0.02

Table 2: Multilevel Regression Analysis of Happiness and Life Satisfaction in 41 Countries (continued)

Country Characteristics						
Political Freedom (High-Low)	0.01	0.02	0.03	0.01	0.03	0.00
GNP*1000	0.01**	0.00	0.10	0.02*	0.01	0.07
Gini-Index (Low-High)	0.01**	0.00	0.07	0.01	0.01	0.03
Growth of GDP (Low-High)	0.01**	0.01	0.09	0.05**	0.01	0.10
R^2_{macro}	0.820			0.953		
R^2_{total}	0.279			0.488		
N	66,456			69,265		

Source: World Value Survey; own calculations. If an item was not asked in a country or not answered by a respondent, a dummy is included but not shown in this table. In both analyses it is controlled for socio-demographic variables and religious denominations as well. For this purpose the same variables as shown in table 1 are included but not shown here.

Only with regard to unemployment are the findings in line with our hypotheses and prior research. Many studies have shown that unemployment leads to a general deterioration of the social situation and the personal mood of those affected by it (Inglehart & Rabier, 1986, p. 20; Frey & Stutzer, 2002, p. 95ff.; Hayo & Seifert, 2003). The unemployed suffer in many regards: Their financial situation is bad, and they have the feeling of being socially "useless", of being hindered to apply and develop further their knowledge and capacities, of lacking a perspective for the future, thus, of having no control over their life circumstances (as shown already by the classical Austrian study by Jahoda et al. (1997), carried out in the 1930ies).

Also occupational status exerts significant effects on happiness. Here, many studies have shown that the semi- and unskilled workers continue to represent a deprived social class: Not only in terms of income and working conditions, but also in terms of little autonomy and influence at the workplace and in society (see Braverman, 1974; Sennett & Cobb, 1972; Hout et al., 1993, p. 263). The opposite is true for the managerial and professional groups. We have seen that they feel to have more freedom of control in their life. Yet, this freedom does not translate into a corresponding higher happiness. These results seem to corroborate those of an Australian study which found "that while high status fails greatly to enhance well-being, low status does generate a sense of ill-being." (Headey et al., 1984, p. 126) Overall, however, subjective well-being clearly does reflect vertical social inequality (see also Noll & Habich, 1990 and Schulz et al., 1988 for similar findings in Germany and Austria).

A variable whose importance for happiness has been stressed particularly by economists is income. In our data, the objective level of income has no significant effect on happiness (see also Frey & Stutzer, 2002, p. 73ff; Myers, 2000, p. 59ff.). However, the subjective perception of the financial situation has the strongest effect on happiness and life satisfaction (see Headey et al., 1984, and Fuentes & Rojas, 2001 for similar findings). Our interpretation of this finding is not, however, in terms of relative deprivation – that people compare themselves only to others who live in similar circumstances. What is more important from our general theoretical point of view is the feeling if an income is adequate for mastering one's daily life. Men who grew up in poor families see that situation not only in terms of material deprivation, but as leading to "chaotic, arbitrary, and unpredictable behavior [...] in other words, as depriving men of the capacity to act rationally, to exercise self-control" (Sennett & Cobb, 1972, p. 22). In fact, this variable of the subjective estimation of one's financial situation had also a strong effect on the feeling of being free and autonomous in one's daily decisions.

The plausibility of this interpretation is confirmed by the finding that the objective level of income can be rather low without affecting happiness negatively. Two additional aspects may be relevant here. First, changes in income over time (Saris, 2001). An individual adapts himself to a certain level of income and therefore clearly feels a loss or an improvement at this level. Biswas-Diener and Diener (2001) carried out an interesting study on three very poor groups in Calcutta (slum dwellers, prostitutes and homeless individuals living on the streets); they found that these people were not as unhappy as one could expect; their life also included several positive aspects, such as rewarding families or religious commitments, the feeling of being "good (moral) people". Thus, the element of self-determination and freedom comes in here again. A second factor explaining the lack of an association between level of income and happiness has to do with attitudes toward income. People with materialistic orientations are less happy (Ryan & Dziurawiec, 2001). The striving toward becoming rich has no in-built limit and the psychic efforts and time investment necessary for it may turn away energies from other, more directly satisfying behavior patterns and styles of life.

Subjective life situation and evaluation as determinants of happiness. In table 2 three variables have been included in this regard: subjective class placement, subjective feeling of health, and satisfaction with the financial situation of the household. We have already seen that all these dimensions are highly relevant from the perspective of the individual feeling of freedom of decision. It turns out, that they also exert significant effects on happiness and life satisfaction. The effects of the subjective financial and health situation are by far the strongest of all variables in this analysis (for similar findings concerning health see Headey et al., 1984; Fuentes & Rojas, 2001). Finally, also the variable of freedom of decision as such has significant positive effects both on happiness and life satisfaction. Thus, the findings corroborate our central hypothesis also in this immediate regard.

In the foregoing section, we found that the perception of good chances for poor people to escape their lot was significantly related to the feeling of personal freedom. This kind of perception seems to be important for happiness and life satisfaction as well; persons who see their society as offering such chances are also more happy and satisfied with their own life.

Thus, the findings suggest a clear overall interpretation of the findings concerning the effects of the personal situation and the immediate social context on happiness. Both the strong direct effect of freedom as well as of several other associations have shown that the amount of self-control in one's daily life contributes substantially to happiness and life satisfaction. Yet, a high degree of freedom evidently does not automatically lead to happiness (as shown by the only moderate level of happiness among managers), and a moderate or below average level of freedom reduce happiness (as it is evident in the cases of students, housewives and retired people). We have to conclude from these findings that freedom and self-control on the one hand, and happiness and life satisfaction on the other are partly independent human goals and states.

Now, let us look at the effects of the macro-social variables on happiness, controlling for all other influences. The findings in table 2 of the multiple regression analysis provide a further confirmation of the dynamic action-theoretical approach developed in this paper. This approach does not consider the objective ("static") situation of an individual at a certain point in time as the main basis for his or her subjective evaluation of that situation but the way how a person feels to be able to cope with that situation, in view of past experiences and future expectations.

The economic prospects of a country are very decisive, but also the objective level of wealth has an impact on happiness. Here we find several effects. First, while GNP/head had no effect on the feeling of freedom, it has significant positive effects on happiness and life satisfaction. Even more important is the effect of economic growth during the 1990ies: If it was high, people not only felt more free (as shown earlier) but are happier and more satisfied with life as well (see also Hayo & Seifert, 2003).

Let us look at this relationship also in graphic form. Figure 5 shows the scattergram of nations according to GNP/head and the mean level of life satisfaction of their populations. By and large, there is no evidence of a clear linear correlation. The distribution approximates an exponential curve or curvilinear association (Frey & Stutzer, 2002 found a similar association; linear relations, however, are reported in Diener et al., 1995; Schyns, 1998). There exist three different groups: First, the post-communist societies with a rather low GNP/head and low happiness; second, the more developed and rich countries with relatively high levels of happiness; third, the very poor countries with a wide variation in happiness; these include the countries with the lowest (Moldavia) and the highest value in happiness (Colombia) in the whole sample. Thus, affluence seems to guarantee a certain level of satisfaction, but obviously there exist factors beside wealth which lead to happiness.

Figure 5: GNP per Capita and Life Satisfaction in 41 Countries

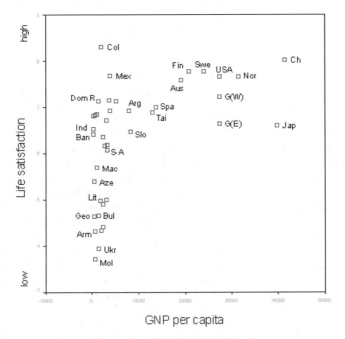

Source: World Value Survey 1995.

The positive effect of national economic wealth on happiness confirms many other studies; it is nevertheless surprising that the effect is not stronger given the extreme variation of standards of living in the countries compared. In Bangladesh and India, GNP/head was less than 400 US-$ in the mid-Nineties, in Azerbaijan, Georgia and Pakistan around 500 $. Switzerland, on the other hand, had a National Product a hundred times as much as these poor countries (41,000 $); in Japan, Norway, Germany and the United States, GNP was around 30,000 $. It is astonishing that these extreme income differences between countries (which, moreover, have increased over the last decades; see Milanovic, 2002) do not correlate more strongly with differences in people's life satisfaction. This clearly proves that pure materialistic-economic explanations of happiness would be wholly incomplete.

Surprising, and contrary to our hypothesis, are the findings concerning the effects of income distribution (measured by the GINI-index). Table 2 shows that it also has no effect on life satisfaction and happiness. This finding becomes plausible when we look at the countries with regard to overall inequality. Far on top in this regard are the South American countries which, at the same time, are characterized by very high levels of happiness; a rather low level of income inequality, however, is typical for the post-communist countries which, at the same time, are characterized by the lowest levels of happiness of their citizens. Our findings in this regard seem to confirm liberal critiques of an excessive and enforced egalitarianism, such as the economist Friedrich Hayek (1960) or the sociologist Helmut Schoeck (1960).

These findings also make sense seen from the perspective of John Rawls' "liberal" theory of justice. This theory asserts that inequality is tolerable if it is combined with positive perspectives for an improvement of all and, thus, also acceptable to the less privileged groups (Rawls, 1972; Methfessel & Winterberg, 1998).

Already in the last sections, we found that the possibility of an improvement of the overall economic situation is a very important fact besides the issues of present poverty and inequality. Table 2 also shows that the growth of the GDP over the Nineties had a significant and rather strong effect on happiness. There exist strong positive and nearly linear associations[8] between economic growth and the feelings of freedom and happiness/life satisfaction at the macro level. Also changes in levels of inflation are correlated significantly with happiness over time (Frey & Stutzer, 2002, p. 111ff.). These correlations probably help to explain the striking result that happiness is rather high in most Latin American countries, but very low in the post-communist Eastern European countries. The Latin American countries had rather high growth rates during the Nineties (between 3 and 8 %). In contrast, the Eastern European countries and the successor states of the former Soviet Union experienced sharp declines in standards of living connected with their transition from centrally planned, state socialist systems to market societies (with decreases of GNP between 3 and 10 %). In a survey on ten post-communist East European countries in the early Nineties, Hayo & Seifert (2003) found that only between 17 % (Poland) and 58 % (Czech Republic) of the respondents considered their economic household situation as satisfactory, compared with 86 % in Austria; only 35-50 % expected an improvement (except Croatia with 70 %). Evidently, the future economic perspectives of a country make people optimistic also about their own situation; they give them the feeling that opportunities are there and it is also in their own discretion how their situation will develop. People in Latin America score highest in the WVS-item "work makes life worth living" as well.

Political freedom is no decisive determinant for individual life satisfaction within the population. Table 2 shows, finally, that the macro dimension of political freedom does not have the expected positive effect on happiness (such an effect did also not turn out with regard to subjectively felt freedom). The consideration was that in stable democratic systems and free market societies, both individual households and enterprises can rely on trustful and reliable relations to other people and organizations, as well as to the state and its officials; this would enhance their individual possibilities of long-term planning. Frey and Stutzer (2002, p. 133ff; see also Schyns, 1998) have argued that instruments of direct democracy, like referenda, can considerably enlarge the real political freedom and influence of the citizens; for Switzerland they show that the degree of participation in the different provinces (cantons) has a significant effect on the happiness of the people living there. Switzerland as a whole occupies a top position among all countries compared in this paper with regard to political and economic freedom and happiness of the population. Yet, in a worldwide sample freedom as such seems not to make a big difference. The individual feeling of being in command of one's life, as well as happiness and life satisfaction, seem to be relatively independent from political circumstances; what counts more is a dynamic economic development in the past and positive economic perspectives for the future.

CONCLUDING REMARKS

Let us first summarize shortly the main findings, relate them to some other studies, and then draw some conclusions about further research. First, it can be said that our general hypothesis could be confirmed clearly, stating that individual happiness depends on the degree of freedom and choice an individual feels to have in his life. This finding is corroborated by earlier studies. Headey and associates (1984, p. 128) found that "personal competence (a feeling that one can control and organise one's life)" related most strongly to indices of positive and negative well-being. In a German study, Schulz et al. (1981), carried out a factor analysis of 42 variables relating to happiness. They found one factor which they called "happiness through freedom"; it included feelings of independence and freedom, the capacity to enjoy life, and to feel light-hearted and carefree.

By and large, our second hypothesis was also confirmed, stating that people will be more happy if they live in personal and societal circumstances providing them with more freedom of individual choice. Strong effects in this regard could be found for subjective health, satisfaction with the personal financial situation and for the perceived chances of an economic improvement of one's own situation in the future. Regarding economic well-being, it seems to be less the objective level of personal income or the objective level of wealth of a nation which is most relevant for happiness, but rather a positive economic development (economic growth) in the past and similar perspectives for the future.

We got only limited support, however, for our third and fourth hypotheses, stating that happiness will be higher in more open, democratic and in less stratified nations. Especially the situation in the Latin American countries contradicts our hypotheses on the relation between equality and happiness. These countries are characterized by the highest degrees of income inequality among all countries in our sample9, but – at the same time – their population is among the happiest around the world.

There exist at least two explanations for these findings. First, we have to differentiate between the situation in the personal life context and in society as a whole. It turns out that satisfaction with one's immediate life circumstances is much higher than satisfaction with the state of a nation as a whole (similar findings were reported for Australia in Eckersley, 2000, and for Germany in Glatzer & Zapf, 1984). In the worldwide *Pew Global Attitudes Project*, which asked about satisfaction with one's own life, one's nation and the world as a whole, the percentages satisfied declined clearly from the lowest to the highest level.[10] This decline of happiness can be explained very well within our framework which sees freedom of decision as an important variable mediating happiness: The smaller and more immediate the social context, the more possibilities an individual has to decide by himself, or herself about ongoing actions and to control the course of events; the larger this context, the less this is the case. Here, we can also refer to the marked tendency of men and women in general, to see one's own performance as being above average (Headey & Wearing, 1988).

Second, it is evident that there must exist other, positive determinants of happiness besides the affluence of a nation and its overall patterns of distribution. Here, we have to mention close personal and social relations whose significance for happiness has been noted by classical writers such as Tocqueville, Durkheim, or Tönnies. Barry Schwartz (2000) has recently argued that there exists an inherent tension between trying to be fully autonomous and free, and the wish for meaningful involvement in social groups. Also the striving for and attainment of material, extrinsic goods must not always increase happiness, but may also lead to new problems, such as envious competition, conflicts of decision, time stress and even depression and suicides (Zahn, 1960; Schoeck, 1960; Inglehart & Rabier, 1986; Etzioni, 1995; Eckersley, 2000; Schwartz, 2000).

From this point of view, an additional explanation can be given for the extremely low level of happiness in the poorer post-communist countries. With its over-emphasis on state intervention and provision, the communist system destroyed many private forms of networks and support and spontaneous, private forms of association. The far-reaching control of public opinion may have created a high level of distrust between citizens (Lewada, 1992). The data of the *World Value Survey* show that active religious participation is lowest in those countries, and people say least frequently that friends are very important. So, these findings point again to the fact that a certain level of individual freedom is indispensable for happiness. In this regard, we can conclude with Ruut Veenhoven (1999, p. 175) that "individualization enhances quality of life" (see also Boudon, 2002). Thus, one of the most interesting questions for research, following from our findings would be: Which are the combinations of individual freedom and social embedding which provide optimal conditions for subjective well-being?

A further promising new line of research would be that of carrying out in-depth studies on the factors that make people quite unhappy in some countries, and which make people very happy in other societies, especially in rather poor countries (such as in Latin America). Such research would be in line with the theoretical argument of a dual structure of happiness and mental health. According to this theory, happiness is more than just the absence of unhappiness or problems; it results only from positive self-concept dimensions and life experiences (Headey et al., 1984; Argyle, 1987; Haller, 1981; Csikszentmihalyi, 1990; Greenspoon & Saklofske, 2001; Vitterso & Nielsen, 2002). Such research would also balance the fact that the social sciences are focusing too much on negative issues and social problems, but neglect the positive factors contributing to growth, development and happiness (Seligman & Csikszentmihalyi, 2000). Finally, the research on the positive factors of happiness in poor countries would be highly relevant from the viewpoint of the most advanced and rich societies themselves. Here, established habits and life styles have to be changed and new ones invented which will be more in line with sustainable societal and ecological development for the world as a whole (Schulz, 1995).

NOTES

1   Thanks are expressed to the researchers who have carried out the World Value Survey in their respective countries as well as all those – especially Ronald Inglehart – who have contributed to the design of this highly valuable data set. Data sets have been delivered to us by the Central Archive, University of Cologne (Germany).
2   In this regard, the *International Social Survey Programme* (ISSP) might be stronger. Its modules, however, are more limited in their substantive range.
3   We tested empirically if this lack of nation-wide sampling made a difference by correlating the scores in the dependent variables "happiness" and "life satisfaction" between the overall samples and the subsamples of only city dwellers in all countries. The correlation coefficients were as high as .99, thus indicating that the differences are negligible.

4   For Spain, for instance, the survey included separately four provinces (Andalusia, Basque country, Galicia, Valencia), for Russia, three subsamples were covered (Russia, Moscow, Tambov).
5   The data are available under http://www.freedomhouse.org.
6   One reader of this paper argued that we should consider additional indicators for freedom at the societal level. We introduced an index of "economic freedom", developed by the Heritage Foundation (Miles et al. 2004). This index varies from 1.94 (Switzerland) to 4.78 (Azerbaijan). Highly rated in economic freedom are West-European and Anglo-Saxon countries; at the bottom (values over 3.50) we find most less-developed post-communist countries, China, India, Bangladesh and Peru. Between this index and GNP/head, however, exists a rather strong connection and if we introduce it into the regression, the effects of either GNP/head or growth of GNP disappear. Thus, we decided not to include this additional index for "economic freedom" into the models in table 1.
7   Concerning freedom, we use here the aggregated mean values from the WVS. In the multivariate analysis, an "external", independent measure is used. (See text below)
8   Pearson correlation coefficients are: growth x freedom: .62; growth x happiness: -.69; growth x life satisfaction: .77.
9   Income inequality, as measured by the GINI coefficient, lies between extremely high values of .45 and .60 in the South American countries, but only between .20 and .40 in most other countries and regions.
10   What the World Thinks in 2002, *The Pew Global Attitudes Project*, Washington, D.C.; see: http://www.people-press.org.

REFERENCES

Arendt, H. (1958): The Human Condition, Chicago: University of Chicago Press.
Argyle, M. (1987): The Psychology of Happiness, London/New York: Routledge.
Bellebaum, A. (ed.) (1992): Glück und Zufriedenheit. Ein Symposium, Opladen: Westdeutscher Verlag.
Biswas-Diener, R. & E. Diener (2001): Making the Best of a Bad Situation: Satisfaction in the Slums of Calcutta, Social Indicators Research 55, 329-53.
Boudon, R. (1999): Le sens de valeurs, Paris: Presses Universitaire de France.
Boudon, R. (2000): Déclin de la Morale? Déclin des valeurs? Québec: Ed. Nota Benel Cefan.
Bradburn, N. M. (1969): The Structure of Psychological Well-Being, Chicago: Aldine.
Braverman, H. (1974): Labour and Monopoly Capital, New York/London: Monthly Review Press.
Bréchon, P. (2002) : Les grandes enquetes internationales. (Eurobarometres, Valeurs, ISSP): Apports et limites, L'Année Sociologique 52, 105-30.
Campbell, A. (1981): The Sense of Well-Being in the America, New York: McGraw Hill.
Campbell, C. (1998): The Myth of Social Action, Cambridge: Cambridge University Press.
Csikszentmihalyi, M. (1990): Flow: The Psychology of Optimal Experience, New York: Harper & Row.
Deci, E. L. & R. M. Ryan (1985): Intrinsic Motivation and Self-Determination in Human Behavior, New York: Plenum Press.
Deeg, D. & R. van Zonneveld (1989): Does Happiness Lengthen Life? R. Veenhoven (ed.): How Harmful is Happiness? Consequences of Enjoying Life or not, Rotterdam/The Hague: Universitaire Pres Rotterdam, 29-43.
Diener, E. (2000): Subjective Well-Being. The Science of Happiness and a Proposal for a National Index. American Psychologist 55, 34-43.
Diener, E., M. Diener & C. Diener (1995): Factors Predicting the Subjective Well-being of Nations. Journal of Personality and Social Psychology 5, 851-64.
Diener, E. & E. Suh (1997): Measuring Quality of Life: Economic, Social, and Subjective Indicators. Social Indicators Research 40, 189-216.
Doi, T. (1973): The Anatomy of Dependence, Tokyo: Kodansha International.
Durkheim, E. (1960): Le Suicide, Paris: Presses Universitaires de France (1st ed. 1897).
Doyle, K. O. & S. Youn (2000): Exploring the Traits of Happy People. Social Indicators Research 52, 195-209.
Eckersley, R. (2000): The State and Fate of Nations: Implications of Subjective Measures of Personal and Social Quality of Life. Social Indicators Research 52, 3-27.
Etzioni, A. (1995): The Spirit of Community. Rights, Responsibilities and the Communitarian Agenda, Hammersmith/London: Fontana Press.
Frey, B. S. & A. Stutzer (2002): Happiness and Economics. How the Economy and Institutions Affect Well-Being, Princeton/Oxford: Princeton University Press.
Fromm, E. (1956): The Art of Loving, New York: Harper.

Fuentes, N. & M. Rojas (2001): Economic Theory and Subjective Well-Being: Mexico. Social Indicators Research 53, 289-314.

Glatzer, W. & W. Zapf (1984a): Lebensqualität in der Bundesrepublik. Objektive Lebensbedingungen und subjektives Wohlbefinden, Frankfurt/New York: Campus.

Goldstein, H. (1995): Multilevel Statistical Models, London: Edward Arnold.

Greenspoon, P. J. & D. H. Saklofske (2001): Toward an Integration of Subjective Well-Being and Psychopathology. Social Indicators Research 54, 81-108.

Gurin, G., J. Veroff & S. Feld (1960): Americans View Their Mental Health, New York: Basic Books.

Haller, M. (1981): Gesundheitsstörungen als persönliche und soziale Erfahrung. Eine soziologische Studie über verheiratete Frauen im Beruf, München/Wien: Oldenbourg/ Verlag für Geschichte und Politik.

Haller, M. (2002): Theory and Method in the Comparative Study of Values. European Sociological Review 18, 139-58.

Haller, M. (2003): Soziologische Theorie im systematisch-kritischen Vergleich, Opladen: Leske & Budrich (2nd ed.).

Haller, M. & M. Hadler (2002): Wer hat von den politischen Reformen der 90er Jahre profitiert? Modernisierungsgewinner und -verlierer in Ost- und Westeuropa und den USA. Europäische Rundschau 30/1, 115-27.

Hayek, F. A. (1960): The Constitution of Liberty, London/Chicago: Routledge & Kegan Paul/University of Chicago Press.

Hayo, B. & W. Seifert (2003): Subjective Economic Well-being in Eastern Europe. Journal of Economic Psychology 24, 329-48.

Headey, B., E. Holmström & A. Wearing (1984): Well-being and Ill-being: Different Dimensions. Social Indicators Research 14, 115-39.

Hout, M., C. Brooks & J. Manza (1993): The Persistence of Classes in Post-industrial Society. International Sociology 8, 259-76.

Inglehart, R. et al. (2000): World Values Surveys and European Value Surveys, 1981-1984, 1990-1993, and 1995-1997, ICPSR – Inter-University Consortium for Political and Social Research, University of Michigan (mimeo).

Inglehart, R. & J.-R. Rabier (1986): Aspirations Adapt to Situations – but Why are the Belgians so Much Happier than the French? A Cross-Cultural Analysis of the Subjective Quality of Life. F. M. Andrews (ed.): Research on the Quality of Life, Michigan: The Survey Research Center/Institute for Social Research, 1-56.

Inkeles, A. (1989): National Character Revisited. M. Haller, H.J. Hoffmann-Nowonty & W. Zapf (eds.): Kultur und Gesellschaft, Frankfurt/New York: Campus, 98-112.

Jahoda, M., P. Lazarsfeld & H. Zeisel (1997): Die Arbeitslosen von Marienthal: Ein soziographischer Versuch über die Wirkungen langandauernder Arbeitslosigkeit, Frankfurt am Main: Suhrkamp.

Kahnemann, D. & E. Diener (eds.) (1999): Well-Being: The Foundations of Hedonic Psychology, New York: Russel Sage Foundation.

Lane, R. A. (2000): The Loss of Happiness in Market Democracies, New Haven/London: Yale University Press.

Lewada, J. (1992): Die Sowjetmenschen 1989-1991. Soziogramm eines Zerfalls, Berlin: Argon (Russ. ed. 1991).

Magen, Z. (1996): Commitment beyond Self and Adolescence: The Issue of Happiness. Social Indicators Research 37, 235-67.

Methfessel, K. & J. Winterberg (1998): Der Preis der Gleichheit. Wie Deutschland die Chancen der Globalisierung verspielt, Düsseldorf/München: Econ.

Michalos, A. C. (1991): Global Report on Student Well-Being. Life Satisfaction and Happiness, Vol. I, New York: Springer.

Miles, M. A. et al. (2004): Index of Economic Freedom, Washington: Heritage Foundation.

Myers, D. G. (1993): The Pursuit of Happiness: Who is Happy and Why? New York: Avon.

Myers, D. G. (2000): The Funds, Friends, and Faith of Happy People. American Psychologist 55, 56-67.

Noll, H.-H. & R. Habich (1990): Individuelle Wohlfahrt: Vertikale Ungleichheit oder horizontale Disparitäten? Soziale Welt, Sonderband 7: Lebenslagen, Lebensläufe, Lebensstile, ed. by P. A. Berger & S. Hradil, 153-88.

Nozick, R. (1989): The Examined Life. Philosophical Meditations, New York: Simon & Schuster.

Przeworski, A. & H. Teune (1970): The Logic of Comparative Inquiry, New York: Wiley.

Rabash, J. et al. (2000): A User's Guide do MlWin, Version d.1d, Centre for Multilevel Modelling, Institute of Education, University of London.

Rawls, J. (1972): A Theory of Justice, London/Oxford/New York: Oxford University Press.

Ryan, R. M. & E. L. Deci (2000): Self-Determination Theory and the Facilitation of Intrinsic Motivation. Social Development, and Well-Being. American Psychologist 55, 68-78.
Ryan, L. & S. Dziurawiec (2001): Materialism and its Relationship to Life Satisfaction. Social Indicators Research 55, 185-97.
Saris, W. E. (2001): The Relationship between Income and Satisfaction: The Effect of Measurement Error as Suppressor Variables. Social Indicators Research 53, 117-36.
Schoeck, H. (1960): Envy. A Theory of Social Behaviour, New York: Harcourt, Brace & World.
Schulz, W. et al. (1981): Glücksvorstellungen, Glückserfüllung, psychische Belastung und deren sozio-strukturelle Variation, Bielefeld: Universität Bielefeld, Fakultät für Soziologie.
Schulz, W. et al. (1988): Subjektive Lebensqualität in Österreich. SWS-Rundschau 28, 162-73.
Schulz, W. (1995): Multiple-Discrepancies Theory Versus Resource Theory. Social Indicators Research 34, 153-69.
Schwartz, B. (2000): Self-Determination. The Tyranny of Freedom. American Psychologist 55, 79-88.
Schyns, P. (1998): Crossnational Differences in Happiness: Economic and Cultural Factors Explored. Social Indicators Research 43, 3-26.
Seligman, M.E.P. & M. Csikszentmihalyi (2000): Positive Psychology. American Psychologist 55, 5-14.
Sen, A. (1999): Development as Freedom, New York: Alfred Knopf.
Sennett, R. & J. Cobb (1972): The Hidden Injuries of Class, New York: Vintage Books.
Sève, L. (1972): Marxisme et théorie de la personnalité, Paris: Editions Sociales.
Tocqueville, A. (1947): Democracy in America, New York: Oxford University Press.
Veenhoven, R. (ed.) (1989): How Harmful is Happiness? Consequences of Enjoying Life or not, Rotterdam/The Hague: Universitaire Pres Rotterdam.
Veenhoven, R. (1993): Happiness in Nations: Subjective Appreciation of Life in 56 Nations 1946-1992, Rotterdam: Erasmus University Press.
Veenhoven, R. (1994): Is Happiness a Trait? Tests of the Theory that a Better Society Does not Make People any Happier. Social Indicators Research 32, 101-60.
Veenhoven, R. (1999): Quality-of-Life in Individualistic Society. A Comparison of 43 Nations in the early 1990's. Social Indicators Research 48, 157-86.
Verkley, H. & J. Stolk (1989): Does Happiness Lead into Idleness? Veenhoven, R. (ed.) (1989): How Harmful is Happiness? Consequences of Enjoying Life or not, Rotterdam/The Hague: Universitaire Pres Rotterdam, 79-93.
Vittersø, J., E. Roysamb & E. Diener (2002): The Concept of Life Satisfaction across Cultures: Exploring its Diverse Meaning and Relation to Economic Wealth. R. Cummins & E. Gallone (eds.), The Universality of Subjective Wellbeing Indicators, Dordrecht: Kluwer Academic Publishers, 81-103.
Vittersø, J. & F. Nielsen (2002): The Conceptual and Relational Structure of Subjective Well-being, Neuroticism, and Extraversion: Once again, Neuroticism is the Important Predictor of Happiness. Social Indicators Research 57, 89-118.

15. SATISFACTION WITH LIFE DOMAINS AND SALIENT VALUES FOR THE FUTURE

Analyses about Children and their Parents

Ferran Casas, Cristina Figuer, Mònica González, and Germà Coenders

Institut de Recerca sobre Qualitat de Vida (IRQV), Universitat de Girona, Spain

ABSTRACT

Within the frame of a cross-cultural project directed to explore how New Information and Communication Technologies (NICTs) affect the life of adolescents, a study of the relationship between life satisfaction domains and salient values for the future, as well as their relation with overall life satisfaction is presented. In order to explore to what extent the different country results could be considered really cross-culturally comparable, two basic topics, sensitive in any research of this kind, such as life domain satisfactions and salient values for the future, have been analyzed in-depth. A Principal Components Analysis (PCA) of each country data and of the total data set have been developed.

The sample is composed of 8,995 adolescents between the ages of 12 and 16 and 4,381 of their parents (48.7 % of the adolescents), from five different geographic regions: Catalonia (Spain), Western Cape (South Africa), Norway, Mumbai (India), and Rio de Janeiro (Brazil).

Results from PCA offer a four-dimensional structure as a good solution for life satisfaction domains and a three-dimensional structure for salient values, which are very similar in all the analyzed regions. Life satisfaction domains have been only explored among children. For salient values, a similar structure for children's and parents' data has been observed throughout all regions. Gender and age differences have been examined. The observed similarity of the structure of these two topics allows us to consider the possibility of comparing data for other topics included within the wider project.

INTRODUCTION[1]

During the past decades, a broad consensus among researchers has emerged, concerning psychological well-being as a key component of quality of life. Some authors call this phenomenon "subjective well-being" (Huebner, 1991; Huebner et al., 1998) or "subjective quality of life" (Cummins & Cahill, 2000). Most of them agree that it is composed of people's satisfaction with certain life domains, and life as a whole, and that it is correlated with other phenomena such as self-esteem, perceived control, perceived social support, and others.

Among these other correlates of well-being, some authors (Diener & Fujita, 1995; Diener, Suh et al., 1998; Csikzentmihalyi, 1997), have recently defended the inclusion of values, especially as a basis to explore psychological well-being in cross-cultural studies.

Value systems have a hierarchical structure, some of them being more nuclear than others (Rokeach, 1973). Although the value system of each individual is rela-

Wolfgang Glatzer, Susanne von Below, Matthias Stoffregen (eds.), Challenges for Quality of Life in the Contemporary World, 233-247.

tively stable, it may change in different social contexts and in different cultural conditions, and it is particularly influenced by the social and political developments within each society (Pinillos, 1982).

Nowadays, satisfaction with life as a whole is understood by many authors as a global evaluation of life (Veenhoven, 1994), in contrast to satisfaction in different domains, and the former is considered to be "something more than" the summing up of the latter. On the other hand, the two types of satisfaction can be explained both through individual and cultural differences (Diener, 1994). As an example, it has been repeatedly observed by Diener and Suh (1997) and Diener et al. (2000) that levels of satisfaction with life as a whole vary by country.

Satisfaction with life as a whole studies have often been conducted from an adult perspective. The study of values in relation to children's and adolescents' psychological well-being has been, compared to adults, even less considered by the research community. In the few occasions that children or adolescents have been explored, they have not always been systematically asked about their own opinions and perceptions (Alsinet, 2000). However, in the last two decades some exceptions can be identified showing that asking children and adolescents about their own life evaluations is of great interest. Consequently, in this paper, adolescents' satisfactions and their values have been explored by asking them directly.

One way of exploring adolescents' values is asking children to what extent they would like to be appreciated for some concrete values, once they get older. We have used this in previous research in order to identify different value structures between parents and adolescents (Casas, Buxarrais, et al., 2004). This same analysis will be extended to samples coming from five different countries.

METHOD

Sample

The data collection has involved questionnaires given to 8,995 boys and girls (aged 12 to 16) and 4,380 of their parents from five different countries (Spain, South Africa, Norway, India, and Brazil, cf. table 1).

The Spanish data have been collected on three different occasions and have been used as different samples. Data for the rest of the samples were obtained between 2000 and 2002.

Gender distribution is around 50 % in all samples, except the Indian one, where the percentage of boys is much higher than that of girls. The whole sample age mean is 13.94 years old (SD=1.18) and is very similar for all country samples. Parents' responses range from 29 % to 68 %, the whole sample percentage being about 48 %.

Instruments

Two questionnaires were designed for this research: one for adolescents and another one for their parents.

The original questionnaires were in Castilian-Spanish and in Catalan languages and had already been tested in previous studies. For the international study, the Spanish version was translated into English and participants from all research teams across the five countries discussed the results at an international meeting, where many cultural and social specific factors were then taken into account. As a result of this discussion, some items of the original questionnaires were changed and a few new ones were added. Then, the English version was translated into all other languages. In the cases of Brazilian-Portuguese and Norwegian, the translations also used the Spanish version, because at least one team member was fluent in Spanish. All translations were tested in each country, and a long e-mail discussion developed among all research teams, until agreement was reached on a new English standard version, and all translated questionnaires were re-adapted to that version.

Table 1: Sample Characteristics

	N	Boys	Girls	Age Mean	Parents
Spain 1999	1,634	792 (48.5 %)	842 (51.5 %)	14.12 (1.13)	666 (40.76 %)
Spain 2001	3,133	1,599 (51 %)	1,534 (49 %)	13.89 (1.24)	1,633 (52.12 %)
Spain 2002	291	127 (43.6 %)	164 (56.4 %)	13.77 (1.17)	143 (49.19 %)
India	1,125	700 (62.2 %)	425 (37.8 %)	13.65 (0.95)	763 (67.82 %)
South Africa	1,002	435 (43.4 %)	567 (56.6 %)	14.49 (1.08)	565 (56.39 %)
Norway	917	466 (50.8 %)	451 (49.2 %)	not available	347 (37.84 %)
Brazil	893	423 (47.4 %)	470 (52.6 %)	13.61 (1.15)	263 (29.45 %)
Total Sample	8,995	4,542 (50.5 %)	4,453 (49.5 %)	13.94 (1.18)	4,380 (48.69 %)

Source: Own calculations.

The questionnaire for adolescents includes closed and open-ended questions aimed at systematically exploring the different activities, perceptions and evaluations of adolescents in regard to different audiovisual media (television, computer and video console), and some of their facilities as well (educational CD-Roms, Internet and games). We have explored to what extent their activities involving these media are addressed in their conversations with parents, siblings, peers, teachers and other people. We also collected information about children's perspectives towards their future related to media use. Some general values, satisfaction with different life domains and overall life satisfaction, self-esteem, mastery and perceived social support have been additionally explored.

The questionnaire for parents includes only closed-ended items, which are very similar to the ones on the children's questionnaire in order to compare answers. Parents were asked about their present interest in NICTs (New Informational and Communication Technologies), the information they have about the above mentioned audiovisual media, their perceptions of how interested and informed their child is, how satisfied they think the child is with conversations about media with different people, and about their own values.

Measures

Most of the questions in the different questionnaire versions are exactly the same, and thus comparison is possible. For the goals of this paper only the following variables have been explored.

Overall life satisfaction
An item on overall life satisfaction measured through a five-point Likert scale, value 1 meaning "very dissatisfied" and 5 "very satisfied", was included.

Life satisfaction domains
Nine items exploring satisfaction with specific domains were included in the questionnaire. Domains are: satisfaction with *school performance*, with *learning*, with *time use*, with *amusement*, with *preparation for future*, with *family*, with *friends*, with *sports*, and with *own body*. In the 1999 and 2001 Spanish samples, this last domain was lacking. These variables are measured through a five-point Likert scale, value 1 meaning "very dissatisfied" and 5 "very satisfied".

Salient values for future
To explore adolescents' expectations they were asked to what extent they would like to be appreciated for some concrete values, when they get older. Parents also were asked to what extent they would like his/her child to be appreciated for the same concrete values, in the future. We have used this technique in previous research in order to identify different value structures between parents and adolescents (Casas, Buxarrais, et al., 2004). For the present study, twelve values were considered: *intelligence, technological skills, social skills, computer knowledge, professional status, family, sensitivity, sympathy, money, power, knowledge of the world* and *own image*. The *family* and *own image* values were not included in the parents' questionnaire for the 1999 Spanish sample. Variables regarding values were measured through a five-point Likert scale, value 1 meaning "not at all" and 5 "very much" (concerned about being appreciated).

PROCEDURE

First of all, school directors and presidents of the mothers and parents association of each selected school were contacted to ask for permission. The next step was to contact teachers responsible for each class-room group in order to establish the days and hours that were best for administering the questionnaires.

The questionnaires were group administered in their regular classroom. One of their usual teachers and one or two researchers were present during the administration and clarified any of the children's questions that arose. The session is usually about one hour long for the youngest children and about 35-40 minutes for the oldest ones.

At the end of the session we give each of the children a letter and a questionnaire for their parents in a sealed envelope, to be delivered by hand. They are asked to return it to the teacher within about one week, also in a sealed envelope. Parents were asked to co-operate in the research with their answers and the questionnaire may be answered by one of them or both together. In their questionnaire, parents are requested to answer with only the child in mind who had answered our school questionnaire. Both questionnaires have a code, so that they can be paired with each other.

RESULTS

Principal Component Analysis of Life Satisfaction Domains across Samples

Principal Component Analysis (PCA), with Varimax rotation, was used to explore how the nine items related to satisfaction with several domains of children's lives are organized in different satisfaction dimensions. The nine items referred to satisfaction with *school performance, learning, amusement, preparation for future, time use, family, friends, sports,* and *own body.* PCA analysis was therefore applied to the 7 available country samples and to the whole sample.[2]

2- and 3-dimensional structures with explained variances ranging from 46 % to 65 % are explored. Two kinds of items have been differentiated according to their loadings, in order to define those dimensions: nuclear and non-nuclear items. Nuclear items are those that consistently have its highest loading in a concrete dimension for all or almost all country samples as well as for the whole sample. Non-nuclear items are those with important loadings in a particular dimension but which also have important loadings in other dimensions and this being not necessarily consistent across samples. In the 2- or 3-dimensional structures it was not always evident how to classify an item into nuclear or non-nuclear, as the structures by samples may vary among each other. So, the decision of using four dimensions was taken in order to clarify the model.

The 4-dimensional structure appears to be conceptually clearer than the 2 or 3-dimensional one. In this new structure we obtained explained variances from 66 % to 75 %. Dimension I was named *Enjoying time satisfaction* and includes nuclear items such as satisfaction with *time use* and with *amusement.* Satisfaction with *school performance, learning* and *preparation for future* are nuclear items for Dimension II, which has been named *Learning related satisfaction.* Dimension III, *Family and friends,* includes satisfaction with *family* and with *friends.* Lastly, nuclear items of Dimension IV, called *Physical activities satisfaction,* are the items satisfaction with *sports* and with *own body* (table 2).

The distribution of nuclear items in the four different dimensions has shown to be the same for all countries and for the whole sample as well. Only few differences have been observed for Norway, where another structure in *Enjoying time satisfaction* and in *Physical activities satisfaction* dimensions is observed. These differences stem from the items of satisfaction with *amusement* and with *own body.*

Table 2: Adolescents' Satisfaction Domains

		Items	E '99	E '01	E '02	IND	SA	N	BR	Total
		N	1,634	3,133	291	1,125	1,002	917	893	8,995
I.	N	Time Use	X	X	X	X	X	X	X	X
		Amusem.	X	X	X	X	X	(2)	X	X
	NN	Sports			(3)				(2)	
		Own Body						X		(2)
		Learning							(2)	
		Prep. for Future	(2)	(2)		(2)	(2)	(3)	(3)	(2)
		Friends	(2)	(2)	(2)		(2)			(2)
II.	N	School Perform.	X	X	X	X	X	X	X	X
		Learning	X	X	X	X	X	X	X	X
		Prep. for Future	X	X	X	X	X	X	X	X
	NN	Time Use		(2)	(2)	(2)				(2)
		Family	(2)	(2)	(2)			(2)	(2)	(2)
III.	N	Family	X	X	X	X	X	X	X	X
		Friends	X	X	X	X	X	X	X	X
	NN	Sports			(2)					
		Amusem.	(2)	(2)				X	(2)	(2)
		Prep. for Future						(2)	(2)	(3)
IV.	N	Sports	X	X	X	X	X	X	X	X
		Own Body				X	X	X		X
	NN	Time Use								(3)
		Prep. for Future			(2)					
Expl. Variance (%)			74.2	74.9	73.6	66.4	67.0	73.5	71.1	68.0

Source: Own Calculations. (2)=Loadings are important but rank in the second place. (3)=Loadings are important but rank in the third place. Note: codes used for each country sample are Spain (E), India (IND), South Africa (SA), Norway (N) and Brazil (BR). Total means the whole sample. Dimensions: I: Enjoying Time; II: Learning Related; III: Family and Friends; IV: Physical Activities; N=Nuclear; NN=Non-nuclear.

Concretely, satisfaction with *own body*, which is a nuclear item of the *Physical activities dimension*, obtains its highest loading on the *Enjoying time* dimension in the case of Norway. And satisfaction with *amusement*, which is a nuclear item of the *Enjoying time* dimension, only ranks in the second place in this same dimension and obtains its highest loading on the *Family and friends* dimension.

Gender and age differences were studied in the whole sample. By gender, we observe significant statistical differences between boys and girls referring to punctuations in the *Learning related satisfaction* (t_{3598}=3.518; $p<0.0005$) and the *Physical activities satisfaction* (t_{3553}=9.552; $p<0.0005$) dimensions. In the first case, girls obtain higher scores than boys, whereas in the second case it is the other way around: Boys' punctuations are higher than girls'.

By age, only the *Enjoying time satisfaction* dimension is not related in any way with children's age.[3] A clear decrease of punctuations in the *Learning related satisfaction* dimension when adolescents grow up ($F_{4,2791}$=25.892; $p<0.0005$) can be observed. In relation with the *Family and friends satisfaction* dimension ($F_{4,2791}$=7.112; $p<0.0005$), the oldest adolescents (16-year olds) score significantly lower than the rest. Finally, in relation to the *Physical activities satisfaction* dimension ($F_{4,2791}$=2.489; p=0.041) 16-year olds obtain the lowest punctuations, whilst the 12-year olds are the ones who obtain the highest punctuations in this same dimension. The rest of boys and girls (13, 14, and 15-year olds) do not differ significantly among themselves or with the 12 and 16-year old adolescents.

Principal Component Analysis of Salient Values for Future: between Adolescents and Parents

The same statistical technique (PCA) was developed for the twelve items included in the questionnaire which measures expectations of values, both children's and parents'. Those values are the following ones: *intelligence, technological skills, social skills, computer knowledge, professional status value, family value, sensitivity, sympathy, money, power, knowledge of the world*, and *own image*. Family and own image values were not included in the first Spanish sample parents' questionnaire (1999), and so this sample is not computed in the whole sample PCA.

In the case at hand, for both children and parents, a 3-dimensional structure appeared and the distribution of nuclear items was consistent enough across samples.

Children's dimensions are the following: Dimension I, which we have called *Materialistic values*, includes as nuclear items money, power and own image. Intelligence, technological skills, computer knowledge, professional status, knowledge of the world and social skills conform the nuclear items of the second dimension, *Capacities and knowledge values*. Dimension III, called *Interpersonal relationship values* is composed by three nuclear items: family, sensitivity and sympathy. The explained variances range from 57 % to 65 % (table 3).

All nuclear items included in both dimensions I (*Materialistic values*) and III (*Interpersonal relationship values*) have their highest loadings on each dimension respectively, and this is true for the 7 samples and the whole sample as well. In contrast, only two items in dimension II (*Capacities and knowledge values*) obtain the highest loading for all samples (by country and whole sample). These two items are *intelligence* and *practical skills*. The other items (*computer knowledge, professional status, knowledge of the world*, and *social skills*) show differences by sample. *Com-*

puter knowledge belongs to dimension I in Norway, *professional status* to dimension I again in Norway and to dimension III in Brazil.

Table 3: Adolescents' Salient Values for Future when They Become 21 Years Old

		Items	E '99	E '01	E '02	IND	SA	N	BR	Total
		N	1,634	3,133	291	1,125	1,002	917	893	8,995
I.	N	Money	X	X	X	X	X	X	X	X
		Power	X	X	X	X	X	(2)	X	X
		Own Image	X	X	X	X	X	X	X	X
	NN	World Kno.	X	X	(2)	(2)	X	(2)	X	(2)
		Prof. Status	(3)					X	(3)	(3)
		Computer Knowledge	(2)	(2)	(2)	(2)	(2)	X		(2)
		Family						(2)		
II.	N	Intelligence	X	X	X	X	X	X	X	X
		Tech. Skills	X	X	X	X	X	X	X	X
		Computer Knowledge	X	X	X	X	X	(2)	X	X
		Prof. Status	X	X	X	X	X	(2)	(2)	X
		World Kno.	(2)	(2)	X	X	(2)	X	(2)	X
		Soc. Skills	(2)	X	X	X	(2)	X	X	X
	NN	Own Image				(2)		(2)		
		Family			(2)	(2)	(2)			(2)
		Power			(2)					
		Sympathy								
III.	N	Family	X	X	X	X	X	X	X	X
		Sensitivity	X	X	X	X	X	X	X	X
		Sympathy	X	X	X	X	X	X	X	X
	NN	Soc. Skills	X	(2)	(2)		X	(2)	(2)	(2)
		Prof. Status	(2)	(2)	(2)	(2)		(3)	X	(2)
		Intelligence	(2)	(2)	(2)					
		Own Image		(2)	(2)					
		World Kno.	(3)							
Expl. Variance (%)			58.8	63.1	62.5	60.3	57.9	64.2	62.3	62.1

Source: Own Calculations. (2)=Loadings are important but rank in the second place. (3)=Loadings are important but rank in the third place. Note: codes used for each country sample are Spain (E), India (IND), South Africa (SA), Norway (N) and Brazil (BR). Total means the whole sample. Dimensions I: Materialistic, II: Capacities and Knowledge Values, III: Interpersonal Relationship Values; N= Nuclear, NN=Non-nuclear; World Kno.=Knowledge of the World.

The *Social skills* value belongs to dimension III in the first Spanish sample (1999) and South Africa. *Knowledge of the world* obtains the highest loadings in dimension I in the case of the first and the second Spanish samples (1999 and 2001), South Africa and Brazil. The decision to consider this last item as part of dimension II was made according to the PCA results obtained with the whole sample.

Gender and age differences were studied in the whole sample. By gender, we observe differences in all three studied dimensions. For the *Materialistic values* ($t_{7969}=15.933$; $p<0.0005$) and *Capacities and knowledge values* ($t_{7966}=7.031$; $p<0.0005$) dimensions, boys obtain higher punctuations than girls, whereas in the *Interpersonal relationships values* dimension ($t_{7938}=19.947$; $p<0.0005$) the findings are the other way around. By age, differences are observed in *Materialistic values* ($F_{4,7218}=9.354$; $p<0.0005$) and in *Interpersonal relationships* ($F_{4,7218}=10.302$; $p<0.0005$). In the former dimension, adolescents from 12 to 14 have significantly higher scores compared to the 16-year olds. In the latter dimension, we observe an increase in the punctuations as adolescents grow up.

Parents' dimensions appear to be the same as children's. Nuclear items included in each dimension are also the same with just one exception: *social skills* which belonged to the *Capacities and knowledge values* dimension for children is now part of the *Interpersonal relationship values* dimension. The variability of variances ranges from 56% to 65% (table 4).

The three items considered nuclear for *Materialistic values* (*money*, *power*, and *own image*) are so for the seven samples and the whole one as well. In relation to the *Capacities and knowledge* dimension, the *professional status* item obtains the highest loading in the *Materialistic values* dimension for Norway and on the *Interpersonal relationships* dimension in the second and third Spanish sample (2001 and 2002), as well as in the whole sample. *Knowledge of the world* obtains the highest loading on the *Interpersonal relationship values* dimension for the first and the second Spanish sample (1999 and 2001).

Related to the *Interpersonal relationship values* dimension, the *family* and *social skills* items show differences by sample. The highest loadings for *Family* are found in the *Materialistic values* dimension for Norway and the *Capacities and knowledge values* dimension in South Africa. Finally, *social skills* highest loadings are detected in the *Capacities and knowledge values* dimension in India and Brazil.

Gender and age of the son or daughter have been studied in the whole sample. Differences are detected in the *Materialistic values* ($t_{3220}=2.503$; $p=0.012$) and *Interpersonal relationship values* ($t_{3132}=2.424$; $p=0.015$) dimensions. Boys' parents score higher than girls' in the first dimension and lower in the second one. By adolescents' age, differences are observed in the same two dimensions: *Materialistic values* ($F_{4,2899}=2.601$; $p=0.034$) and *Interpersonal relationship values* ($F_{4,2899}=3.104$; $p=0.015$). However, the tendency is not clear in any of the cases.

Table 4: Parents' Salient Values for their Children's Future when They Become 21 Years Old

		Items	E '99	E '01	E '02	IND	SA	N	BR	Total
		N	666	1,633	143	763	565	347	263	4,380
I.	N	Money	X	X	X	X	X	X	X	X
		Power	X	X	X	X	X	X	X	X
		Own Image		X	X	X	X	X	X	X
	NN	Family		(3)				X		(3)
		Prof. Status			(2)	(3)		X		(3)
		Computer Knowledge		(2)		(2)	(2)	(2)		(2)
		World Kno.	(3)	(2)		(2)				(2)
II.	N	Intelligence	X	X	X	X	X	X	X	X
		Tech. Skills	X	X	X	X	X	X	X	X
		Computer Knowledge	X	X	X	X	X	(2)	X	X
		Prof. Status	X			X	X	(2)	X	(2)
		World Kno.	(2)	(3)	X	X	X	X	X	X
	NN	Soc. Skills	(2)	(2)	(2)	X		(2)	X	(2)
		Own Image		(2)	(2)				(2)	
		Family		(2)		(2)	X			(2)
		Sympathy							(2)	
		Power					(2)			
III.	N	Family		X	X	X	(2)	(2)	X	X
		Sensitivity	X	X	X	X	X	X	X	X
		Sympathy	X	X	X	X	X	X	X	X
		Soc. Skills	X	X	X	(2)	X	X	(2)	X
	NN	Prof. Status		X	X	(2)			(2)	X
		World Kno.	X	X	(2)			(2)	(2)	(3)
		Tech. Skills			(2)		(2)			
		Own Image		(2)						
		Intelligence					(2)			
		Expl. Variance (%)	61.6	59.7	56.8	64.9	63.2	62.4	58.6	62.1

Source: Own Calculations. (2)=Loadings are important but rank in the second place. (3)=Loadings are important but rank in the third place. Note: codes used for each country sample are Spain (E), India (IND), South Africa (SA), Norway (N) and Brazil (BR). Total means the whole sample. Dimensions I: Materialistic, II: Capacities and Knowledge Values, III: Interpersonal Relationship Values; N= Nuclear, NN=Non-nuclear; World Kno.=Knowledge of the World.

Children's and parents' dimensions of values were also correlated among each other. All correlations are significant but not very high. They are displayed in table 5:

Table 5: Correlations of the Different Value Dimensions between Parents and Adolescents

Value Dimensions	Pearson Correlations	*p*-Value
Materialistic	0.295	<0.0005
Capacities and Knowledge	0.176	<0.0005
Interpersonal Relationship	0.185	<0.0005

Source: Own Calculations.

Correlations among Overall Life Satisfaction, Life Domains Satisfaction and Salient Values for Future

Overall life satisfaction correlates positively and significantly with all four life domains satisfaction dimensions:
-    Enjoying time satisfaction ($r=0.313$; $p<0.0005$).
-    Learning satisfaction ($r=0.292$; $p<0.0005$).
-    Family and friends satisfaction ($r=0.318$; $p<0.0005$).
-    Physical activities satisfaction ($r=0.255$; $p<0.0005$).
It also correlates positively and significantly with 2 out of 3 value dimensions with:
-    Capacities and knowledge values ($r=0.094$; $p<0.0005$).
-    Interpersonal relationship values ($r=0.134$; $p<0.0005$).
Correlations among life domains satisfaction dimensions and value dimensions are displayed in table 6.

Table 6: Correlations among Life Domains Satisfaction Dimensions and Salient Values Dimensions

		Value Dimensions		
		Materialistic	Capacities and Knowledge	Interpersonal Relationship
Satisfaction Dimension	Enjoying Time	$r=0.088$ $p<0.0005$	$r=0.080$ $p<0.0005$	$r=0.091$ $p<0.0005$
	Learning	-	$r=0.089$ $p<0.0005$	$r=0.077$ $p<0.0005$
	Family and Friends	-	$r=0.063$ $p<0.0005$	$r=0.146$ $p<0.0005$
	Physical Activities	$r=0.037$ $p=0.036$	-	-

Source: Own Calculations. -: non statistically significant (p>0.05).

When exploring correlations among all of these measures and the sample place, we observe a high number of coincidences and few differences across countries. The most important differences are the following:

Overall life satisfaction does not correlate with the *Capacities and Knowledge values* dimension in the Spain (2002), Norway, and India samples.

The *Learning satisfaction* dimension correlates significantly and negatively with the *Materialistic values* dimension in the Spain (2001) sample, while it does not correlate with the *Capacities and Knowledge values* dimension in the South Africa, India and Brazil samples. Also, no correlations could be found within the *Interpersonal relationship values* dimension in the Spain (2002), South Africa and India samples.

While the *Enjoying time satisfaction* dimension does not correlate with any value dimension in the Spain (2002) sample, it does correlates positively with the *Materialistic values dimension* in the South Africa and India samples as well as the *Materialistic* and *Interpersonal relationship values* dimensions in the Brazil sample. A positive correlation with the *Materialistic* and *Capacities and knowledge values* dimensions can also be observed in the Norway sample.

The *Family and friends satisfaction* dimension correlates significantly and negatively with the *Materialistic values* dimension in the 2001 and 2002 Spanish samples; while it does not correlate with the *Capacities and knowledge values* dimension in Spain (1999 and 2002), Norway, and India.

The *Physical activities satisfaction* dimension does not correlate with the *Materialistic values* dimension in Norway and Brazil; whereas a significant and positive correlation with the *Capacities and knowledge values* dimension can be found in the Spain 1999 and 2001 samples.

Although the Pearson correlation coefficients are generally not very high in absolute value, it is worth mentioning that country sample correlations are generally higher than whole sample ones.

DISCUSSION

In this paper, relationships between life satisfaction domains and salient values for the future, as well as their relation with overall life satisfaction have been explored in a sample of 8,995 adolescents and 4,381 of their parents from five different countries.

In regard to overall life satisfaction and life satisfaction domains, some observations can be made. As expected, different life domains are related positively with overall life satisfaction, indicating that life as a whole is not simply the summing up of the several life domains (see, e.g., Veenhoven, 1994). Interestingly, a similar satisfaction domains structure among each country sample has been observed. This suggests that a common understanding among adolescents of the items assessing life satisfaction domains – beyond the individual and cultural differences generally attributed to them (Diener, 1994) – can be inferred. However, and according to Cummins (1996), it would be desirable to explore more satisfaction domains in the future in order to achieve more depth in the life satisfaction domains structure, especially in those dimensions with fewer items.

The analysis of the results by gender for the *Learning related satisfaction* dimension show higher mean scores for girls than for boys, whereas for the *Physical ac-*

tivities satisfaction dimension it is the other way around. Throughout all samples, such differences seem to confirm common stereotypes. The oldest (16-years-old) boys and girls show lower punctuations in satisfaction related to the *Learning* dimension, to the *Family and friends* dimension, and to the *Physical activities* dimension than the youngest ones (12-years-old). Such results may be explained by their different stages in adolescence. In relation to this, Verdugo and Sabeh (2002) state that age is one of the parameters that should be taken especially into account when studying life satisfaction in non-adult populations.

A future improvement of this research approach should include asking parents about the satisfaction with the same domains than adolescents and about their overall life satisfaction. This would be very helpful to show coincidences between generations, as we have noticed in the case of values.

When analyzing results both from parents and adolescents about salient values for the future, despite of the high similarity of value structures among samples, explanations are not as clear as they have been in the case of life satisfaction domains because some items have loadings in different dimensions and the distribution of these loadings is not the same in all the studied countries.

As expected, the comparison between parents' and adolescents' values has turned out to be very interesting. The high similarity between adolescents' and their parents' value structure, which seems to question the so called *Generation Gap*, was more unexpected. These results are, however, in line with the ones obtained by Astill, Feather et al. (2002) with a sample of 1,239 Australian adolescents. In accordance with the authors, the higher influence in the process of adolescents' value acquisition seems to arise from parents' beliefs and values, besides those defended by peers. Differences between adolescents' and their parents' values are also minimal in the study conducted by Thomson and Holland (2002) in the United Kingdom. For instance, both generations highlighted the importance of family values.

Once again and according to gender stereotypes, girls obtain higher scores in the *Interpersonal relationships values* dimension than boys, and lower in the *Materialistic values* and *Capacities and knowledge values* dimensions. This same pattern can be identified in parents' answers: Girls' parents get higher punctuations in *Interpersonal relationships values* than boys' parents, and lower in *Materialistic values*.

By age, younger adolescents give more importance to *Materialistic values* and less to *Interpersonal relationships values* than the older ones. These differences and unclear tendencies in parents' answers related to the age of their son or daughter, lead us to think that they should be deeply explored in future studies to search for explanations.

It is worth mentioning that the *Materialistic values* dimension is the only value dimension that does not correlate with overall life satisfaction, in contrast to the negative relationships found by Ryan and Dziurawiec (2001). Oishi, Diener et al. (1999) think that weak relationships among materialistic values and well-being in general, could be due to the fact that people defending these kinds of values are less likely to reach the objectives they want to reach.

Correlations between life domain satisfaction and value dimensions are generally low and in some cases statistically non significant. These results seem to be in agreement with those of Sagiv and Schwartz (2000).

Finally, the observed similarity of the structure of the two topics explored in this paper (satisfaction domains and salient values) allows us to consider the possibility of comparing data of other topics included within the wider project. The obtained results can be thus understood as a first descriptive stage that opens the door to more accurate statistical analysis. However, the exploration of other values, so important in understanding today's societies (as tolerance, personality or solidarity), is still to be done.

NOTES

1   Acknowledgements are due to the country project directors and their associates: Per Egil Mjaavatn (Norwegian University of Science and Technology, Trondheim, Norway), Usha Nayar (Tata Institute of Social Sciences, India), Irene Rizzini (Pontifícia Universidade Católica do Rio de Janeiro, Brazil), Rose September (Western Cape University, South Africa) and Ferran Casas (Catalan Network of Child Researchers – XCIII – in co-operation with the University of Girona, Spain) for permitting us to use part of their project and to Childwatch International, Oslo, for sponsorship.
2   PCA for whole sample does not include 1999 and 2001 Spanish samples because *own body* item was not included in the questionnaire.
3   Norway is not included in this analysis because age of each subject was only collected as an interval in this country sample.

REFERENCES

Alsinet, A. (2000): El Benestar en la Infància, Lleida: Pagès editors.
Astill, B.R., Feather, N.T. & Keeves, J.P. (2002): A multilevel analysis of the effects of parents, teachers and schools on student values. Social Psychology of Education 5, 345-63.
Csikzentmihalyi, M. (1997): Finding Flow: The Psychology of Engagement with Everyday Life, New York: Basic Books.
Casas, F., M. R. Buxarrais, C. Figuer, M. González, J. M. Rodríguez, A. Tey & E. Noguera (2004): Los Valores y su Influencia en la Satisfacción Vital de los Adolescentes entre los 12 y los 16 Años: Estudio de Algunos Correlatos'. [Values and their Influence in the Life Satisfaction of Adolescents between 12 and 16 Years Old: A Study of some Correlates]. In press.
Cummins, R. (1996): The domains of life satisfaction: an attempt to order chaos. Social Indicators Research 38, 303-28.
Cummins, R. & J. Cahill (2000): Avances en la Comprensión de la Calidad de Vida Subjetiva [Advances in Subjective Quality of Life comprehension]. Intervención Psicosocial 9 (2), 185-98.
Diener, E. (1994): El Bienestar Subjetivo [Subjective well-being]. Intervención Psicosocial 3 (8). 67-113.
Diener, E. & F. Fujita (1995): Resources, Personal Strivings, and Subjective Well-being: A Nomothetic and Idiographic Approach. Journal of Personality and Social Psychology 68, 926-35.
Diener, E.; C. L. Gohm, E. Suh & S. Oishi (2000): Similarity of the Relations between Marital Status and Subjective Well-being across Cultures. Journal of Cross-cultural Psychology, 31 (4), 419-36.
Diener, E. & E. Suh (1997): National Differences in Subjective Well-being. D. Kahneman, E. Diener and N. Schwartz: Well-being: The Foundations of Hedonic Psychology, New York: Russell Sage Foundation.
Diener, E., E. Suh & S. Oishi (1998): Recent Studies on Subjective Well-being. Indian Journal of Clinical Psychology 24, 25-41.
Huebner, E. S. (1991): Correlates of Life Satisfaction in Children. School Psychology Quaterly 6, 103-11.
Huebner, E. S., J. E. Laughlin, C. Asch & R. Gilman (1998): Further Validation of the Multidimensional Student's Life Satisfaction Scale. Journal of Psychoeducational Assessment 16 (2), 118-34.
Oishi, S., Diener, E.F., Lucas, R.E. & Suh, E.M. (1999): Cross-cultural Variations in Predictors of Life Satisfaction: Perspectives from Needs and Values. Personality and Social Psychology Bulletin 25 (8), 980-90.
Pinillos, J. L. (1982): El Cambio de los Sistemas de Valores en las Sociedades Desarrolladas y en las Sociedades en Desarrollo [Change in Value systems in Developed and Developing Societies]. Reunión Internacional sobre Psicología de los Valores, Policopied.
Rokeach, M. (1973): The Nature of Human Values, New York: The Free Press.
Ryan, L. & S. Dziurawiec (2001): Materialism and its Relationship to Life Satisfaction. Social Indicators Research 55, 185-97.

Sagiv, L. & Schwartz, S.H. (2000): Value priorities and subjective well-being: Direct relations and congruity effects. European Journal of Social Psychology 30, 177-98.

Thomson, R. & Holland, J. (2002): Young people, social change and the negotiation of moral authority. Children & Society 16, 103-15.

Veenhoven, R. (1994): El Estudio de la Satisfacción con la Vida [The study of Life Satisfaction]. Intervención Psicosocial 3 (9), 87-116.

Verdugo, M.A. & Sabeh, E.N. (2002). Evaluación de la percepción de calidad de vida en la infancia [Child's Perception of Quality of Life Assessment]. Psicothema 14 (1), 86-91.

16. PARENTAL DIVORCE AND THE WELL-BEING OF ADOLESCENT CHILDREN

Changes between 1984-1999 in the Netherlands

Anna Lont and Jaap Dronkers[1]

University of Amsterdam, The Netherlands,
and European University Institute in San Domenico di Fiesole, Italy

ABSTRACT

In this paper we address the question: "Have the negative correlations between particular aspects of the well-being of children and parental divorce changed during the 1984-1999 period in the Netherlands?" We used the NIBUD school-surveys of 1984, 1990, 1992, 1994, 1996, and 1999 to compare for every year (aspects of) the well-being of adolescents living in complete families with that of their peers living in single-mother- or single-father-families. The results indicate that there are no significant differences between single-parent families and complete families in the late 1990s compared to the situation in the 1980s. A comparison of the early and late 1990s between single-parent families and complete families also shows hardly any significant differences, except for the amount of money children received from their parents in single-parent families (get less in single-mother families than in single-father families) and the expected age children expect to leave their parental home in single-father-families (at a higher age in the 1990s), so approximating the situation in complete families.

INTRODUCTION

To date, Dutch research on the correlations between parental divorce and the well-being of their children shows that it is not so much the divorce itself but the quarrelling that goes with divorce (both before and after) that has the greatest negative effects on the well-being of the children concerned (Bosman, 1993: Borgers, Dronkers & van Praag, 1996; Dronkers, 1996, 1997; Spruyt & de Goede, 1997; Fischer & de Graaf, 2001; for a divergent but incorrect interpretation of the research results: van Gelder, 2000). American research (Amato & Keith, 1991; Amato, 2001) mainly points in that direction too.

This Dutch research study is limited to a measurement, as precise as possible, of these effects and the mechanisms and processes involved. The question whether these effects vary in different cohorts cannot be answered by the greater part of these studies, because the data they contain almost always concerns only one cohort. However, the question on the different correlations between parental divorce and their children's well-being in the case of different cohorts is important for the interpretation of those correlations and for the relevance to be attributed to them. This article attempts to establish, for the successive generations of secondary schoolchil-

Wolfgang Glatzer, Susanne von Below, Matthias Stoffregen (eds.), Challenges for Quality of Life in the Contemporary World, 249-270.
© 2004 Kluwer Academic Publishers. Printed in the Netherlands.

dren in the 80s and 90s of the twentieth century, how far these correlations have shifted.

The negative correlations between parental divorce and the well-being of their children can develop in two opposite directions: becoming stronger or weaker. Amato (2001, p. 362-365), in his meta-analysis on American research, found that a curvilinear relation existed between the effects of single-parent families on the well-being of their children and the decennium in which these effects were measured: These effects (good school results, behavior, psychological well-being and self-image) became less significant in the course of the 1970s and 80s, but increased again in the course of the 80s and 90s. Amato gives two possible explanations for this curvilinear relation: (1) A change in the nature of divorce, whereby recent divorces increasingly concern relationships wherein the ex-partners were only marginally (instead of extremely) unhappy in their marriage. And indeed divorces with relatively little conflict between parents are particularly hard for the children to understand, which leads to more frustration and thus to a lower well-being of the children. (2) Complete families benefited more than single-parent families from the prosperity in the 1990s, so that the latter are lagging increasingly further behind. Similar arguments are addressed by South (2001) for consideration in this connection on the possible contrasts in changes in the effect of working women on their divorce chances.

There are three reasons leading to the assumption that the negative correlations between parental divorce and the well-being of their children have diminished in the case of more recent cohorts in the Netherlands.

1.   compared to the 1960s and 70s, the number of divorces involving children has markedly increased. Although it is true that this increase leveled off in the 80s and 90s, the current number of divorces certainly shows that the phenomenon of divorce involving children has become much more common and thus easier to accept. Because of the increase in acceptance, parents divorcing seem to be less stigmatized and better able to continue to be functioning parents. Moreover, children of divorced parents form much less of an exception and tend to be better accepted by their peers and even supported by them. This greater level of acceptation and support by peers seems to lessen the negative effects on their well-being.

2.   The *de facto* juridical handling of divorce appears to have become more flexible in the course of the 1980s and 90s, because divorces involving children became more common and were better accepted. This might mean that there was a lower intensity of tension and conflict between partners divorcing, and that these conflicts were not fought out so much on the back of the children. Nowadays people divorce "more rationally" than before. This means that the children involved are less subject to tension and therefore that there are less negative consequences for their well-being. Moreover, there is nowadays a lot more mediation between divorcing parents instead of a lengthy court case in which the divorce is "threshed out".

3.   A third possible cause of the decrease in negative correlations between parental divorce and children's well-being is the increase in "co-parenthood": Divorced parents nowadays more frequently have joint custody over their children. In this way, the parents remain in (good) contact with each other, and the children continue to see both parents and are brought up by both of

them. Moreover, upbringing by both parents becomes more effective and the well-being of the children suffers less damage.

There are, however, also three reasons leading to believe that the negative correlations between parental divorce and children's well-being have increased in the case of more recent cohorts.

1. In the second half of the twentieth century, the number of divorces involving children increased markedly. Taking for granted that the portion of bad marriages during the twentieth century remained more or less constant, this increase shows that nowadays the average divorce has different reasons than it had in the past. De Graaf & Kalmijn (2001, p. 25) show that the reasons for divorce in the second half of the twentieth century changed and also became less weighty. In the 50s, the explanation "sexual infidelity of the man" had a role in over 54 % of divorces, in the 80s only in 38 % (infidelity of the woman 35 %, resp. 28 %). The particularly weighty grounds for divorce, "physical violence", were less frequently mentioned with the passing of the decades. This could mean that the rare divorce cases in the 1960s and 70s often brought conscious relief to the children involved because divorce led to termination of an untenable situation. The more frequent divorces in the 80s and 90s, on the other hand, more often resulted in a lack of understanding and a state of confusion in the children, because they could not see the need for the divorce. The fact that they had more and more difficulty in understanding their parents' divorce could have an increasingly negative influence on the children involved in more recent divorces.

2. De Graaf and Kalmijn (2001, p. 26) also find that women in recent divorces more often use the reason of "growing apart", "lack of attention" and "not being able to talk to each other properly" than was the case in divorces during previous decades. Of the women who divorced in the period 1949-1972, 69 % named the grounds for divorce as not being able to talk, while that percentage in more recent cases of divorced women increased to 80 %. The importance for children of a good psychological relationship between their parents is certainly present, but it may have less weight than maintenance of the parental marriage, because, for children, an upbringing as undisturbed as possible is more important than a good relationship between their parents. If the number of divorces on the grounds of a bad psychological relationship increases, this means that the negative effects of an average divorce on children also increase.

3. According to De Graaf and Kalmijn (2001: 27) women more and more frequently name the grounds "former partner spends too much time at work" and the "division of housekeeping tasks" as reasons for separation. Too much work was mentioned by 8 % of women divorcing in the 1950s and 60s, compared to 28 % in divorces during the 80s; and problems concerning division of tasks were mentioned by 15 %, resp. 30 %. It may be in the children's interest for their parents to have a more emancipated relationship, but this interest may be slighter than that of their parents remaining married, because for children it is more important to have an upbringing as undisturbed as possible then a more emancipated role division between their parents. If the number of divorces on the grounds of too little emanci-

pation in the division of gender roles increases, this could mean that the negative ef of the average divorce on children increases.

It is of course possible that no changes will be found in the well-being of children in consequence of a divorce in the 1984-1999 period. This would mean that both the above-mentioned developments balance each other out.

Given these apparently contradictory developments and the current stage of research, the main question in the context of this research study is in the first place descriptive: *Have the negative correlations between certain aspects of children's well-being and parental divorce diminished during the 1984-1999 period?*

The data available allow this main question to lead to two specific sub-questions that can contribute to a better understanding of changes, or of no changes, in the negative correlations.

1. *In the 1980s and 90s, did the negative effects of single-father families on the children's well-being increase more than the effects of single-mother families on the children's well-being?* Previous Dutch research (Borgers, Dronkers & van Praag, 1996; Dronkers, 1996, 1997) showed that the well-being of children in single-mother families was negatively influenced by divorce, while that was not the case in single-father families. These authors explained this phenomenon by assuming that the fathers who after divorce had full custody of the children formed a special group. Moreover, there was more social support for the category of single-fathers than for single-mothers. However, due to a marked increase in single-father families during the 80s and 90s, the category of fathers taking care of their children became less exceptional. More fathers took on full custody of their children so that the negative consequences of divorce on their children's well-being was no longer compensated for to such a degree by their particular capacities or by extra social support.

2. *In the 1980s and 90s, were there any differences in the negative effects on the well-being of children in single-mother families depending on the mother's educational status?* In previous Dutch research (Borgers, Dronkers & van Praag, 1996) no difference was found between the well-being of children in single-mother families with a higher educated mother and the well-being of children in single-mother families with a lower educated mother, while according to American research such a difference can be found. This difference in results can be explained by the fact that in the Netherlands, until the 70s, divorce was not customary, and hence it was mostly women endowed with perseverance and intelligence (Dronkers, 2002) who were in a condition to push a divorce through. For less perseverant women the threshold was much higher: divorce procedures were difficult and unfamiliar, and they preferred not to risk it. During the 80s and 90s the category of women forming single-mother families became less selective. Since divorce had become quite normal and divorce procedures were simpler and more common, it may be assumed that divorced mothers were no longer predominantly women endowed with a high degree of perseverance and intelligence (see for an analogous argument Goode, 1962). This change in the composition of categories of divorced mothers from the viewpoint of perseverance and intelligence could be the reason why differences in well-being between children in single-mother

families with a higher educated mother and children in single-mother families with a lower educated mother increased throughout the 1980s and 90s.
The selective category of divorced women in the 70s neutralized, thanks to
their greater intelligence and perseverance, the difference in resources of
women with a lower and higher education by comparison with complete
families. Since during the 80s and 90s the category of women forming single-mother families became less selective, the difference in resources of
lower and higher educated divorced women was more evident for instance
in the well-being of their children.

DATA

The article by Borgers, Dronkers en van Praag (1996) addresses the well-being of
secondary schoolchildren at the beginning of the 1990s. The School Surveys used by
them were, however, put together in a more or less comparable way at different
times during the 80s and 90s. For this reason, these School Surveys are suitable for
the purpose of answering our questions. For the present article we have been able to
use data from the 1984, 1990, 1992, 1994, 1996 and 1999 NIBUD[2] School Surveys.
These School Surveys can be considered to be representative of a specific year's
secondary schoolchildren from all classes and types of school education. They consist of written questionnaires distributed via the school and collected during school
time. The schoolchild and the type of family he/she lives in is the independent variable. The well-being of the schoolchildren is the dependent variable. We have limited the group under study to schoolchildren of Dutch nationality in order to exclude
the confusing influence of different cultures.[3] Moreover, we have only included
schoolchildren below eighteen years of age in our research population, in order to
avoid distortion caused by changes in the indexes of older students. The schoolchildren were asked to give their opinion on a great number of aspects of their lives,
without, however, connecting this with the divorce of their parents. All the data we
used for this secondary analysis of the NIBUD data consist therefore of the self-
assessments of the schoolchildren questioned. Secondary schoolchildren orphaned
of one parent were also removed from the analysis data, in order to avoid confusion
between widowed/orphaned families and divorced families (see Borgers, Dronkers
& van Praag, 1996).

From the questionnaires, we selected the questions providing an indication of the
different aspects of schoolchildren's well-being. We had to limit ourselves to using
those indicators of well-being that had been measured in a comparable manner during the 1980s and 90s. Because of these limits, the range of our indicators of well-
being is not as broad as that of Borgers, Dronkers & van Praag (1996). Since the
extent of conflicts between parents was only quantified during the 90s, we could not
include this control variable in our analysis. For the purpose of our investigation the
omission of this control variable with regard to the extent of conflicts between parents before and after divorce means that we may overestimate the decrease in negative relations between parental divorce and their children's well-being, since we
cannot account for the presumed increase of 'rational' divorces during the 80s and
90s. However, if we do not find that these negative correlations have diminished,
that result will not be due to the omission of control for the extent of conflicts between parents before and after divorce.

We can now analyze the following aspects of secondary schoolchildren's well-being:

- *Parents' financial contributions to the children.* It is frequently seen that in divorced families there is a greater degree of poverty (Hoff, Dronkers & Vrooman, 1997). That implies that children in divorced families have less money available than children in complete families. At the same time, divorced parents might (temporarily) devote less time and attention to their children, and compensate for this with a greater financial contribution. We are using three indicators: the amount of pocket money per week; the amount of extra money per week, divided into clothing allowance and travel allowance. These sums of money have not been adjusted for inflation or price level. Due to inflation in the 80s, this could lead to an overestimation of the rise in financial contributions from parents during this period of time.

- *Schoolchild's health problems.* The tension resulting from parental divorce (both before and after) can also have consequences on the state of health of the schoolchildren. Supervision by parents can also diminish during the divorce period, so that their health is threatened. The indicator is the number of times the student has been home on sick leave during the last month.

- *Undesired negative behavior.* The tension brought about by parental divorce (both before and after) can also have consequences on the degree of undesired negative behavior manifested by the children. Supervision by parents can also diminish during the divorce period, so that there are more opportunities for undesired negative behavior. The indicator is a scale of 10 questions to the schoolchild concerning the amount of quarrels, fights and petty criminality per year, such as vandalism and theft, etc. The Cronbach Alpha of this scale is 0.80.

- *Planning future independence and role division.* The tension caused by parental quarrelling and divorce may lead the children to want to leave their parental home earlier and to live independently in order to be no longer disturbed by the fighting and tension. Parental divorce can also cause children of divorced parents to aspire to a more emancipated domestic role division in their own relationships. Moreover, following their parents' divorce, children of divorced parents more frequently see their father and/or mother fill the role of the other parent, so that the chance of a more balanced domestic role division is more realistic. There are two indicators: (1) the age the schoolchild wishes to leave the parental home and live independently. (2) a scale of five questions concerning the future task division in upbringing and caring for children, cooking, earning money and domestic chores, whereby we have reformulated the questions in such a way that it is mostly the traditional role division of man and women that scores the highest points in this scale. The Cronbach Alpha of this scale is 0.72.

The averages, standard deviations and numbers relating to these indicators of well-being are shown in the last two rows of Table 1. In the 1984 School Survey, the variables 'bad health', 'undesired negative behavior' and 'future role division in upbringing and care of children' was not measured. For these indicators we can only establish a shorter trend, (1990-1999) instead of 1984-1999.

Differences in the well-being of secondary schoolchildren between single-parent and complete families and the possible changes that took place in the 1984-1999 period may also be caused by changes in background features. In fact, due to the increased number of divorces, the composition of the categories of divorced parents changed, and consequently also their characteristics in relation to the category of non-divorced parents.

Table 1: Average Scores of Schoolchildren in Complete Families, Mother Families and Father Families on the Various Indicators for Well-being for the Years 1984, 1990, 1992, 1994, 1996, and 1999 (in Brackets the Standard Deviations)

Table 1a:Average Amount of Pocket Money per Month

	1984	1990	1992	1994	1996	1999	Total	N
Complete Family	46.55	62.03	49.52	50.34	49.81	48.19	50.98	59,061
	(34.54)	(56.12)	(45.54)	(42.21)	(51.29)	(41.87)	(45.61)	
Single-Parent Family, Mother	53.10**	75.45**	59.31**	56.15**	50.97	55.63**	58.72	4,961
	(42.16)	(69.11)	(54.88)	(47.14)	(35.87)	(53.13)	(52.55)	
Single-Parent Family, Father	55.01**	70.87*	66.10**	63.48*	57.52	56.08*	62.10	882
	(34.36)	(56.86)	(70.30)	(52.72)	(37.09)	(47.72)	(54.61)	
Total	47.11	63.22	50.61	50.93	49.92	48.88	51.72	64,904
	(35.16)	(57.34)	(47.01)	(42.77)	(50.33)	(42.93)	(46.37)	
N	9,830	10,041	12,360	13,360	7,803	10,917	64,904	

Table 1b: Average Amount of Clothing Allowance per Month

	1984	1990	1992	1994	1996	1999	Total	N
Complete Family	83.60	113.32	118.84	113.84	98.23	100.74	107.16	19,330
	(43.04)	(62.06)	(64.81)	(55.91)	(42.21)	(51.72)	(56.74)	
Single-Parent Family, Mother	85.19	120.36*	122.36	113.03	102.03	107.82	111.55	2,226
	(44.36)	(68.74)	(76.22)	(58.26)	(55.52)	(67.19)	(65.23)	
Single-Parent Family, Father	88.82	119.89	122.74	130.33	90.94	101.88	112.26	386
	(46.59)	(74.36)	(75.40)	(65.05)	(31.90)	(56.61)	(65.95)	
Total	83.84	114.20	118.96	113.92	98.56	101.43	107.70	21,942
	(43.24)	(63.11)	(66.32)	(66.32)	(43.65)	(53.20)	(57.85)	
N	2,668	4,018	4,502	4,924	2,547	3,283	21,942	

Table 1c: Average Amount of Travel Allowance per Month

	1984	1990	1992	1994	1996	1999	Total	N
Complete Family	54.10	65.07	49.04	63.89	46.72	52.13	57.57	8,492
	(49.86)	(70.76)	(41.14)	(58.13)	(46.75)	(48.41)	(56.85)	
Single-Parent Family, Mother	49.11	61.78	46.90	60.14	41.82	61.07	55.34	957
	(43.74)	(56.20)	(37.49)	(46.00)	(30.67)	(52.12)	(47.50)	
Single-Parent Family, Father	50.74	53.16*	45.17	65.48	41.20	62.50	54.40	181
	(52.73)	(40.76)	(40.37)	(66.87)	(18.36)	(71.76)	(53.15)	
Total	53.66	64.50	48.70	63.47	46.20	53.40	57.29	9,630
	49.47)	(68.99)	(40.69)	(56.96)	(45.28)	(49.81)	(55.93)	
N	2,180	2,560	1,392	1,915	596	987	9,630	

Table 1d: Average Age at which the Schoolchild Wishes to Leave Home

	1984	1990	1992	1994	1996	1999	Total	N
Complete Family	20.76	20.05	20.32	20.55	20.15	17.50	19.85	62,867
	(2.06)	(3.33)	(2.84)	(2.81)	(2.31)	(8.92)	(4.73)	
Single-Parent Family, Mother	20.63	19.42**	20.03**	20.25**	19.88**	17.55	19.62	5,683
	(2.19)	(4.19)	(2.84)	(2.75)	(2.03)	(8.52)	(4.58)	
Single-Parent Family, Father	20.48	19.05**	20.27	19.85**	18.82**	17.56	19.18	981
	(2.19)	(4.83)	(2.49)	(2.53)	(1.83)	(7.76)	(5.12)	
Total	20.74	19.98	20.29	20.51	20.12	17.50	19.82	69,540
	(2.08)	(3.44)	(2.83)	(2.80)	(2.29)	(8.87)	(4.73)	
N	10,598	11,052	13,275	15,413	6,132	13,070	69,540	

Table 1e: Average Scale Scores on Futures Role Division as Seen by the Schoolchild

	1990	1992	1994	1996	1999	Total	N
Complete Family	8.81	8.69	8.62	8.55	8.69	8.67	54,107
	(1.32)	(1.45)	(1.51)	(1.49)	(1.66)	(1.50)	
Single-Parent Family, Mother	8.74	8.53**	8.54**	8.45	8.55**	8.56	4,867
	(1.13)	(1.27)	(1.33)	(1.20)	(1.52)	(1.31)	
Single-Parent Family, Father	8.78	8.71	8.50	8.54	8.68	8.66	820
	(1.31)	(1.31)	(1.29)	(1.47)	(1.65)	(1.48)	
Total	8.80	8.67	8.61	8.54	8.68	8.66	59,794
	(1.31)	(1.43)	(1.50)	(1.47)	(1.65)	(1.48)	
N	9,730	14.063	15,976	8,148	11,877	59,794	

Table 1f: Average Number of Times at Home on Sick Leave during the Last Month

	1990	1992	1994	1996	1999	Total	N
Complete Family	1.60	0.68	0.86	1.07	1.43	1.09	53,743
	(1.04)	(1.98)	(2.16)	(2.32)	(5.56)	(3.04)	
Single-Parent Family, Mother	1.92**	1.11**	1.34**	1.54**	1.78**	1.48	4,897
	(1.27)	(2.71)	(2.38)	(2.70)	(4.43)	(2.85)	
Single-Parent Family, Father	1.77	1.02*	0.93	1.54	1.61	1.38	819
	(1.20)	(2.51)	(2.04)	(2.37)	(3.03)	(2.43)	
Total	1.63	0.73	0.91	1.10	1.46	1.13	59,459
	(1.07)	(2.07)	(2.18)	(2.35)	(5.44)	(3.02)	
N	10,193	13,704	15,305	8,572	11,685	59,459	

Table 1g: Average Scale Scores on Undesired Negative Behavior Manifested by the School-child

	1990	1992	1994	1996	1999	Total	N
Complete Family	0.62 (1.75)	0.61 (2.03)	0.53 (1.57)	0.45 (0.96)	0.93 (4.51)	0.63 (2.48)	44,632
Single-Parent Family, Mother	0.88** (2.26)	0.77* (2.12)	0.68** (1.78)	0.54* (1.06)	0.87 (2.30)	0.75 (2.01)	4,058
Single-Parent Family, Father	0.76 (1.55)	0.74 (2.08)	0.70 (1.49)	0.84 (1.90)	1.01 (2.56)	0.83 (2.07)	641
Total	0.64 (1.79)	0.62 (2.04)	0.55 (1.60)	0.45 (0.97)	0.93 (4.35)	0.64 (2.44)	60,247
N	10,916	13,295	15,716	8,735	11,585	60,247	

Source: School Surveys 1984, 1990, 1992, 1994, 1996, 1999. *=p<0.01; **=p<0.05 (t-test of comparison with complete family).

This is why we check for the following variables: type of school the schoolchild attends (from lower to higher levels: lbo, mavo, havo, mbo and vwo); schoolchild's age; schoolchild's gender (women score higher); religious belief of the student (five dichotomous variables: Roman Catholic, Protestant, Reformed, Islam, other belief; no belief as a reference category); highest type of parental education (distinguished between mothers and fathers, from lower to higher: from primary school to university level). Table 2 shows how far the most important features of complete families, mother families and father families have shifted in the period from 1984 to 1999.

The education level of the father and mother were not measured in the 1984 School Survey. Therefore, we cannot take into account the parents' education level over the period 1984-1999. Only in the comparisons over 1990-1999 do we use the parents' education level as a control variable. Since in all comparisons relating to the period 1984-1999 the education level of the schoolchild was checked, we believe that the consequences of the lack of data on parental education level in the 1984-1999 comparisons is not disastrous for the purpose of identifying a possible trend.

Schoolchildren in single-mother families less often provide information on the education level of the father who left the home, while children in single-father families often do not mention the education level of the mother who left. In the multivariate comparisons relating to single-mother families we only used the education level of the mother as a control variable, while in the case of single-father families we only used the father's education level. Inclusion of the education level of both parents in the comparisons leads to distortion of results relating to single-parent families, since in that case we would have to take account only of the single-parent families in the comparisons, in which children have more frequent contact with the parent who left home, and hence are aware of his/her education level.[4]

Table 2: The Most Relevant Background Features of Complete families, Mother Families and Father Families during the years 1984, 1990, 1992, 1994, 1996, and 1999 (in Brackets the Standard Deviations)

	1984	1990	1992	1994	1996	1999	Total
% Mother Families	7.1	8.0	8.7	9.2	7.4	7.6	8.1
% Father Families	1.3	1.7	1.6	0.7	0.5	2.2	1.4
Average Type of School Complete Families	2.96 (1.33)	2.89 (1.36)	3.06 (1.26)	3.00 (1.35)	3.20 (1.41)	3.47 (1.35)	3.07 (1.35)
Average Type of School Mother Families	2.88 (1.33)	2.88 (1.41)	2.95^{**} (1.29)	2.85^{**} (1.32)	3.24 (1.43)	3.47 (1.32)	3.01^{**} (1.36)
Average Type of School Father Families	2.92 (1.40)	3.00 (1.36)	2.92 (1.27)	2.38^{**} (1.18)	2.44^{**} (1.31)	3.31 (1.38)	2.94^{**} (1.35)
Average Education Level Father in Complete Families		2.74 (1.44)	3.01 (1.54)	3.08 (1.41)	3.29 (1.48)	3.24 (1.45)	3.05 (1.48)
Average Education Level Father in Father Families		3.10^{**} (1.68)	3.13 (1.60)	3.07 (1.68)	3.50 (1.69)	3.55^{**} (1.43)	3.25^{**} (1.59)
Average Education Level Mother in Complete Families		2.20 (.96)	2.46 (1.17)	2.83 (1.15)	2.97 (1.25)	3.00 (1.23)	2.69 (1.19)
Average Education Level Mother in Mother Families		2.29^{**} (1.16)	2.66^{**} (1.37)	2.95^{**} (1.22)	3.22^{**} (1.34)	3.04 (1.31)	2.81^{**} (1.31)
% Roman Catholic Complete Families	38	35	29	30	28	21	30
% Roman Catholic Mother Families	36	25^{**}	24^{**}	24^{**}	21^{**}	18^{**}	24^{**}
% Roman Catholic Father Families	37	24^{**}	24^{*}	16^{**}	33	16	23^{**}
% Protestant Complete Families	18	21	19	18	18	17	18
% Protestant Mother Families	12^{**}	15^{**}	11^{**}	10^{**}	9^{**}	7^{**}	10^{**}
% Protestant Father Families	8^{**}	19	13^{**}	19	15	7^{**}	13^{**}

Source: School Surveys 1984, 1990, 1992, 1994, 1996, 1999. $^{*}=p<0.01$; $^{**}=p<0.05$ (t-test or χ^2 by comparison with complete family).

The average type of school attended by children in single-mother families was only significantly lower than the type attended by children from complete families in the years 1992 and 1994. In the years 1984 and 1990, although it was lower than was the case for children in complete families and in the years 1996 and 1999 equivalent or even higher, the differences are not significant. The average type of school attended by children in single-father families was of a significantly lower level in the years 1994 and 1996 than was the case for children in complete families. In the years 1984, 1992 and 1999, although the level was lower than for children in complete families (and in 1990 higher), these differences are not significant. In general, the average type of school attended by children from both single-mother and -father families is of a significantly lower level than the average type of school attended by children in complete families.

The average education level of fathers in single-father families was significantly higher in the years 1990 and 1999 than the average education level of fathers in complete families. In the other years (with the exception of 1994) the average education level of fathers in single-father families was in fact higher than that of fathers in complete families, but these differences are not significant. In general, the average education level of fathers in single-father families was significantly higher than the average education level of fathers in complete families. The average education level of mothers in single-mother families was, in the years ranging from 1990 through 1996, significantly higher than the average education level of mothers in complete families. This also goes for the year 1999, but this difference is not significant. In general the average education level of mothers in single-mother families was significantly higher than the average education level of mothers in complete families.

Children in single-parent families were less often members of a Catholic or Protestant church than children in complete families. This was, however, less evident in the 1980s than in the 90s, and less evident with regard to children in single-father families than to children in single-mother families.

These results in table 2 clearly show that taking account of changed background features of the categories of divorced and not divorced parents can be important for a correct assessment of the changed effects of single-parent families on the well-being of their children.

DIFFERENCES IN WELL-BEING BETWEEN SCHOOLCHILDREN FROM COMPLETE AND DIVORCED FAMILIES

Table 1 shows the differences for each year in the well-being of schoolchildren in complete and divorced families. In this way we obtain a first answer to our main question.

Mothers in single-mother households gave significantly more pocket money to their children compared to parents in complete families. In 1984 children in single-mother families received f 6.55 more (f 53.10-f 46.55), in 1999 the difference was f 7.44 (f 58.72-f 50.98). No clear trend can be established in the course of years, but it can be concluded that by comparison with 1984 this difference in the amount of pocket money only increased in 1999. With regard to fathers in single-father households the result in the course of years concerning pocket money was somewhat more inconsistent, but in this category too, albeit to a lesser degree, it can be seen that a significantly higher amount of pocket money was given to the children. Here too no clear trend can be established, the differences in amount show great fluctuations in the different years.

Concerning the amount of clothing allowance and travel allowance no significant differences were found between complete families and single-mother and -father families.

The average age when a schoolchild in a single-mother family wants to live independently was significantly different in the years ranging from 1990 to 1996 than was the case for schoolchildren in complete families (0.63 year in 1990 and 0.27 year in 1996). This desire to leave the family earlier was, according to previous research, actually fulfilled: Children in divorced families left home at a younger age than children in complete families. This difference in age between children in single-mother families and children in complete families decreased from 1990 to 1996, indicating a trend specific for that time. For children in single-father families the same significant difference can be seen in the age the child considered leaving home during the years 1990 through 1996, with the exception of the year 1992 (1.00 year in 1990 and 1.33 years in 1996). However, no trend can be established between these differences through the years as it can be for children in single-mother families compared to children in complete families. The 1999 data show a deviating image with regard to the data of previous years, and this is valid for all types of family. In this year no significant differences between types of family could be found.

A more emancipated future role-division was expected significantly more often by children in single-mother households than by children in complete families during the years 1992, 1994 and 1999. This was not the case for children in single-father families compared with children in complete families.

Staying sick at home was found significantly more often for children in single-mother families than for children in complete families. The difference amounted to 0.32 in 1990 and 0.35 in 1999, and no clear increase or decrease was found in the differences in the course of years. For children in single-father households the same significant difference appears only in the year 1992 (difference: 0.34) in the frequency of staying at home on sick leave during the last month.

Undesired negative behavior was observed to a significantly greater degree for children in single-mother families than for children in complete families (difference 0.25 in 1990 and 0.09 in 1996), with the exception of the year 1999 during which data show a deviating image. It is clear that the difference in undesired negative behavior between children in single-mother families and children in complete families diminished from 1990 through 1996. In 1999 children in single-mother households manifested a lesser degree of undesired negative behavior than children in complete families. No significant difference was found with regard to children living in single-father families.

In general, we did not find a much lower degree of significant differences in the late 90s between children in single-parent families and children in complete families compared to the 80s or early 90s, but the year 1999 does appear at times to form an exception. That would make the answer to our main question negative: The negative correlations between certain aspects of the well-being of children and parental divorce appear to have hardly diminished during the period 1984-1999, with the sole positive exception of undesired negative behavior.

However, changes in background features, such as those shown partially in Table 2, may play a role, since they neutralize any possible decrease of negative effects. We shall look at this in the following paragraphs with the help of multivariate regression. We shall do this first for the indicators of well-being over the whole

1984-1999 period, and then separately for single-mother and -father families. Next, we will look at all the indicators of well-being over the 1990-1999 period, and here we can also check the education level of parents. Finally, we will check whether in the 1990-1999 period the differences in well-being between children with higher educated divorced mothers and children with lower educated divorced mothers increased.

Table 3: Effects of Mother Families and Father Families (Both by Comparison with Complete Families) on the Various Indicators for Well-being Checked for Different Background Features, in the 1984-1999 Period

	Pocket Money	Clothing Allowance	Travel Allowance	Age Of Leaving Home
Mother Families				
Mother Family	0.04^{**}	0.01^{*}	-0.01	-0.02^{**}
Year	0.09^{**}	0.10^{**}	0.07^{**}	-0.11^{**}
Gender	-0.07^{**}	-0.03^{**}		-0.09^{**}
Age	0.25^{**}	0.06^{**}	0.13^{**}	0.11^{**}
Type of School	-0.08^{**}	-0.09^{**}	-0.18^{**}	-0.08^{**}
Roman Catholic				0.06^{**}
Protestant	-0.08^{**}	-0.07^{**}		0.05^{**}
Islam	0.04^{**}	0.03^{**}		0.02^{**}
Other Belief	-0.01^{**}			0.01^{**}
Mother Family*year	n.s.	n.s.	n.s.	n.s.
Adjusted R2	0.08	0.02	0.05	0.05
Father Families				
Father Family	0.03^{**}	0.02^{*}	-0.02	-0.02^{**}
Year	0.09^{**}	0.10^{**}	0.06^{**}	-0.12^{**}
Gender	0.08^{**}	-0.03^{**}		-0.09^{**}
Age	0.25^{**}	0.06^{**}	0.13^{**}	0.11^{**}
Type of School	-0.08^{**}	-0.08^{**}	-0.19^{**}	-0.09^{**}
Roman Catholic				0.05^{**}
Protestant	-0.08^{**}	-0.08^{**}		0.05^{**}
Islam	0.04^{**}	0.03^{**}		0.02^{**}
Other Belief	-0.01^{**}			
Father Family*year	n.s.	n.s.	n.s.	n.s.
Adjusted R2	0.08	0.02	0.05	0.05

Source: School Surveys 1984, 1990, 1992, 1994, 1996, 1999. $^{*}=p<0.05$; $^{**}=p<0.01$.

TRENDS IN THE 1984-1999 PERIOD

In the multivariate regression analysis shown in Table 3, the variables 'type of family' (mother and father family) and 'year of investigation' are taken up regardless of whether they have a significant effect or not. The other variables are shown according to the 'stepwise' method, that is, only the variables with significant effects are shown. Finally, the variable on the interaction 'type of family*year' gives an indication of whether there is a significant increase or decrease in the course of successive years.[5] The interaction variable is also only shown where it is relevant.

Single-Mother Families in the 1984-1999 Period

Children in single-mother families received significantly more pocket money than children in complete families, as shown in Table 3. In the course of successive years the amount of pocket money received by all children regardless of the type of family they live in increases; in 1999 children received more pocket money than in 1984, but this can be explained by the inflation during the 1980s. There is, however, no significant interaction effect, that is, there is no significant increase or decrease in the effect of single-mother families in the course of successive years on the variable 'pocket money'.

Clothing allowance for children in single-mother households was significantly higher than that of children in complete families. The amount of clothing allowance received increased significantly too for all children in the course of successive years. There is, however, no significant increase or decrease in the effect of single-mother families in successive cohorts on the variable 'clothing allowance'.

Children in single-mother households did not receive significantly less travel allowance than children in complete families. In successive years all children received significantly more travel allowance. There is no significant interaction effect of the effect of single-mother families during successive years in the variable 'travel allowance'.

Leaving home at a lower age was more desired by children in single-mother families than their peers in complete families. During the 90s all children, regardless of the type of family they belonged to, wanted to leave home earlier than children during the 80s.[6] There is, however, no significant increase or decrease to be seen in the effect of single-mother households in the course of successive years on the variable 'age of leaving home'.

There are, therefore, no significant differences in the late 1990s between children in single-mother families and children in complete families as compared to the 80s, if we take into account the available background features.

Single-Father Families in the 1984-1999 Period

Children in single-father families received significantly more pocket money than children in complete families, as shown in Table 3. There was, however, no significant interaction effect, that is, there was no significant increase or decrease in the effect of single-father households in successive years on the variable 'pocket money'.

Clothing allowance of children in single-father families was significantly higher than that of children in complete families. There was no significant increase or decrease in the effect of father families in successive cohorts on the variable 'clothing allowance'.

Children in single-father households did not receive significantly less travel allowance than children in complete families. There was no significant interaction effect on the variable 'travel allowance'.

Leaving home at a lower age was desired more by children in single-father families than by their peers in complete families. There was, however, no significant increase or decrease in the effect of single-father families in the course of years on the variable 'home-leaving age'.

There are, therefore, no significant differences in the late 1990s between children in father families and children in complete families by comparison with the early 80s, if we take account of the available background features.

TRENDS IN THE 1990-1999 PERIOD

In the multivariate regression analysis shown in Tables 4 and 5 the family type variable (single-mother and -father family) and year-of-investigation variable are shown, regardless of whether they have a significant effect or not. The other variables are shown according to the 'stepwise' method, that is, only the variables with significant effects are shown. Besides the interaction variable 'type of family*year', the interaction terms 'single-mother family*mother's education level'[7] and 'single-mother family*mother's education level*year appear, if they are significant'[8]. The second interaction term indicates whether there is a significant difference in well-being between children in single-mother families with a mother having a higher or lower level of education other than the normal difference in well-being between children with parents with a higher and lower education level. The third interaction term indicates whether this difference in well-being between children in single-mother families having a mother with a higher or lower level of education in successive years significantly increases or decreases. These three interaction variables are only shown where they are significant.

Single-Mother Families in the 1990-1999 Period

Children in single-mother families received significantly more pocket money than children in complete families, as shown in Table 4. The increase in pocket money received from 1990 to 1999 by all children, regardless of the type of family they belonged to, is not significant, as opposed to the 1984-1999 period. The effect of single-mother households on the pocket money variable, however, diminishes significantly in the course of successive years, as opposed to the 1984-1999 period. That means in this case that children in single-mother families between 1990 and 1999 received less and less pocket money as compared to children in complete families, so that the difference in the amount of pocket money received between children in single-mother families and children in complete families diminished.

Table 4: Effects of Mother Families (by Comparison with Complete Families) on the Various Indicators for Well-being Checked for Different Background Features in the 1990-1999 Period

	Pocket Money	Clothing Allowance	Travel Allowance	Age of Leaving Home	Future Role Division	At Home on Sick Leave	Negative Behavior
Mother Family	0.09**	0.01	-0.00	-0.02**	-0.04**	0.03	0.02
Year	0.01	-0.07**	0.01	-0.08**	0.05**	0.02**	0.02**
Gender	-0.08**			-0.09**		0.03**	-0.09**
Age	0.23**	0.06**	0.13**	0.09**	-0.08**	0.02**	-0.04**
Type of School	-0.08**	-0.08**	-0.19**	-0.09**	-0.08**	-0.05**	-0.06**
Mother's Education		0.03**		-0.02**	-0.06**	0.01**	0.02**
Roman Catholic				0.05**	0.03**	-0.02**	-0.04**
Protestant	-0.08**	-0.09**		0.05**	0.09**	-0.02**	-0.05**
Islam	0.02**	0.03**		0.01*	0.01**	0.05**	0.03**
Other Belief				0.01*		0.03**	0.01**
Mother Family*Year	-0.06**	n.s.	n.s.	n.s.	n.s.	n.s.	n.s.
Mother Family*Mother's Education	n.s.	n.s.	n.s.	n.s.	n.s.	n.s.	n.s.
Mother Family*Mother's Education*Year	n.s.	n.s.	n.s.	n.s.	n.s.	n.s.	n.s.
Adjusted R²	0.08	0.02	0.05	0.05	0.03	0.01	0.02

Source: School Surveys 1984, 1990, 1992, 1994, 1996, 1999. *=$p<0.05$; **=$p<0.01$.

In single-mother households, children did not receive significantly more clothing allowance than children in complete families. There was no significant increase or decrease in the effect of single-mother families in the course of successive years on the clothing allowance variable.

There was no difference in the amount of travel allowance received by children in single-mother families and children in complete families. There is no significant interaction effect between year and single-mother family.

Leaving home at a lower age was more desired by children in single-mother families than by their peers in complete families. There is no significant interaction effect between year and single-mother family, indicating no change in this difference between 1990 and 1999.

In single-mother households, children expected a significantly less traditional role division with their future partners than their peers in complete families. There is no significant interaction effect between year and single-mother family.

Staying sick at home happened more frequently for children in single-mother families than for children in complete families. All children, regardless of the type of family they belonged to, were more frequently home on sick leave during the 90s. There is no significant interaction effect between year and single-mother family, indicating that this difference didn't change between 1990 and 1999.

Children in single-mother families manifested significantly more undesirable behavior than children in complete families. The amount of undesirable behavior manifested by all children, regardless of the type of family they belonged to, increased significantly in 1999, as compared to 1990. There is no significant interaction effect between year and single-mother family.

In general, we do not find a much less significant difference in the late 1990s between children in single-mother families and children in complete families compared to the early 1990s, when we take into account the available background features. And in this respect the answer to our main question is negative: the negative correlations between certain aspects of the well-being of children and parental divorce have, during the period 1990-199, hardly diminished, with the positive exception of the amount of pocket money.

Nor have we found any significant difference in the well-being of children in single-mother families having a mother with a higher or lower education level, and hence no significant increase or decrease in that effect in the 1990-1999 period.

Single-Father Families in the 1990-1999 Period

Children in single-father families did not receive significantly less pocket money in comparison to children in complete families, as shown in Table 5. In the course of successive years all children, regardless of the type of family they belonged to, received a comparable amount of pocket money. However, in the course of successive years, the effect of single-father households on the pocket money variable did increase significantly. That is, children in single-father families during the 90s received more and more pocket money by comparison with children in complete families. That shows a difference when comparing it to the results from the 1984-1999 period.

Children in single-father families, compared to children in complete families, did not receive significantly more clothing allowance. There is no significant increase or decrease in the effect of single-father families in the course of successive years on the clothing allowance variable.

Children living in single-father households did not receive significantly less travel allowance than children in complete families. There is also no interaction effect between year and single-father family.

Leaving home at an earlier age was significantly more often expected by children in single-father families than by children in complete families. There was an increase in the effect of single-father families on the age at which their children wish to leave home between 1990 and 1999. That means that children in single-father households in the course of the 90s wanted to leave home at an increasingly later age.

Table 5: Effects of Father Families (by Comparison with Complete Families) on the Various Indicators of Well-being Checked for Different Background Features

	Pocket Money	Clothing Allowance	Travel Allowance	Age of Leaving Home	Future Role Division	At Home on Sick Leave	Negative Behavior
Father Family	-0.01	0.02	-0.02	-0.06**	-0.01	0.01*	0.01*
Year	0.00	-0.07**	0.03	-0.09**	0.02**	0.02**	0.03**
Gender	-0.07**	-0.02*		-0.09**	-0.02**	0.02**	-0.09**
Age	0.24**	0.05**	0.14**	0.09**	-0.08**	0.02**	-0.04**
Type of School	-0.08**	-0.09**	-0.20**	-0.08**	-0.07**	-0.05**	-0.06**
Father's Education		0.05**	0.04*	-0.06**	-0.06**		0.02**
Roman Catholic				0.04**	0.03**	-0.03**	-0.04**
Protestant	-0.08**	-0.09**		0.04**	0.09**	-0.03**	-0.06**
Islam	0.03**				0.01*	0.06**	0.03**
Other Belief						0.02**	0.01*
Interaction Father Family*Year	0.04*	n.s.	n.s.	0.05**	n.s.	n.s.	n.s.
Adjusted R^2	0.08	0.03	0.05	0.05	0.03	0.01	0.02

Source: School Surveys 1984, 1990, 1992, 1994, 1996, 1999. $^{*}=p<0.05$; $^{**}=p<0.01$.

Children in single-father families did not see a significantly less traditional role division in their own future relationships than children in complete families. There was no significant increase or decrease of the effect of single-father families on the variable 'future role division' in the course of successive years.

Staying home on sick leave happened significantly more frequently for children in single-father families than for their peers in complete families. There was no significant interaction effect between year and single-father family.

Undesirable negative behavior was found significantly more often for children in single-father families than for children in complete families. There was no significant increase or decrease in the effect of single-father families in the course of the 90s on the undesirable behavior variable.

In general, we did not find less difference in the late 90s between the well-being of children in single-father families and children in complete families as compared to the early 90s, if we take into account the available background characteristics. Respectively, the answer to our main question is negative: the negative correlations between certain aspects of the well-being of children and parental divorce have hardly diminished in the 1990-1999 period, with the positive exception of the amount of pocket money and the age at which children expect to leave home.

CONCLUSION AND DISCUSSION

What do the above results now mean in the context of our investigation?

In the first place, it is apparent that, in general, the assumption that the negative correlations between parental divorce and the well-being of their children have diminished during the 1984-1999 period cannot be confirmed. In order to establish differences in the degree of well-being between children in single-parent families and children in complete families in the 1984-1999 period, we have had to confine ourselves to the sole well-being in terms of *financial maintenance* and the *age at which schoolchildren considered leaving home*. No significant effects were found on the basis of these indicators on the well-being of secondary schoolchildren in either single-mother or -father families in the course of successive years. There was no difference between the well-being of children in single-parent families and the well-being of children in complete families in the late 90s compared to the 80s.

Measuring the shorter trend, that is, 1990-1999, the negative correlations between parental divorce and the well-being of children change either hardly or not at all. There are, however, two indicators of well-being showing changes between the early and late 1990s. The effect of single-mother families on the pocket money variable diminished significantly during this period. Children in single-mother households received, in the course of successive years, less and less pocket money in comparison to children in complete families, so that the original difference in the amount of pocket money received between children in single-parent families and children in complete families diminished. This could point to a decrease in ′buy-off behavior′ in single-mother families, caused by their paying less attention to their children and/or to compensate for the more difficult family situation. Single-mother families became more common during the 90s, because of this possible decrease in 'buy-off behavior', and in this sense became more similar to complete families.

The effect of single-father families did instead increase significantly during this period, which means that children in single-father families in the course of successive years received more and more pocket money as compared to children in complete families. This points to an increase in 'buy-off behavior' in single-father families, which came about because single fathers with custody became less exceptional in the course of the 1990s. In this sense, single-father families became more and more comparable to the old-fashioned single-mother families, where children received more pocket money than those in complete families. For single-father households there was, moreover, an increased effect in the course of successive years on the age at which children considered leaving home. This means that children in single-father families during the 90s considered leaving home at an increasingly later age than children in complete families. This could mean that children living in single-father families find life in a single-parent family more positive and therefore want to continue living at home for a longer period of time.

In the introduction we also posed two specific sub-questions. The assumption that in the 1980s and 90s the negative effects of single-father families on the well-being of their children seem to have increased to a greater degree than the negative effects of single-mother families on their children cannot be confirmed. There were no more significant negative effects in the course of successive years for children in single-father than for those in single-mother families. The category of fathers forming single-father families probably did not become more selective. We see that the average education level of fathers in single-father families in 1999 was significantly higher than that of fathers in complete families, just as it was significantly higher in 1990.

The assumption that in the 1980s and 90s the negative effects of divorce on the well-being of children were smaller if the divorced mother had a high level of education compared to divorced mothers with a low education can also not be confirmed. Apparently, the negative marks of divorce do not depend on the amount of available educational resources of divorced mothers.

The conclusion to this research study is that the negative consequences of divorce and life in a single-parent family during the late 1990s hardly diminished in comparison to the 80s and early 90s. However, this does not necessarily mean that the trend commonly assumed does not play a role. The time span of fifteen and/or nine years may be too short to be able to set such a trend. It would be preferable if analyses could be made over a greater number of years in order to be able to establish trends over a longer period of time. In our research, we made use of all School Surveys carried out in a more or less similar way during the 80s and 90s. There are, however, no similar Dutch research data available covering longer periods of time. Moreover, the different indicators of well-being in the various School Surveys were not measured in a comparable way. This makes it harder to make comparisons over longer periods of time. Therefore, we are of the opinion that, despite these methodical restrictions, the measuring of possible changed effects of single-parent families, addressed in this article, for the moment cannot be carried out in a better way in the Netherlands.

The conclusion that the negative consequences of divorce and life in a single-parent family during the late 1990s hardly diminished compared to the 80s and early 90s has consequences in two opposing directions. In the first place, it does not support the notion that divorce can become a normal and harmless feature of a modern and enlightened society, such as was hoped during the 70s and 80s. In the second place, however, this conclusion does not support the notion that the increased number of divorces might be responsible for the rapid increase in undesired features of modern society (for example, increase in violence by young people), as the neo-conservatives now assert. The effects of divorce and the growth in the number of divorces with children are too slight for this to be feasible (see Table 2, first two rows). Above all, our analyses show that the increase in undesirable behavior in young people during the 90s (more negative behavior, more often sick, more traditional views on role division) appeared in all children regardless of the type of family they belonged to at the time.

No scapegoats or cheap and fast solutions exist for undesired features of societies, and neither can classical institutions like marriage and family be changed at will or denied without damage being caused.

NOTES

1   Anna Lont is a doctoral student of pedagogy at the University of Amsterdam. She wrote this article in the context of the course on 'research experience' given by the second author, who was at the time professor of empirical sociology at the same university. Our thanks go to the NIWI, where the various School Surveys were stored, and to the NIBUD, for allowing us to use this data. Jaap Dronkers is currently professor of Social stratification and inequality at the European University Institute in San Domenico di Fiesole. Correspondence should be addressed to the second author; EUI, Department of

270 ANNA LONT AND JAAP DRONKERS

Political and Social Sciences, Via dei Roccettini 9, I-50016 San Dominico di Fiesole. E-mail: jaap.dronkers@iue.it.
2 Data available at NIWI Amsterdam under catalogue numbers P1446, P1447, P1448, P1449, P1450 and P1495.
3 That does not, however, mean that changes in correlations between single-parent family, ethnical origin and well-being of secondary schoolchildren is not interesting or important. It does, however, require a separate study, that would go beyond the scope of this article.
4 Analyses not appearing in this article show that the variances within the dependent variables are smaller in the case of single-parent families whereby schoolchildren are aware of the education level of both parents.
5 This interaction term is 0 in the case of a complete family, 1 in the case of a mother family in the year 1984 and 15 in the case of a mother family in the year 1999.
6 This result seems contradictory to the tendency in the 80s and 90s, when adolescents in fact lived longer in the parental home. What is meant is not actual behavior but an expectancy. The decreasing age at which these schoolchildren expect to leave their parental home expresses rather their greater independence within the parental household.
7 This interaction term is 0 in the case of a complete family and increases with the education level of the mother in a mother family.
8 This interaction term is 0 in the case of a complete family and increases with the education level of the mother in a mother family and with the year of investigation.

REFERENCES

Amato, P. R. (2001): Children of Divorce in the 1990s: An Update of the Amato and Keith (1991). Meta-analysis. Journal of Family Psychology 15, 355-370.
Amato, P. R. & B. Keith (1991): Parental Divorce and Adult Well-being: A Meta-analysis. Journal of Marriage and the Family 53, 43-58.
Borgers, N., J. Dronkers & B. van Praag (1996): Verschillen tussen kinderen uit twee- en eenoudergezinnen in hun welbevinden op de middelbare school. Nederlands Tijdschrift voor Opvoeding, Vorming en Onderwijs 12, 350-365. English version in: Social Psychology of Education 1:147-169.
Bosman, R. (1993): Opvoeden in je eentje. Een onderzoek naar de betekenis van het moedergezin voor de onderwijskansen van kinderen, Lisse: Swets & Zeitlinger.
Dronkers, J. (1996): Het effect van ouderlijke ruzie en echtscheiding op het welzijn van middelbare scholieren. Comenius 16, 131-147. English version in: European Sociological Review 15:195-212.
Dronkers, J. (1997): Het effect van contact met de vader na echtscheiding op het welzijn van middelbare scholieren. Recht der Werkelijkheid 18, 119-137.
Dronkers, J. (2002): Bestaat er een samenhang tussen echtscheiding en intelligentie? Mens en Maatschappij 77, 25-42.
Fischer, T. & P. M. de Graaf (2001): Ouderlijke echtscheiding en de levensloop van kinderen: negatieve gevolgen of schijnverbanden? Sociale Wetenschappen 44, 138-163.
Gelder, K. van (2000): Mamma, is het waar? Positieve en negatieve aspecten van het leven in een-ouder-gezinnen, Utrecht: Verwey-Jonker Instituut.
Goode, W. J. (1962). Marital satisfaction and instability: A cross-cultural class analysis of divorce rates. In R. Bendix & S. M. Lipset (eds.), Class, status, and power (377-387) New York: The Free Press.
Graaf, P. M. de & M. Kalmijn (2001): Scheidingsmotieven in Nederland sinds de jaren vijftig. Sociale Wetenschappen 44, 16-33.
Hoff, S. J. M., J. Dronkers & J. C. Vrooman (1997): Arme ouders en het welzijn van kinderen. G. Engbersen, J. C. Vrooman & E. Snel (eds.): De kwetsbaren. Tweede jaarrapport armoede en sociale uitsluiting, Amsterdam: Amsterdam University Press, 123-141.
South, S. J. (2001): Time-Dependent Effects of Wives' Employment on Marital Dissolution. American Sociological Review 66, 226-245.
Spruijt, E. & M. de Goede (1997): Het welbevinden van jongeren uit verschillende gezinstypen. Comenius 17, 99-116. English version in: Adolescence, 32: 897-911.

17. BELIEF IN VALUES AND THEIR PERCEIVED REALIZATION AS DETERMINANTS OF QUALITY OF LIFE

The Case of Kibbutz Members

Uriel Leviatan

University of Haifa, Israel

ABSTRACT

This paper demonstrates that "belief in personal values" – kibbutz unique social and collectivistic values – and the "perceived level of realization of these values in one's community (kibbutz)," strongly determine the level of subjective quality of life among kibbutz members. Their effect is over and above what is determined by members' satisfaction with their major domains of life ("fulfilments of aspirations and fit with abilities", "feeling of belonging", "work," "material standard of living", and "social relations"). The subjective QOL indicators are four: "satisfaction with life in general", "satisfaction with one's kibbutz life", "psychological commitment to one's kibbutz life", and a "global" indicator composed of all three. The analyses were multiple regressions which demonstrated that the "values" variables contributed about a third of the mean *explained variance* across the four indicators (ranging from 5 % to 31 % of the variance), while the "domains satisfaction" contributed about two thirds (with a range of 18 % to 46 %). Demographic variables (gender, age, education, and social position) played an insignificant role in explaining variance in the indicators of subjective quality of life. However, age and gender showed a conditioning position affecting the relative importance of "values" for different subgroups: "Values" were more important for males, and for some age groups, in particular the 71-80 and 51-60 age groups. "Satisfaction with one's kibbutz life" and "psychological commitment to one's kibbutz life" were also shown to serve as intervening variables between the independent variables of "values" and "domains satisfaction" and the outcome of 'satisfaction with life in general". Further analyses reported in the "summary" section show that the same conclusions hold for individuals who are low in their belief in values and therefore it is suggested that the findings should be generalized into other populations.

INTRODUCTION

Level of need satisfaction in life domains is commonly used to explain variance in indicators of quality of life. As a consequence, research seeks to find the level of individual's need satisfaction in various domains of life and relate it to some global measure(s) of well-being, and subjective quality of life. Cummins and his research collaborators (e.g., Cummins et al., 2002) furnish an illustrative example. They question their respondents about their level of satisfaction with life domains such as (personal aspects) standard of living, health, achievement in life, safety, feeling part of community, future security; and level of satisfaction with (national aspects) the economic situation in respondents' respective society, state of natural environment,

Wolfgang Glatzer, Susanne von Below, Matthias Stoffregen (eds.), Challenges for Quality of Life in the Contemporary World, 271-294.
© *2004 Kluwer Academic Publishers. Printed in the Netherlands.*

social conditions, government, business, and national security. Variability in these responses is then related to the global measure of "satisfaction with life as a whole". Similarly do Veenhoven and his collaborators in their pursuit after the explanation of variance in "happiness" in life (e.g., Veenhoven, 1997).

However, the literature on quality of life that focuses on "life satisfaction as a whole" or similar indicators as outcome variables, demonstrates scarcity on two accounts: First, a scarcity of research with reference to respondents' personal values. Second, when values are used as predictors of life satisfaction studies (or happiness or other quality of life indicators) (e.g., Yetim, 2002), they tend to ignore the more common measures of domain satisfaction. The list of papers presented at the ISQOLS conference 2003 (cf. Stoffregen, 2003) offers a typical illustration for these two missing characteristics of research about quality of life: Out of about two hundred presentations, I could identify only seven that dealt, at least somewhat, with values as contributors to quality of life; of these only two referred to both values and needs as contributors to a global indicator of subjective quality of life.

Yet, is it really justifiable to view "needs" in life domains, and their level of satisfaction, as a sole contributor to "life satisfaction" or to the level of other general indicators of subjective quality of life? Should not these indicators be influenced also by the *meaningfulness* people give to their life as it results from their personal values expressed both by (1) the existence of values as part of a person's self-identity and (2) as the perceived level of the realization level of these values?

It is odd that this question has at all to be asked when one recalls that psychologists have for more than thirty years considered values people hold as the most central shapers of attitudes about self and environment, of behaviors, and as major contributors to self-identity in all its dimensions (e.g. Rokeach, 1973; Shamir, 1990; Hofstede, 1991, 1998; Schwartz, 1994a, 1994b; Triandis, 1994; Mayton et al., 1994; Sverke & Kuruvilla, 1995). Given this background, should values not be considered also central in shaping self-evaluation of one's life in the form of "satisfaction with life as a whole?"

In this paper, I want to demonstrate how (1) the extent of individual commitment to personal values; and, (2) the degree of their perceived realization in individuals' own society/community – contributes to well-being *independently* of the contribution accounted for by "satisfaction with specific life domains". However, since this study deals with kibbutz communities in Israel[1], it offers an opportunity to gauge the contribution of satisfaction with life domains, level of value conviction, and extent of value realization – not only to the explanation of variance in "life satisfaction" but also to the explanation of variance of two other global expressions of subjective well-being: (1) satisfaction with one's life in a kibbutz; and (2) extent of psychological commitment to – or psychological identification with – kibbutz life. I consider these two indicators as additional expressions of global levels of well-being in the kibbutz context, because of some of the kibbutz' unique characteristics as I will explain in the next paragraph.

One of the kibbutz communities' unique features is being – for their members – all engulfing with respect to most life domains. Members' roles within all major life domains (such as work, leisure, health, civic, education, family, etc.) are performed within the framework of their kibbutz social boundaries, if not its physical boundaries. Therefore, when members relate to their "satisfaction with their kibbutz life" it probably captures for them most life domains and serves as a different perspective of their relatedness to "life as a whole". Similar is the case with psychological commitment to, or psychological identification with, (which is a major component of organizational commitment; Mowday et al., 1982) kibbutz life. This is so because being a kibbutz member is at least initially an expression of free choice. Consequently, since, as said before, such membership engulfs all major social roles and therefore relates to a major part of one's self-identity – psychologically not identifying with this life must express a low level of well-being and the opposite when identification is high.

Thus, I use in this study indicators of members' "satisfaction with their kibbutz life" and members' "psychological commitment to their kibbutz life" as additional indicators of general subjective quality of life. These two indicators should stand somewhat independently from global indicators such as "satisfaction with life in general". But because kibbutz life does not encompass *the whole* spectrum of domains and perspectives of life, these two more concrete expressions serve, to an extent, also as intervening variables, in the statistical sense, between satisfaction with specific life domains, belief in relevant values, and the perception of their realization, and between the most global expression – satisfaction with life in general.

Translated into formal hypotheses, the study reported here suggests the following (figure 1) relationships among its variables:

Figure 1: Hypothesized Relationships among the Groups of Variables in the Study

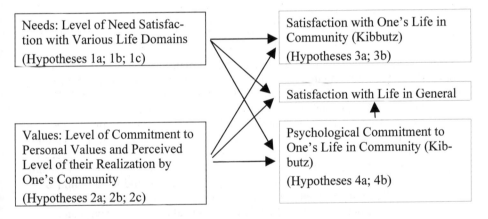

Hypothesis 1: Level of satisfaction with various life domains is positively related (a) to satisfaction with one's life in community (kibbutz); (b) to psychological commitment to one's community (kibbutz) life; (c) to satisfaction with life in general.

Hypothesis 2: Extent of commitment to personal values, and perceived level of their realization in one's community, is positively related (a) to satisfaction with one's life in community (kibbutz); (b) to psychological commitment to one's community (kibbutz) life; (c) to satisfaction with life in general.

Hypothesis 3: Satisfaction with one's life in community (kibbutz) (a) is positively related to satisfaction with life in general; (b) serves also as an *intervening variable* between satisfaction with life domains, commitment to values, and their perceived level of realization, on the one hand, and satisfactions with life in general on the other.

Hypothesis 4: Psychological commitment to one's community (kibbutz) life (a) is positively related to satisfaction with life in general; (b) serves also as an *intervening variable* between satisfaction with life domains, commitment to values, and their perceived level of realization, on the one hand, and satisfactions with life in general on the other.

KIBBUTZ COMMUNITIES AS SITES OF THE STUDY

Kibbutzim (plural of "kibbutz") are communal communities. The first was established in 1909 and currently they number about 270 with a total population of about 115,000. A major defining characteristic of kibbutz communities is the centrality taken by social values as expressed in their "Kibbutz regulations" (1973) (kibbutz by-laws). In its first paragraph it states:

> "The kibbutz is a free association of people for the purpose of the […] existence of a communal society based on principles of public ownership of property, […] equality and participation in all domains of production, consumption and education. The kibbutz […] sees itself as a leader of the [Jewish] national insurrection and aims at establishing in Israel a Socialist society based on principles of economic and social equality…
>
> Kibbutz Goals [among others] are…:
>
> To develop and promote friendship and fraternity among its members.
>
> To develop and promote members' personality, personal ability and collective ability in the spheres of economy, social, culture, science, and art."

These passages at once indicate the values that formally should govern kibbutz life: collectivistic values with emphasis on equality, partnership, solidarity among members, and influencing the Israeli society in directions of social and economic equality – combined with individualistic values with a strong emphasis on realization and development of members' unique potentials. At the same time it emphasizes in its opening sentence the freedom of choice individual members have to join or not to join kibbutz life. One has to assume, therefore, as I argued in the previous section, that both satisfaction with one's life in a kibbutz as well as psychological commitment to it, and therefore satisfaction with life in general, should be determined also by the level of conviction members have with their expressed values and with their judgment as to the degree of the realization of those values by their community.

General Aims of the Current Study – Relevancy of Past Kibbutz Research and What it Lacked

Past research has shown Israeli kibbutz members to enjoy a high level of quality of life. A glaring example is the kibbutz population's high level of life expectancy as demonstrated in table 1.

Table 1 shows how life expectancy at birth and at age 50 in kibbutzim surpasses that of Israeli Jews by about three years at every measuring period. It is also higher than life expectancy levels in most industrial societies (e.g., National Research Council, 2001, p. 48).

Past research dealt with contributors to this high level of life expectancy and demonstrated that it comes about first and foremost because of the unique social arrangement kibbutzim adopt for their aged members in all important life domains. It has also shown that those arrangements stem from the kibbutz unique social values as summarized in the "kibbutz regulations" (1973).

Table 1: Life Expectancy at Birth and at Age 50 of Kibbutz Permanent Population and Israeli Jews in Three Years — 1977, 1984, and 1995 (by Gender)

Gender	Year	Life Expectancy at Birth		Life Expectancy at Age 50	
		Kibbutz	Israeli Jews	Kibbutz	Israeli Jews
Males	1977	74.4	71.9	28.3	25.7
	1984	76.7	73.5	29.6	26.5
	1995	78.1	75.9	30.8	28.3
Females	1977	79.0	75.4	31.0	28.0
	1984	81.3	77.1	33.4	29.2
	1995	82.5	79.8	33.8	31.2

Source: Reproduced from Leviatan (2003). Data for the Jewish Population in Israel are taken from the Statistical Abstracts of Israel, Central Bureau of Statistics, 1979; 1986; 1997.

This meant that similar to other societies, life expectancy results in major part from satisfaction with both life domains and with life in general. For instance, in a longitudinal (twelve years difference) analysis of data from research with kibbutz elderly (Leviatan, 1999) – both "satisfaction with life domains" and "satisfaction with life in general" differentiated between those who survived and those who passed away within twelve years of the original data collection. Additionally, "satisfaction with one's kibbutz life" contributed over and above the contributions of satisfaction with specific life domains to explaining variance in "life satisfaction in general" and this was also the case with "commitment to kibbutz life" (Leviatan et al., 1981). Thus, contributions of domains' satisfaction to the explained variance in general indicators of well-being, were established in the kibbutz population.

Other research (Leviatan, 1998) has shown that *both* satisfaction with life domains and level of realization of kibbutz social values contribute to satisfaction with, and commitment to, one's kibbutz life. And that contribution accounts for about a fourth of the explained variance as estimated in multiple regression analyses.

Still other research on kibbutz society (Leviatan & Rosner, 2001) has shown a certain degree of belief in social values such as collectivism (vs. individualism) and social equality (vs. inequality) to be major contributors to the level of commitment to one's life in a kibbutz.

Thus, while all the different variables portrayed in figure 1 have each appeared in different studies, missing is a study that would combine all groups of independent variables (satisfaction with life domains, degree of values' conviction, perceived level of their realization) into one study and aim at explaining variance not only in commitment to, and satisfaction with, one's kibbutz life, but also in global indicators of well-being such as "life satisfaction in general" as an outcome variable. This is one aim of the current study.

Another aim of this study is to exploit structural changes that many kibbutzim currently go through. These structural changes are expressed in abandonment of many of the social arrangements that were based on kibbutz unique social values and transform the kibbutzim to be more similar to the outside world (Leviatan, 2003). In addition, many members give up on the kibbutz unique values, e.g. collectivism, equality, solidarity, and contribution to the larger society (cf. Leviatan & Rosner, 2001; Leviatan, 2003). This situation allows to raise the following research question: Are the beliefs in social values and the extent of their perceived realization by one's community still important as contributors to explaining variance in global indicators of well-being; even when both the extent of the belief in these values and the level of values' realization are low and more similar to life outside kibbutz communities?

RESEARCH METHODS

Study Design, Population, and Sample

This study investigated 29 kibbutzim, as whole communities, rather than subparts of them (such as, for instance, their industrial organizations). It is a secondary analysis of data originally collected by survey methods from a larger number of kibbutzim (during the years 1993-2001), for the purpose of organizational diagnostics. These 29 kibbutzim are included in the current analyses because only in their surveys I asked about respondents' "satisfaction with life in general". Members of these kibbutzim offered data via self-administered written, anonymous questionnaires. About 70 % of all members in these kibbutzim responded to the questionnaires. Under-representation of the samples appeared in the youngest ages (18-25) and the oldest (65+). The average size of the samples of respondents in the kibbutzim studied was 162 (Median=145) with a range of 46-333. The entire sample of respondents from the 29 kibbutzim consists of about 4,700.

Instruments and Variables

The self-administered questionnaire asked, among other questions, about demographic details, attitudes, states, and perceptions about self and kibbutz. All questions besides the demographics were on a five category scale transformed for this paper to 1=least positive (or lowest degree), 5=most positive (or highest degree). Some of the variables were indexes calculated – following factor analyses – as means across several items.

1. Dependent variables
- Satisfaction with life in general; a single item.
- Satisfaction with one's kibbutz life; a single item.
- Psychological commitment to one's kibbutz life; an index of 4 items – trust in kibbutz future; choosing again kibbutz life if given such a choice; selecting kibbutz life (from a list of possible different kinds of life) as the most desired; recommending kibbutz life to a young, loved, person.

2. Independent Variables: Expressions of Personal Values
- Wishes life of solidarity, partnership, and equality in most desired place of living; an index of 5 items: Desired is life in a society that practices communal ownership of means of production, communal production, qualitative equality, no connection between contribution and remuneration, full mutual solidarity.
- Social (collectivistic) values highly important; an index of 4 items – high importance attached to: acting for realization of social ideals, feeling that one contributes to shaping a better society, ideological considerations guide one's life, be active and have influence.
- Individualistic values highly important; an index of 4 items – high importance attached to: reaching a high material standard of living, be oneself in any role one holds, encounter challenges and develop initiatives, have a job that demands a lot of responsibility.

3. Independent Variables: Satisfaction with Value Realization
- Extent of personal values realized in kibbutz life; an index of 4 items – satisfaction with own kibbutz' life: contribution to building a more just society in Israel, fit with own values, expression of equality among members, expression of social ideals.

4. Independent Variables: Satisfaction with Life Domains
- Satisfaction with extent of fit between kibbutz life and one's ability and aspirations; a single item.
- Satisfaction with extent of feeling at home and belonging in kibbutz; a single item.
- Satisfaction with material standard of living and economic state of kibbutz; an index of 5 items – satisfaction with: material standard of living, level of housing, level of consumption, current economic state, future economic security.
- Satisfaction with work domain; an index of 4 items – satisfaction with: work, social relations at work, opportunity to use one's skills, knowledge, and experience, influence at the work place.
- Satisfaction with social relations in the kibbutz; an index of 2 items – satisfaction with: interpersonal relations, intergenerational relations.

5. Demographics
Gender, age, years of formal education, highest level of managerial office held during five years prior to data collection.

FINDINGS

Descriptive Findings

Table 2 presents characteristics of all variables in the study for the total sample (Means, SDs, Ns). The four right columns show the first-order coefficients of correlations among the dependent variables and correlations of all independent and demographic variables with the dependent variables. Given the strong relationships among the three original dependent variables, I created a fourth variable – an index called "global measure of well-being" – calculated as the Mean across the three original indicators. Its first-order-correlation levels with all other variables, is portrayed in the right most column.

Table 2: Descriptive Characteristics of the Variables and Indices in the Study and First-order Correlations of Variables in Group (1) "Subjective Indicators of Quality of Life" among themselves, and with the Other Variables

Variable	Mean	SD	First Order Correlations with...			
	(N=3,910- 4,690)		1. LS	2. KS	3. KID	4. GLB
1. Subjective Indicators of Quality of Life						
Satisfaction with Life in General (LS)	3.38	.97	-	.546	.417	.777
Satisfaction with One's Kibbutz Life	3.47	.88		-	.551	.710
Psychological Commitment to One's Kibbutz Life	3.28	.99			-	.797
Global Measure (Mean across the Three above) (GLB) (α=.75)	3.39	.80				-
2. Expressions of Personal Values						
Wishes of Life of Solidarity, part-nership, and Equality in Most De-sired Place of Living (5 Variables, α=.85)	3.59	1.05	.202	.345	.569	.436
Social, Collectivistic Values (4 Variables, α=.81)	3.62	.85	.052	NS	.156	.105
Individualistic Values (4 Variables, α=.71)	3.89	.81	-.068	-.160	-.179	-.151
3. Satisfaction with Value Realization						
Satisfied with Kibbutz Realization of Social/Ideology Values (4 Variables, α=.71)	2.27	.74	.421	.575	.447	.574

Table 2: Descriptive Characteristics of the Variables and Indices in the Study and First-order Correlations of Variables in Group (1) "Subjective Indicators of Quality of Life" among themselves, and with the Other Variables (continued)

4. Satisfaction with Life Domains in Kibbutz

Satisfied with Fit of Kibbutz Life to Own Aspirations and Abilities	3.21	.97	.430	.588	.490	.580
Satisfied with Feeling of "Belonging" and "at Home" in Kibbutz	3.64	1.01	.434	.590	.445	.799
Satisfied with Material Standard of Living (5 Variables, α=.74)	3.09	.79	.405	.533	.421	.503
Satisfied with Work Domain (4 Variables, α=.80)	3.86	.76	.311	.293	.173	.329
Satisfied with Interpersonal Relations in Kibbutz (2 Variables, α=.71	3.29	.78	.395	.553	.403	.660

5. Demography

Gender (1=Males; 2=Females)	1.53	.50	.074	.044	.132	.109
Years of Study (1= up to 12; 2=13; 3=15, 16; 4=17 and More)	2.06	1.00	.052	-.048	NS	NS
Age	48.22	16.08	.052	.130	.155	.109
Holding Central Office during the Last Five Years (1=None; 4=Top Office)	2.28	.99	.060	NS	NS	.064

Source: Own Calculations. All scales: 1=highest or most positive; 5= lowest or least positive; 3=middle level. All shown correlations are significant at the $p<.001$ level.

Table 2 lends itself to the following summary: (a) All three subjective indicators of quality of life are above the middle level, signifying a relatively positive level of subjective well-being. As an illustration of this point in percentage distribution: 8.7 % stated that they were "very satisfied with their life" (category 5), 41.4 % were "satisfied" (category 4); 5.1 % were "very unsatisfied" (category 1), 11.0 % "unsatisfied" (category 2); 33.8 % chose 3, the middle category. (b) The mean levels of the five variables denoting domain satisfaction are also above the middle level but satisfaction with the domain of "standard of living" is close to this middle score and is lowest among the domain satisfaction measures. (c) The three variables denoting conviction with values, are all above the middle category, as is also demonstrated in the percentage of respondents holding strong belief in them – 60.6 % "wish life of solidarity, partnership, and equality" (a much lower percentage than in previous times; e.g. Leviatan & Rosner, 2001); 75.8 % hold to social, collectivistic values; 79.0 % hold to individualistic values. Yet, the level of satisfaction with realization of those values is very low (only 20.9 are "satisfied" or "very satisfied" with their kibbutz realization of these values). This finding attests to the changes experienced in kibbutzim as mentioned earlier. (d) Both independent groups of variables – those that denote "satisfaction with life domains" and those that denote holding to values and evaluation of their realization level, positively relate to the three indicators of well-being: "life satisfaction in general", "satisfaction with one's kibbutz life", and "psychological commitment to one's kibbutz life". However, indicators of domains' satisfaction have a stronger relationship than both groups of the "value" variables. (e) As a rule, the relationships of "domains' satisfaction" with the more specific measures of "kibbutz life" ("satisfaction" and "commitment") are stronger than their relationships with the general measure of "satisfaction with life in general". (f) Satisfaction with the work domain is the only independent variable that shows stronger relations to the general measure. (g) The demographic variables seem to be very weakly related to any of the dependent variables. (h) The "global measure of well-being" shows in its first order correlations with the independent variables, a level that is about average of its three original components. This is expected and since creating an index composed of three variables increases its reliability, it is also statistically desired. An exception shows in the correlation with the variable "satisfied with feeling of 'belonging'..." where "global" is correlated $r=.799$. This correlation is very high, almost too high, and I am not sure about the interpretation of this number. It may suggest, perhaps, that "feeling 'belonging' and 'at home'" captures most of the content and expression of the "global" indicator of well-being and almost fully overlaps it; as if this is what is meant by the combination of "satisfaction with life; satisfaction with one's kibbutz life; and identification with one's kibbutz life". Anyway, this strong overlap would prevent the use of "satisfaction with 'belonging'..." as part of a group of independent variable in analyses where "global" is the dependent variable.

Testing the Hypotheses

I employ multiple regression and partial correlation analyses as major tools to test the hypotheses. I now add to the original formulation of the hypotheses the new variable: "Global indicator of well-being".

Hypothesis 1: Level of satisfaction with various life domains is positively related (a) to "satisfaction with one's life in kibbutz"; (b) to "psychological commitment to one's kibbutz life"; (c) to "satisfaction with life in general"; (d) to the "global" indicator.

Hypothesis 2: Extent of commitment to personal values, and perceived level of their realization in one's community, is positively related (a) to "satisfaction with one's life in kibbutz"; (b) to "psychological commitment to one's kibbutz life"; (c) to "satisfaction with life in general"; (d) to the "global" indicator.

Hypothesis 3: "Satisfaction with one's kibbutz life" (a) is positively related to "satisfaction with life in general"; (b) serves also as an *intervening variable* between satisfaction with life domains, commitment to values, and their perceived level of realization, on the one hand, and satisfactions with life in general on the other.

Hypothesis 4: "Psychological commitment to one's kibbutz life" (a) is positively related to "satisfaction with life in general"; (b) serves also as an *intervening variable* between satisfaction with life domains, commitment to values, and their perceived level of realization, on the one hand, and satisfactions with life in general on the other.

Test of these hypotheses with their subparts is presented in the summary tables 3-7. The pattern of presentation in all tables is similar. For instance, table 3 has "satisfaction with one's kibbutz life" as its dependent variable and tests hypotheses 1(a) and 2(a). The table presents several models, each in a separate column, of multiple regressions – the first three models are one for each of the "predictor" groups of variables ("values," "domain satisfaction," "demographics") to "explain" variance in "satisfaction with one's kibbutz life". The fourth model combines all predictors in one analysis. Entries in the table are standardized *betas* of the regression analysis. However, the last right most column (column 5) offers more exact estimates of the relative contribution (in %), of each "predictor" variable, to the explained variance in the outcome variable.

Table 3: Models of Multiple Regression Analyses to Explain Variance in "Satisfaction with One's Kibbutz Life". Separate Analyses for Three Groups of Predictors (Values, Domain Satisfaction, Demographics) and one for All Combined

Predictors	Multiple Regression Analyses, "Satisfaction with One's Kibbutz Life" Dependent Variable; Standardized βs.				
	Values	Do-main Satisf.	Demo graph-ics	All Three Com-bined	Esti-mated %
Expressions of Personal Values					
Wishes Life of Solidarity, Partnership, and Equality in Most Desired Place of Living	.195	-	-	.074	2.6
Social, Collectivistic Values	.068	-	-	.029	0.0
Individualistic Values	-.076	-	-	NS	NS
Satisfaction with Values Realization					
Satisfaction with kibbutz realization of social/ideological values	.512	-	-	.217	12.6
Satisfaction with Life Domains in Kibbutz					
Satisfied with Fit of Kibbutz Life to Own Aspirations and Abilities	-	.280	-	.216	12.7
Satisfied with Feeling of "Belonging" and "at Home" in Kibbutz	-	.267	-	.278	16.4
Satisfied with Material Standard of Living	-	.250	-	.209	10.8
Satisfied with Work Domain	-	.043	-	.043	1.2
Satisfied with Interpersonal Relation-ships in Kibbutz	-	.114	-	NS	NS

Table 3: Models of Multiple Regression Analyses to Explain Variance in "Satisfaction with One's Kibbutz Life". Separate Analyses for Three Groups of Predictors (Values, Domain Satisfaction, Demographics) and one for All Combined (continued)

Demography					
Gender (1=Males; 2=Females)			.040	NS	NS
Years of Study (1= up to 12; 2=13; 3=15, 16; 4=17 and More)			.035	.033	0.1
Age			-.120	NS	NS
Holding Central Office during the Last Five Years (1=None; 4=Top Office)			NS	NS	NS
R^2	.372	.532	.018	.565	
F (all significant at the $p<.000$ level)	495	900	25	4,460	

Source: Own calculations. Since $R^2= beta_1*r_1 + beta_2*r_2 +...+ beta_n*r_n$. Therefore, $beta_n*r_n / R^2 * 100$ gives an estimate in % of the contribution of predictor n to the explained variance in the dependent variables. This is true as long as the major $beta_n$s and r_ns carry the same sign. When this condition does not hold, and the *beta* and r that are involved are large, the formula is difficult to interpret.

The points illuminated by table 3 are the following: (a) Both "values" (model 1) and "domain satisfactions" (model 2), when used as predictors by themselves explain a sizable part of the variance in the dependent variable (R^2=.372; .532 respectively) while the demographics are negligible as "predictors" (R^2=.018). (b) "Value realization" and "wishes life..." have the highest *betas* in model 1 while the two other variables offer relatively low *betas*. Yet the collectivistic values are positively related to the outcome variable while the individualistic values have negative relationship. (c) Among the domain satisfaction variables, the first three ("fit", "belonging" and "standard of living") are of relatively similar (and high) importance as "predictors" while "work" and "relations" are much lower in importance. (d) Model 4 combines all predictors into one regression formula. It shows an R^2=.565 and the "domains satisfaction" group as a much stronger predictor of the outcome variable. This is particularly true for the first three "predictors" but "value realization" appears also to be on the same order of magnitude. (e) When I attribute estimated relative percentages of explained variance to each group of predictors (see description to table 3 for explanation) the "values" explain 15.2 % of the variance (about 27 % of explained variance) while the "domain satisfaction" group explains 41.1 % (about 73 % of the explained variance).

Table 4 has "psychological commitment to one's kibbutz life" as its dependent variable and tests hypotheses 1(b) and 2(b). Its structure is analogous to that of table 3.

Table 4: Models of Multiple Regression Analyses to Explain Variance in "Psychological Commitment to One's Kibbutz Life". Separate Analyses for Three Groups of Predictors (Values, Domain Satisfaction, Demographics) and on for All Combined

Predictors	Multiple Regression Analyses; "Psychological Commitment to One's Kibbutz Life" Dep. Variable; Standardized βs.				
	Values	Domain Satisf.	Demogr.	All Three Combined	Estimated %
Expressions of Personal Values					
Wishes Life of Solidarity, Partnership, and Equality in Most Desired Place of Living	.435	-	-	.376	21.4
Social, Collectivistic Values	.153	-	-	.130	1.7
Individualistic Values	.150	-	-	-.121	2.5
Satisfaction with Value Realization					
Satisfaction with kibbutz realization of social/ideological values	.306	-	-	.131	5.8
Satisfaction with Life Domains in Kibbutz					
Satisfied with Fit of Kibbutz Life to Own Aspirations and Abilities	.306	-	-	.131	5.8
Satisfied with Feeling of "Belonging" and "at Home" in Kibbutz	-	.283	-	.136	6.6
Satisfied with Material Standard of Living	-	.220	-	.160	7.1
Satisfied with Work Domain	-	-.033	-	NS	NS
Satisfied with Interpersonal Relationships in Kibbutz	-	.049	-	NS	NS
Demography					
Gender (1=Males; 2=Females)			.123	.103	1.5
Years of Study (1= up to 12; 2=13; 3=15, 16; 4=17 and More)			NS	-.029	0.0
Age			-.152	.045	-1.6
Holding Central Office during the Last Five Years (1=None; 4=Top Office)			NS	NS	NS
R^2	.426	.333	.040	.504	
F (all significant at the $p<.000$ level)	647	409	87	288	

Source: Own calculations. See description to table 3.

Table 5 has "life satisfaction in general" as its dependent variable and tests hypotheses 1c and 2c and hypothesis 3a and 4a.

Table 5: Models of Multiple Regression Analyses to Explain Variance in "Satisfaction with Life in General". Separate Analyses for Three Groups of Predictors (Values, Domain Satisfaction, Demographics), for "Satisfaction with One's Kibbutz Life" and "Psychological Commitment to One's Kibbutz Life", and One for All Predictors Combined

| Predictors | Multiple Regression Analyses; "Satisfaction with One's Life in General" Dependent Variable; Standardized βs. | | | | | | |
	1	2	3	4	Est. %	5	6
Expressions of Personal Values							
Wishes Life of Solidarity, Partnership, and Equality in Most Desired Place of Living	.096	-	-	NS	NS	-	-.074
Social, Collectivistic Values	.052	-	-	.047	0.2	-	NS
Individualistic Values	NS	-	-	NS	NS	-	-.034
Satisfaction with Value Realization							
Satisfied with Kibbutz Realization of Social/Ideology Values	.389	-	-	.115	4.8	-	NS
Satisfaction with Life Domains in Kibbutz							
Satisfied with Fit of Kibbutz Life to Own Aspirations and Abilities	-	.177	-	.158	6.8	-	.080
Satisfied with Feeling of "Belonging" and "at Home" in Kibbutz	-	.193	-	.178	7.6	-	.081
Satisfied with Material Standard of Living	-	.205	-	.202	8.4	-	.137
Satisfied with Work Domain	-	.151	-	1.39	4.3	-	.130
Satisfied with Interpersonal Relationships in Kibbutz	-	.046	-	NS	NS	-	NS

Table 5: Models of Multiple Regression Analyses to Explain Variance in "Satisfaction with Life in General". Separate Analyses for Three Groups of Predictors (Values, Domain Satisfaction, Demographics), for "Satisfaction with One's Kibbutz Life" and "Psychological Commitment to One's Kibbutz Life", and One for All Predictors Combined (continued)

Demography							
Gender (1=Males; 2=Females)	-	-	.075	.060	0.5	-	0.46
Years of Study (1= up to 12; 2=13; 3=15, 16; 4=17 and More)	-	-	-.055	-.051	0.3	-	.061
Age	-	-	NS	.043	0.2	-	.036
Holding Central Office during the Last Five Years (1=None; 4=Top Office)	-	-	.036	NS	NS	-	NS
Satisfaction with One's Kibbutz Life	-	-	-	-	-	.453	.287
Psychological Commitment to One's Kibbutz Life	-	-	-	-	-	.169	.155
R^2	.180	.311	.011	.326		.319	.374
F (all significant at the $p<.000$ level)	252	362	15	150		1,014	147

Source: Own calculations. See description to table 3.

Its structure is analogous to that of tables 3 and 4 but is a bit more complex. In addition to the models that are the same as in tables 3 and 4, model 5 includes as predictors "satisfaction with one's kibbutz life" and "psychological commitment to one's kibbutz life" and model 6 runs all predictors (inclusive of the last two) in one regression analysis.

Findings in table 5 could be summarized in this way: (a) Again, both "values" (model 1) and "domain satisfactions" (model 2), when used as predictors by themselves, explain a sizable part of the variance in the dependent variable (R^2=.180; .311, respectively) which means that the "domains satisfaction" group is more important as contributor to explaining variance in the outcome variable. In this table as in tables 3 and 4, the demographics are negligible (R^2=.011). (b) "Value realization" has the highest *beta* in model 1 without a rival. As in tables 3 and 4, collectivistic values are positively related to the outcome variable while the individualistic values are not included in the regression formula. (b) In model 2, among the domain satisfaction variables, the first three ("fit," "belonging", and "standard of living") are of relatively similar (and high) importance as "predictors"; "work" takes a close second place, and "relations" are negligible in importance. (c) Model 4 combines the three groups of predictors into one regression formula. It shows an R^2=.326 and the "domains satisfaction" group as a much stronger predictor of the outcome variable. (d) When I attribute estimated relative percentages of explained variance to each of the three group of predictors (see description to table 3 for explanation) the "values" explain 5.0 % of the variance (about 15 % of explained variance) while the "domain satisfaction" group explains 27.1 % (about 83 % of the explained variance). (e) When the variables "satisfaction with one's kibbutz life" and "psychological commitment to one's kibbutz life" are used as the sole predictors (model 5) the level of explained variance reaches $R^2=.319$. This is a very similar level to the variance explained by model 4 and a clear support of hypotheses 3(a) and 4(a). This finding hints to the possibility that the two predictors indeed take an intervening role as suggested by hypotheses 3(b) and 4(b). I will perform a more detailed investigation of these two hypotheses by table 7. (f) Model 6 includes all variables (inclusive of model 4 and model 5) and the level of explained variance does increase to $R^2=.374$, about 5 % over model 4 and 5 % over model 5 – meaning that model 5 and model 4 pull their explained variances in the outcome variable from at least somewhat different perspectives. Yet model 5 is the major contributor as can be judged by the level of *betas* of its two variables in comparison of the level of the *betas* for the other variables.

Table 6: Models of Multiple Regression Analyses to Explain Variance in "Global Measure of Well-being." Separate Analyses for Three Groups of Predictors ("Values", Domain Satisfaction, Demographics). Model 4 Includes All Predictors. Analyses Exclude "Feeling of 'Belonging'"

Predictors	Multiple Regression Analysis; "Global Measure of Well-being" Dep. Variable. Standardized βs.				
	Values	Do-main Satisf.	De-mogr.	All Three Comb.	Esti-mated %
Expressions of Personal Values					
Wishes Life of Solidarity, Partnership, and Equality in Most Desired Place of Living	.276	-	-	.172	7.4
Social, Collectivistic Values	.123	-	-	.105	0.9
Individualistic Values	-.096	-	-	.118	1.1
Satisfaction with Value Realization					
Satisfied with Kibbutz Realization of Social/Ideology Values	.486	-	-	.118	6.7
Satisfaction with Life Domains in Kibbutz					
Satisfied with Fit of Kibbutz Life to Own Aspirations and Abilities	-	.265	-	.186	10.8
Satisfied with Feeling of "Belonging" and "at Home" in Kibbutz	-	-	-	-	-
Satisfied with Material Standard of Living	-	.196	-	.144	7.4
Satisfied with Work Domain	-	.065	-	.083	2.7
Satisfied with Interpersonal Relationships in Kibbutz	-	.450	-	.390	25.9
Demography					
Gender (1=Males; 2=Females)			.099	.080	1.0
Years of Study (1= up to 12; 2=13; 3=15, 16; 4=17 and More)			NS	NS	
Age			-.100	.058	-0.6
Holding Central Office during the Last Five Years (1=None; 4=Top Office)	-	-	.034	NS	NS
R^2	.419	.575	.024	.633	
F (all significant at the $p<.000$ level)	627	1,412	34	113	

Source: Own calculations. See description to table 3.

Table 6 has the "Global indicator of well-being" as its dependent variable and tests hypotheses 1(d) and 2(d). Its structure is analogous to that of tables 3 and 4. However, given the strong first order correlation of the "global" measure with the "predictor" "feeling of 'belonging'..." (r=.799) and how I interpreted it, I run the combined regression analysis (model 4) with that "predictor" excluded.

(a) Again both "values" (model 1) and "domains satisfaction" (model 2), when used as predictors by themselves, explain a sizable part of the variance in the dependent variable (R^2=.419; .575, respectively), though it is much stronger for the "domain satisfaction" group. The demographics keep to their minor explaining role as in the other tables (R^2=.024). (b) As explained earlier, the "satisfaction with 'belonging'..." is not included in the analyses. We see that its place is taken by the variable of "satisfaction with interpersonal relations" in both the unique (model 2) and in the combined model (4). This is not surprising when one considers that the correlation between the two variables is r=.770. (c) Model 4 tests for the relative importance of "values," "domain satisfaction," and "demographics" when all are combined into one regression formula. The total explained variance is R^2=.633. When I attribute estimated relative percentages of explained variance to each of the three groups of predictors in model 4 (see description to table 3 for explanation), the "values" explain 16.1 % of the variance (about 25 % of explained variance) while the "domain satisfaction" group explains 46.8 % (about 74 % of the explained variance). (d) Remember that the "values" group of "predictors" consists of two kinds of relatedness to values: "level of value conviction" – denoted by degree of belief in the first three expressions in the table – and extent of "satisfaction with value realization in one's kibbutz". While both groups contribute independently to the explained variance in the outcome measure, it is the level of "value conviction" that is the stronger contributor – by about a third more.

Table 7 tests for the intervening role of "satisfaction with one's kibbutz life" and "psychological commitment to one's kibbutz life" (call them variables B1 and B2) between the independent variables of "domains satisfaction" and levels of "value conviction" and "values' realization" (call it A) and "satisfaction with life in general" (call it C) – hypotheses 3(b) and 4(b). I perform this test according to the following rationale: If variables B1 & B2 have an intervening position between variables A and C, than, when controlling for variables B1 & B2 (holding them constant by a procedure such as partial correlation), the statistical relationship between A and C should be strongly reduced compared to the level of the original relationship between them. Since it is also possible that contrary to hypotheses 3(b) and 4(b), variable C serves as an intervening variable between A and B1 & B2 – a test should be performed where variable C is controlled and each of the ensuing statistical relationships of A and B1 & B2 are compared to the original relationship between them.

The results of these analyses with the data at hand are shown in table 7 for the nine independent variables (A). These variables are listed in the first (left) column in nine rows – the first four rows are the "values" variables, and the next five rows are for the "domains satisfaction" variables. The second column represents entries of first-order correlations of "Satisfaction with life in general" (C) with the independent variables (A) while the third column lists entries for partial correlations of same variables. Here both "satisfaction with one's kibbutz life" (B1) and "psychological commitment to one's kibbutz life" (B2) are statistically controlled. Columns 4 and 5 in the table show results of similar analysis for the first-order correlations between the independent variables (A) and "satisfaction with one's kibbutz life" (B1) and partial correlations between these variables while "satisfaction with life" (C) is controlled. Similar is the case in columns 6 and 7, this time with "psychological commitment to one's kibbutz life".

The last row table 7 shows summary calculations of comparing for each variable (B1 & B2) and (C) the two columns and summarizing across the nine independent variables. I have done it by subtracting the squared partial correlation for each analysis from the squared original correlation (but paying attention to sign). In fact, a calculation that shows the reduction in the common statistical variance for two variables when a third variable is statistically controlled by a partial correlation.

This last row summarizes the major findings in support of hypotheses 3(a) and 4(a). It is clear that when variables B1 and B2 are held constant in a partial correlation analysis, the mean reduction in strength of relationship between variables in group (A) is very sizeable –93.4 %, while the reduction in strength of relationship between variables in group (A) and variables (B1) & (B2), when (C) is held constant, is much smaller: 37.1 % and 40.6 % respectively. These results indicate that B1 and B2 are indeed intervening in the relationship between A and C but that C is intervening in the relationship between A and B1 & B2 only to a small extent.

Table 7: "First-order" and "Partial" Correlations between Independent Variables (A) and "Satisfaction with Life in General" (C), "Satisfaction with One's Kibbutz Life" (B1), and Psychological Commitment to One's Kibbutz Life" (B2). Variables (B1 & B2) Are Controlled for Partial Correlations of (A) with (C). Variable (C) is Controlled for Partial Correlations of (A) with (B1 & B2)

Independent Variables (A):	Satisfaction with Life in General (C)		Satisfaction with One's Kibbutz Life (B1)		Psychological Commitment to One's Kibbutz Life (B2)	
	1st Order Corr. (Partial Corr., Variables B1 & B2 Contr.)		1st Order Corr. (Partial Corr., Variable C Contr.)		1st Order Corr. (Partial Corr.; Variable C Contr.)	
Wishes Life of Solidarity, Partnership, and Equality in Most Desired Place of Living	.202	(-.074)	.345	(.278)	.569	(.545)
Social Values – Highly Important	.052	NS	.040	NS	.156	(.148)
Individualistic Values – Highly Important	.068	(-.042)	.160	(.147)	-.179	(-.166)
Satisfied with Kibbutz Realization of Social/Ideology Values	.421	(.128)	.575	(.455)	.447	(.329)
Satisfied with Fit of Kibbutz Life to Own Aspirations and Abilities	.430	(.125)	.588	(.467)	.490	(.379)
Satisfied with Feeling of Belonging and Feeling of Home in Kibbutz Life	.434	(.140)	.590	(.467)	.445	(.322)
Satisfied with Material Standard of Living	.405	(.135)	.533	(.407)	.421	(.303)
Satisfied with Work Domain	.311	(.189)	.293	(.154)	.173	(.050)
Satisfied with Interpersonal Relations in Kibbutz	.395	(.112)	.553	(.439)	.403	(.285)
Mean Reduction in % of Explained Variance	93.4 %		37.1 %		40.6 %	

Source: Own Calculations.

SUMMARY AND DISCUSSION

Test of Hypotheses 1(a-d); 2(a-d): Models of type (2) as separate regression analyses in tables 3-6, demonstrate sizeable levels of the "domains satisfaction" contributions to the explained variance in each of the four indicators of subjective quality of life as suggested by hypotheses 1(a-d) (Range of R^2s is .310 - .575, and an average level of .437). Models of type (1) show the same for the "values" contribution, and hypotheses 2(a-d), though at a somewhat lower levels of R^2s (.180 to .426, and an average of .349). Looking through the perspective of models of type (4) and their accompanied columns of "% estimations of variance attributed to each predictor" in tables 3-6, where I combined all "predictors" in each of the multiple regression analyses, shows a similar pattern. The independent level of explained variance taken by the "domains satisfaction" is 36.3 % to 83.1 %, with an average of 66.5 %. The corresponding percentages of the explained variance taken by "values" are 15.3 % to 62.3 %, with an average of 32.5 %. The contribution of the "demographics" in each analysis of models of type (3) and models of type (4) of the tables is always insignificant.

Thus, it is clear that both hypotheses 1(a-d) and 2(a-d) are strongly supported – separately and together. Both satisfaction of needs in various life domains as well as belief in values and their perceived realization, are strong independent contributors to levels of quality of life as used in the current study. Their combined explained variance across the four indicators of quality of life ranges from 32.6 % to 63.3 %, with an average of 50.7 %.

The analyses in tables 3-6 hint to the reason why so many researchers in the field are satisfied with their results of explaining variance in "life satisfaction," or other general indicators of quality of life, by level of need satisfaction only. Comparing the level of explained variance – as expressed by R^2s – in models of type (2) to that of models (4), shows that models (2) by themselves capture almost all explained variance (an average of .507 for models (4) and .437 for model of type (2)). It is difficult to see that such results conceal more complex findings. But, models of type (4), the combined regressions, demonstrate that a major part of the variance expressed by "domain satisfactions" belongs, in fact to the "values" section. Once the "values" are included in the analyses, the explained variance is dissected to give each contributor group its right share.

Tests of Hypotheses 3(a) and 4(a) suggest the strong relationship of "satisfaction with one's kibbutz life," and "psychological commitment to one's kibbutz life," with "life satisfaction in general". Indeed this is the case as can be easily seen in table 2 and model 5 in table 5. Hypotheses 3(b) and 4(b) suggest that these two variables also serve as intervening variables between the "predictors" ("values" and "domain satisfactions") and "life satisfaction in general." These hypotheses are supported by the findings of model 6 in table 5 where these two variables account for the major part of the explained variance. But the results of table 7 offer an even clearer support for these hypotheses: When the two hypothesized intervening variables are held constant (in partial correlation analyses), the level of correlation between the "predictors" and "satisfaction with life" is reduced by 93.4 % of variance explained.

Different perspectives on "values": Throughout this paper I referred to two separate aspects of the "values" group of "predictors": level of belief in, or conviction of, personal values, and perceived extent of the values' realization in one's kibbutz community. Are these two aspects really different from each other? The answer is clearly positive. Level of *belief in values* is portrayed by three variables – "wishes life of solidarity...," belief in "social, collectivistic, values," and belief in "individualistic" values. Level of "satisfaction with realization of kibbutz unique values" is expressed by one variable. Models of type (4) in tables 3-6 show that, on average, the "realization" variable contributes about 60 % of the explained variance of the combined "value" group of "predictors" while the "belief" variables account for about 40 %. We should conclude, therefore, that individuals' subjective quality of life are affected by degree of belief in values but also by the extent that these values are expressed and realized in their relevant social environments.

Another important conclusion from the findings in the analyses is that "collectivistic" and "individualistic" beliefs contribute independently to the explained variance of the outcome indicators of quality of life. Even though their separate relations to the outcome variables are in the opposite direction – "social/collectivistic" belief are in positive relation with subjective quality of life, while "individualistic" belief stand in negative relation. Therefore, it is not (only) the content of the values that matters for subjective quality of life, but also the intensity of belief in them.

Outcomes for "low beliefs" in values: Do the conclusions I reached about the importance of "values" in determining various indicators of subjective quality of life hold for populations who care less about values? After all, many kibbutz members joined (freely) their kibbutzim due to their personal belief in the kibbutz unique values. Perhaps values make a difference for subjective quality of life only in populations for whom ideology is a major component of life? Answering this question is important also because it may indicate the extent of possible generalization from this study to other populations. I tested for an answer by running regression analyses of the model (1) type (only "value variables" as "predictors") for the four indicators of subjective quality of life but only for those that were below the median level of (1) wishes life of solidarity..." and (2) "satisfaction with kibbutz realization of values". I compared the resulting R^2s of the eight analyses with those of models of type (1) in tables 3-6. Indeed, the findings of the comparison show a reduction in R^2 – on average: from $R^2=.349$ in the original analyses to an average of $R^2=.281$, still a level of explained that is very high. Also, one has to keep in mind that in these two analyses I used – by definition –samples of restricted range on the very variables in the center of analysis. Thus, it seems that the importance of values for well-being and quality of life is true not only for those with strong ideological conviction. I suggest, therefore, that "values" are important contributors to subjective quality of life in all populations.

The position of "demographics": A striking finding throughout all analyses is that "demographics" are not significant in determining level of any of the indicators of quality of life. Yet, could demographic characteristics, such as gender or age, act as mediators / conditioners for the regression formulas? I tested for this possibility by running regression analyses similar to model 4 in table 6 (the dependent variable was the "global measure") separately for males and females and then separately for six age groups (-30; 31-40; 41-50; 51-60; 61-70; 71-80). In each analysis I calculated the estimated percentage of variance in the dependent variable that could be attributed to the "values" group. The results support the suggestion of a mediating role for these demographic variables. The "values" "predictors" account for more variance in the analysis of males (19.8 % vs. 13.5 %). Results for the different age groups do not have an immediate interpretation, as there is no linear change across the age groups. "Values" account for 16.5 % of the variance in the -30 age group; 18.7 % for the 31-40 group; 25.8 % for the 41-50 group; 29.2 % for the 51-60 group; 22.7 % for the 61-70 group, and 42.5 % for the 71-80 group. Thus, it is clear that the "demographics" have a role in determining the pattern of "predictors" contributions to indicators of subjective quality of life. Their exact role and why they operate in the way they do is still open for further analyses that is beyond the framework of the current paper.

I believe that while the findings of this study are of general importance, they are of particular importance for the kibbutz society. They demonstrate the values members hold, and the extent of the actual realization of the kibbutz' formally defined ideology, and are important for the enhancement of subjective quality of life among members. They are also important for the enhancement of psychological commitment and identification with kibbutz life. Since for members their kibbutz life is a free choice – such commitment is a must for membership growth and survival.

NOTES

1   In the next section I give relevant kibbutz background for the current study but in very general statements. I am assuming the readers have a general knowledge of what are the kibbutz communities. For English readers who are less familiar with the kibbutz phenomenon, I recommend a recent publication that covers major domains of kibbutz life both at present and as compared to their past manifestation (Leviatan, Oliver and Quarter, 1998); and an historical presentation in two volumes (Near, 1992; 1997).

REFERENCES

Central Bureau of Statistics, Israel (1979; 1986; 1997): Statistical Abstracts of Israel, Jerusalem.
Cummins. R. A., R. Eckersley, J. Pallant, J.Van Vugt & R. Misajon (2002): Developing a National Index of Subjective Well-being: The Australian Unity Well-being Index. Social Indicators Research 64, 159-90.
Diener, E. & M. Diener (1995): Cross Cultural Correlates of Life Satisfaction and Self-Esteem. Journal of Personality and Social Psychology 68, 653-63.
Hofstede, G. (1991): Cultures and Organizations: Software of the Mind, London: McGraw-Hill.
Hofstede, G. (1998): Attitudes, Values and Organizational Culture: Disentangling the Concepts. Organization Studies, 19 (3), 477-92.
Kibbutz Regulation (Kibbutz By-Laws) (1973), Kibbutz Artzi, Tel-Aviv.
Leviatan, U. (1998): Second and Third Generations in the Kibbutz – Is the Survival of the Kibbutz Society Threatened? U. Leviatan, H. Oliver & J. Quarter (eds.): Crisis in the Israeli Kibbutz. Meeting the Challenge of Changing Times, Westport, Conn.: Praeger, 81-96.
Leviatan, U. & M. Rosner (2001): Belief in Values and the Future of Kibbutzim, Institute for Social Research of the Kibbutz, 174 (Hebrew).
Leviatan, U. (1999): Contribution of Social Arrangements to the Attainment of Successful Aging – the Experience of the Israeli Kibbutz. Journal of Gerontology: Psychological Sciences, 54b: 205-13.
Leviatan, U. (2003): Is it the End of Utopia? The Israeli Kibbutz at the Twenty-First Century. Center for Study of Co-operatives, University of Saskatchewan, Saskatoon.
Leviatan, U., A. Am-Ad & G. Adar (1981): Aging in the Kibbutz: Satisfaction with Life and its Determinants, Hakibbutz, 8: 16-60 (Hebrew).
Mayton, D. M., S. J. Ball-Rokeach & W.E. Loges (1994): Human Values and Social Issues: Journal of Social Issues, 50 (4), 1-8.
Mowday, R. T., L. M. Porter & R. M. Steers (1982): Review and Reconceptualization of Organizational Commitment. Academy of Management Review 10 (3), 465-76.
National Research Council (2001): Preparing for an Aging World: The Case for Cross National Research, Panel on a Research Agenda and New Data for an Aging World, Committee on Population and

294 URIEL LEVIATAN

Committee on National Statistics, Division on Behavioral and Social Sciences and Education. Washington D. C.: National Academic Press.

Near, H. (1992): The Kibbutz Movement: A History, Vol 1. Oxford: Oxford University Press.

Near, H. (1997): The Kibbutz Movement: A History, Vol 2. Oxford: Oxford University Press.

Rokeach, M. (1973): The Nature of Human Values, NY: The Free Press.

Schwartz, S. H. (1994): Beyond Individualism/Collectivism. U. Kim, H. C. Triandis, C. Kagitcibasi, S. C. Choi & G. Yoon (eds.): Individualism and Collectivism: Theory, Methods, and Applications, Thousand Oaks, Ca.: Sage Publications, 85-119.

Schwartz, S. (1994): Structure of Human Values. Journal of Social Issues 50 (4), 18-45.

Shamir, B. (1990): Calculations, Values, and Identities: The Sources of Collective Work Motivation. Human Relations, 43 (4), 313-32.

Stoffregen, M. (ed.) (2003): Challenges for Quality of Life in the Contemporary World: 2003, 5th Conference of the International Society for Quality of Life Studies (ISQOLS), July, 20-24, 2003, Abstract Brochure, Frankfurt/Main, Germany.

Sverke, M. & S. Kuruvilla (1995): A New Conceptualization of Union Commitment: Development and Test of an Integrated Theory. Journal of Organizational Behavior, 16, 505-532.

Triandis, G. (1994): Theoretical and Methodological Approaches to the Study of Collectivism and Individualism. U. Kim, H. C. Triandis, C. Kagitcibasi, S. C. Choi & G. Yoon (eds.): Individualism and Collectivism: Theory, Methods, and Applications, Thousand Oaks, Ca.: Sage Publications, 41-51.

Triandis, H. C. (1995): Individualism and Collectivism, Boulder, Co.: Westview Press.

Veenhoven, R. (1997): Advances in Understanding Happiness. Revue Quebecoise de Psychologie, 18, 29-74 (English Version).

Yetim, U. (2002): The Impacts of Individualism/Collectivism, Self-esteem, and Feeling of Mastery on Life Satisfaction among the Turkish University Students and Academicians. Social Indicators Research 61, 297-317.

PART V:
OPTIONS AND RESTRICTIONS
FOR QUALITY OF LIFE

18. QUALITY OF LIFE IN A DIVIDED SOCIETY

Valerie Møller

Rhodes University, Grahamstown, South Africa

ABSTRACT

Quality-of-life studies of the 'counting' variety were launched in America and Europe in the 1960s. Since then it is primarily research based on populations in developed countries that has informed our knowledge of quality-of-life measurement and substantive issues pertaining to life quality. In the first section, the paper states that developing country studies are increasingly finding space in leading scientific quality-of-life journals and thereby afford opportunities to expand the global knowledge base. The paper then focuses on quality-of-life studies in divided societies, taking South Africa as example of a deeply divided society – ethnically and socio-economically. It is argued that disaggregation of social indicators along the fault lines in society leads to a deeper understanding of the complexities in the social fabric which are masked by country-level statistics.

INTRODUCTION

When Professor Wolfgang Glatzer invited me to participate in this opening session, he made it clear that he regarded me as a representative of quality-of-life researchers in developing countries. I feel greatly honored to represent the strong contingent of researchers from developing countries at this conference and elsewhere, who are contributing to our knowledge of well-being.

Wolfgang Glatzer also made it abundantly clear that he did not want me to talk exclusively about South Africa, my home country for the past 27 years. So, this evening I would like to wear two hats, the first one of a scholar from a developing society and then switch hats and wear the one of a scholar from South Africa. When wearing my South African hat, I would like to explore with you in greater detail the challenge of studying quality of life in a divided society.

The main theme of this paper will be *difference* – the difference underlying social divides in the world and their impact on quality of life.

This paper is divided into four parts: In the *first* I explore the inclusiveness of contemporary quality-of-life research. In the *second* I focus on a particular dimension of 'difference' at the global level, that of rich and poor. In the *third* part, I ask whether national entries in our quality-of-life databases might not mask important within-country differences. The *fourth* part looks at quality of life trends in South Africa as a case study of a divided society where within-country differences matter.

Wolfgang Glatzer, Susanne von Below, Matthias Stoffregen (eds.), Challenges for Quality of Life in the Contemporary World, 297-310.

QUALITY OF LIFE STUDIES IN GLOBAL PERSPECTIVE

We quality-of-life scholars from developing countries owe an enormous debt to the developed world in the sense that quality of life and social indicators research of the modern, 'counting' variety originated in Western and developed countries. Two distinct traditions of quality of life and living levels research emerged in America and Europe (Vogel, 1997). Many of us from the global periphery studied in the West or learnt the tools of our trade from mentors in Europe or America.

One of the first exercises newcomers to quality-of-life research from developing countries undertake is to explore the meaning of the good life and of the key concepts of well-being in their own country. This is precisely what we did in South Africa in the late 1970s when I joined the quality-of-life research fraternity. And I have observed that colleagues from other non-Western and developing countries have taken the same course. This curiosity of scholars from far-flung places has resulted in a growing number of monographs that chart the range and salience of quality-of-life issues in different cultures around the world.

In 2000 the editor of Mapi's *Quality of Life Newsletter*, which addresses mainly health-related quality-of-life issues, put a question to his readers: Does QOL research pay enough attention to quality of life in the Third World. The question was repeated last year because the editor had received so few replies (Joyce, 2002; Fielding, 2003).[1] To get a tentative answer to the question, I attempted a count of articles based on quality-of-life research in 'developed' and 'developing' contexts, or to use Huntington's (1998) crude distinction in his book on the clash of civilizations, in countries of the 'West' and the 'rest'. The exercise produced the following results:

I counted close on 200 (196 to be exact) articles published in *Social Indicators Research* since 1990 – excluding one special issue devoted to methodology issues. Approximately half of the articles included a country-specific reference in title or abstract.[2]

Focusing only on the country-specific contributions with labels of origin, *Social Indicators Research* appears to be doing a good job of encouraging the global production of quality-of-life studies by disseminating reports on developing countries. Among the articles with country labels, I counted some 98 studies from developed countries and only a slightly lower number, 89, from developing ones. A similar exercise for the *Journal of Happiness Studies* since inception in 2000 yielded 7 developed country articles and 6 developing country articles while the bulk of articles discussed more general issues of quality of life or were based on cross-cultural or international studies.

This counting exercise was initially prompted by a personal grumble of mine. I have often resented, that as a researcher from the periphery, I feel compelled to identify the study context in the title of my papers while colleagues from the developed center feel free to simply present their work without a label of origin.[3] However, as you see, I seem to be mistaken. The majority of colleagues in both the 'West' and the 'rest' do mention social context if not in the title then at least in the abstract of their reports. In other words, they believe 'difference' does matter. By reporting social context boldly, we are better able to detect cultural variations in quality of life dynamics.

In all, I thought that about 13 % of articles published since 1998 in *Social Indicators Research* might have made mention of context in title or abstract. In support of my original hypothesis, I came across only few daring researchers from developing countries who felt sufficiently confident to dispense with labels of origin. Actually two such authors were based in Africa. One writer reported on consumer satisfaction with public service delivery in the Cameroon. Another was a South African author whose paper on 'measuring quality of life in rural development' had missed my attention. The latter case serves as example that missing labels might be counterproductive in that they hinder the exchange of local knowledge among neighbors.

In short, in response to the editor of the Mapi quality-of-life newsletter, as the counting exercise demonstrates clearly, our quality-of-life journals have made it their business to support the internationalization of quality-of-life research. They are providing a good forum for researchers in developing countries to report their work.

FROM NATIONAL TO INTERNATIONAL: THE GLOBAL DIFFERENCE

Quality-of-life studies may have started off as parochial national studies in the West. We often turn to the most familiar and to our backyard to satisfy intellectual curiosity. However, as the journal count illustrates, quality-of-life research has grown from being a national business to become an international enterprise. Many of the articles with no country labels were international studies. Increasingly, we are turning to cross-country databases to explore global differences in quality of life.

In the new millennium, we realize how interconnected the world is and at the same time how divided we are, as events of the new millennium such as September 11, which occurred shortly before our last meeting in 2001, and more recently, the Second Gulf War and the SARS epidemic make abundantly clear.

In national studies, it might be correct to say that quality-of-life researchers tend to underplay difference. Possibly, having established that in stable Western societies biographical or demographic factors such as age, gender, and education explain such a small proportion in the variance of life satisfaction (Michalos, 1991, among others), most quality-of-life researchers have moved on.

There is one exception, however. Quality-of-life researchers seem to be obsessed and intrigued with income, which has emerged as one of the most powerful divides within and *between* societies. This preoccupation is shared by colleagues all over the world from a wide spectrum of disciplines ranging from psychologists, to political scientists, to economists. Friends and colleagues in South Africa have a habit of sending me newspaper clippings with headings – to quote a few: "Healthy, wealthy and unhappy"; "Rising prosperity does not make people feel more contented – economists want to know why" ; "Richer Britain gets depressed"; "An affluent but more anxious society". Of course the reference is to fairly affluent social contexts such as the United States or the United Kingdom. Obviously, it makes my less affluent South African colleagues feel better when they send me these reminders of trivial pursuits in happiness research!

Starting with Richard Easterlin's work in the 1970s (Easterlin, 1974; 1995; 2002), the role of income in enhancing life quality has fascinated many researchers including colleagues Ed Diener and family and colleagues (Diener et al., 1993;

Diener & Diener, 1995; Diener & Oishi, 2000; and Diener & Biswas-Diener, 2002); Wolfgang Glatzer (2002) with his edited volume on rich and poor; Ruut Veenhoven, Peggy Schyns, Willem Saris and colleagues in the Netherlands and Russia (Veenhoven, 2002; Saris & Andreenkova, 2001; Schyns, 2001); and Bob Cummins (2000) and his Australian colleagues; and many others. In a world subscribing to capitalism, income is *the* ultimate resource, which allows people to access all other resources, to cushion stress when their happiness set-level is under threat or has experienced a dip. Income will assist in restoring happiness to its normal set-level when it has been dragged down. In this sense, income plays an important role in bolstering individual capabilities, referring to the quality-of-life concept made popular by economist Nobel laureate Amartya Sen (1999).

The Income/Satisfaction Curve

One of the strongest images we have of international 'difference' and of a divided world is the curve that plots life satisfaction against individual or national income for developed and developing countries (Inglehart & Klingemann, 2000). This compelling picture of global quality of life is the product of cross-national research that is increasingly including a larger number of developing countries. Typically, the curve rises sharply from the origin at the bottom left and then flattens at top right. In short, at bottom left in the graph we see a strong correlation between income and satisfaction in poorer developing and transition countries. The higher the income or wealth of nations, the flatter the curve becomes at top right. Increasing income has a lesser impact on perceived quality of life in richer developed countries.

There are different ways of interrogating this image of the global divide between rich and poor.

The image reflects the global distribution of power. In many ways, it makes one of the strongest cases for the supremacy of economic growth, free markets and democracy. Quality-of-life researchers may have difficulties in disentangling the effects of factors which correlate with high satisfaction levels such as high living standards, education, wealth, democracy and intangibles including human rights, freedom of expression, and social equality. However, in countries of the South – the non-Western countries, the trappings of modernity, consumer goods, are often viewed as synonyms of Western capitalism and the developed world. Westernization is regarded as the embodiment of everything modern. As Diener and Biswas-Diener remark, it may be that well-off people around the world serve as models of consumption for others, even people in poorer nations (2002: p 149).

Certainly, the Afrobarometer (2002) conducted in a dozen Southern African countries found that ordinary citizens expect democracy to deliver, if not consumer goodies, then at least the basic necessities of life such as food, water, shelter and education. Citizens in new democracies are predisposed to judge the performance of democracy primarily in terms of improving living standards rather than abstracts such as regular elections, competing political parties, and freedom to criticize governments.

How long will it take for poorer nations to catch up on their consumption and satisfaction deficit? Ronald Inglehart, referring to the wealth of nations/life satisfaction curve, observes that historically Protestant societies have had a head start in reaping the material rewards of capitalism that appears to have translated into life satisfaction. According to Claus Kernig (1999: p. 41), transition from a traditional to modern society in western capitalist society took place over a long rather than a short period of time and a large part of the social conflicts in the period of transition were externalized. In contrast, capitalism in the transition countries came as a shock and has yet to meet the material aspirations of citizens as quality-of-life research in Eastern Europe and Russia demonstrates (see Schyns, 2001, among others).

Referring to the flattening of the income/life satisfaction curve for richer countries, Inglehart's classic explanation is that once basic needs have been met, it is the intangibles; the post-materialist or higher order needs that enhance subjective well-being. Diener & son drawing on the literature on income and well-being offer this recipe for achieving happiness: "Avoid poverty, live in a rich country and focus on goals other than material wealth!" (Diener & Biswas-Diener, 2002: p. 161).

I would venture to say that in poorer countries, higher order needs find their expression or – more often – their suppression through the basics. For instance, in South Africa, poorer people have told us researchers that access to basic needs such as water, electricity, or a basic state pension have afforded dignity, feelings of freedom, increase in life choices, and a sense of equality. On the other hand, South Africans in dire economic straits, such as the long-term unemployed, have told us that there can be no happiness without money. Those who have lost their jobs know firsthand that "You even lose your friends when you lose your income" and "Money is everything" (Møller, 1993).

WITHIN-COUNTRY DIFFERENCE

I should like to explore another aspect of the income/satisfaction curve so familiar to us. The third part of my talk poses the question: "Do our national statistics mask within-country difference?"[4] It is important to address this question in order to better understand the study of quality of life in a divided society such as South Africa.

As in so many other cross-cultural studies, the units of analysis in the income/satisfaction graph are nation states. The question is whether nations are pitched at the right level to capture nuances in quality-of-life dynamics. We know that nations are recent and arbitrary creations. This is certainly the case for many countries in Africa where there was complete disregard for ethnic and territorial identities straddling national borders. In recent years some nation states have split up in ways to better reflect ethnic/racial identities and visions for the future welfare of their people. Recent examples include Yugoslavia and Czechoslovakia. Since the collapse of the USSR, quality-of-life researchers have automatically accepted a host of smaller units for their cross-country comparisons. More than a decade after unification, the two Germanys still feature separately in European databases.

'Territorial' indicators are hardly a new idea. Back in the 1970s Knox (1974) was an early advocate of so-called 'territorial indicators' that broke down statistics along spatial divisions. Other differences, which might or might not overlap with territory, may be equally important. In so-called conflict or divided societies, class, ethnicity or religious factors may play a decisive role in shaping quality of life.

When I see a country value for South Africa, I often wonder, *which* South Africa is captured in the data knowing fully well that the differences are so stark, ranging from First to Third World living conditions and a mix of cultures. In fact, the historian Paul Johnson (1996: p. 728) may have been among the first to express the idea that South Africa is "one world in one country".

The United Nations Development Programme realized the importance of delving deeper into the South African case. For the first time in 1994, the year which saw all South Africans voting for the first time, the United Nations Development Programme saw fit to report Human Development Index indicators disaggregated for racial groups in South Africa. They noted that disparities between blacks and whites in South Africa were four times larger than in the United States (UNDP, 1994: p 98). Since this time, university-based researchers and Statistics South Africa follow suit and break down the HDI by race as well as region.

Theodor Hanf (1999), an international scholar of cultural difference and conflict resolution, argues that economic criteria are not the sole pole around which individuals aggregate their interests. Once a group that is defined in terms of a cultural marker gains power, it is able to distribute power and privilege in terms of its defining cultural marker that is disproportionately in its own favor. The conflict faults always run between the 'haves' and 'have-nots', between those who want to maintain the existing distribution of resources and power and those who want to change it. And divisions in society tend to run deeper when they follow differences of origin, language, and religion, all of which embrace and express socio-cultural values.

Hanf (1999) identifies five ideal-type patterns of conflict resolution, from the most extreme solution of partition to more amicable solutions such as power-sharing or syncretism which often occurs under the motto of "unity in diversity". For example, Switzerland might be regarded as a model of peaceful co-existence of different language and religious groups.

We now turn to the fourth and last part of this paper – to quality of life in a divided society focusing on the case of South Africa (Møller, 1999a).

QUALITY OF LIFE TRENDS IN DIVIDED SOUTH AFRICA

South Africa is often called the "land of miracles". In recent times South Africa has become known as a prime example of a nation that is coming to terms with difference. South Africa may be unique in that the ruling white minority voluntarily renounced its position of power in favor of a democratic power-sharing solution with the disenfranchised black majority. The "big" miracle occurred in 1994 when all South Africans went to the polls in long snaking queues to cast their vote for the new democratic government. Since that time the eyes of the world have been trained on South Africa to follow the course of developments.

In 1994, the new beach-towel flag became a firm favorite. The new founding myth of the "rainbow people" captured the imagination of ordinary South Africans from all walks of life. The new South Africans burst with pride when they won the Rugby World Cup in 1995 with a solitary black player to make up the "rainbow" team.

A decade later, in 2003, South Africa is looking ahead to its third open national elections in a year's time. The appeal of the founding myth, which celebrates diversity and regards people of all colors as equal, has faded in time. Although less obvious than the "big" miracle of 1994, smaller miracles of peaceful co-existence occur in everyday life when ordinary South Africans try to live up to the ideals of the "rainbow nation". Quite remarkable is the manner in which formerly oppressed black South Africans continue to express their goodwill towards fellow citizens while waiting patiently to harvest the fruits of democracy.

South Africans have been remarkably patient when seeking to rebuild post-apartheid society. However, history has a long memory. It will take time to erase the legacy of apartheid in so many aspects of life. Reality is that the country is still divided into rich and poor, a divide which coincides with color as under the apartheid regime which engineered caste-like ethnic divisions and distribution of power and privilege among four officially designated population groups, whites, Indians/Asians, colored people of mixed race, and Africans/Blacks. South Africa's social indicators tell the full quality-of-life story only if they are broken down by ethnicity.

Given its unique history, the cultural diversity of its peoples, and its extreme wealth differentials[5], South Africa serves as a social laboratory for quality-of-life studies. The *South African Quality of Life Trends Project,* managed by Rhodes University's Institute of Social and Economic Research in Grahamstown, has tracked the satisfaction and happiness of South Africans against the backdrop of changes occurring in society before and after the coming of democracy (Møller & Schlemmer, 1983; Møller, 1997; 1998; 2001).

Figure 1. South African Quality of Life Trends: Percentages of South Africans Happy, Satisfied with Life, and Seeing Life as Getting Better or Worse

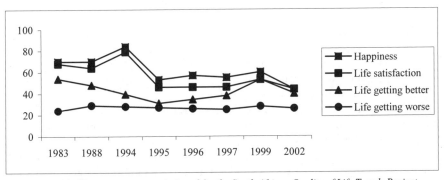

Source:MarkData surveys commissioned for the South African Quality of Life Trends Project

Results are striking. Citizen satisfaction peaked in 1994 in the month after the first open democratic elections (Figure 1). Under apartheid, levels of life satisfaction and happiness reflected the imposed racial hierarchy of power and privilege with whites mostly satisfied, blacks mostly dissatisfied, and Indian and colored people falling somewhere in between. In May 1994, a month after the first open elections, black and white and rich and poor were equally satisfied with life for the first time. South African levels of satisfaction reached ones generally found in Western and democratic societies; approximately four in five South Africans stated they were satisfied with life overall and happy. However, post-election euphoria was short-lived. Satisfaction levels have since returned to ones reminiscent of those under the former regime (Møller, 1998).

In the last survey undertaken for the *South African Quality of Life Trends Study* in mid-2002, only some 44 % of all South Africans stated they are satisfied with life. Some 68 % of whites are satisfied, 65 % of Indians, 58 % of colored, and only 37 % of blacks (Figure 2). Levels of dissatisfaction are particularly pronounced in the domains of income, social security, and access to jobs.

Figure 2. South African Quality of Life Trends: Percentages Satisfied with Life-as-a-whole

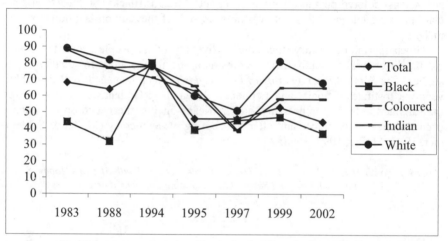

Source: MarkData surveys commissioned for the South African Quality of Life Trends Project.

What would make ordinary South Africans happy? An earlier 1999 survey undertaken for the South African Quality of Life Trends Study posed this question. Poorer respondents thought they would be happier if their material living conditions improved and cited wants such as access to jobs and livelihoods, housing, infrastructure services – water, electricity, sanitation, and education, In short, poorer South Africans listed the ingredients of the elections promises and South Africa's ambitious Reconstruction and Development Programme. In contrast, safety and security issues – "less crime"[6], and a strong economy featured more prominently in the wish lists of richer South Africans (Møller, 1999b).

The conclusions to be drawn from these quality-of-life trends are clear-cut. Now that South Africans have achieved political freedom, it is "bread and butter" issues, such as lack of income security and unemployment, that eclipse other life concerns among the black majority, which according to the latest census make up 79 % of the country's population of close on 45 million in 2001.

Characteristics of South African Quality of Life

There are four striking features of quality of life in South Africa:
1. There is a vast discrepancy between the levels of satisfaction of black and white and of rich and poor in society.
2. Optimism correlates negatively with current happiness. Black and poor South Africans expect to be more satisfied with life in future, albeit from a low satisfaction base, while better-off whites and Indians tend to be more pessimistic.
3. There is a close match between objective and subjective indicators, that is, between perceived well-being and standards of living.
4. Overall life satisfaction and domain satisfactions appear to be sensitive to changing circumstances in society. Importantly, satisfaction seems to increase with rising living levels.

Bridging the Divides

What then are the prospects of bridging the gap between the racial divisions in quality of life?

The majority of youth under apartheid were willing to forego education for liberation. Contemporary South African youth take political freedom for granted and crave the trappings of consumerism and modernity of the Western world they know from television. The new government is acutely aware of the need to underpin the country's fragile democracy with material rewards. True to its election promises of 1994, the democratically-elected African National Congress government built a million houses by the turn of the century and is in the process of building the next half million as part of the country's Reconstruction and Development Programme. It has brought clean water and electricity to poorer households throughout the country. Under discussion are ways to increase social security benefits for poor households through a mix of employment opportunities and increased government transfers. Free basic electricity and water will make mainly urban household incomes stretch further in future.

One of South Africa's greatest achievements since 1994 has been the adoption of a sound macro-economic policy, which has resulted in economic stability to finance nation building. Noteworthy is that the disposition of optimism and quiet patience among South Africa's poor has bought time for the new government to maintain fiscal discipline while seeking to fulfill its Reconstruction and Development Programme obligations to the poor.

Another major achievement signifying the triumph of human rights has been the adoption in 1996 of one of the most progressive constitutions in the world that guarantees equality for all. Nevertheless, some sectors of South African society believe the country's economic policy has failed the poor. In spite of economic stability, South Africa has achieved only jobless growth. The official unemployment rate is currently estimated at some 30 % (30.5 %), and up to some 40 % (41.8 %) if discouraged workers are included (SAIRR, 2003: p. 5). The HIV/AIDS epidemic, which has yet to peak in South Africa, will retard economic growth. Latest estimates are an HIV prevalence rate of 15.6 % in the total population rising to 28 % among

25-29 year olds and people living in the informal urban housing areas (Shisana and Simbayi, 2002).

Social Comparison in Divided Societies

Identifying the nature of social comparisons in divided societies proves to be a tricky business in many instances.

It is fairly evident that poorer South Africans feel entitled to a better deal under democracy. Politically emancipated citizens are aware of their rights under the new constitution and are not afraid to voice their grievances if they feel short-changed. This sense of entitlement as social comparison factor may account for some of the satisfaction deficit among black South Africans. Equity considerations most certainly act as social comparison factors here (Michalos, 1985).

Disentangling the effects of individualist and collectivist tendencies (Triandis, 2000) in shaping social comparisons becomes more difficult in a society which includes mainly individualist whites and mainly collectivist blacks. Thus there is no central cultural script for South Africans to follow to enhance personal well-being in line with person-environment fit theory (Kitayama & Markus, 2000). The question is whether poorer blacks should follow the script of the more economically privileged individualists to optimize well-being rather than remaining true to their own group's collectivist ideals.

On the other hand, attuning to collectivist ideals might enhance well-being among white Afrikaans speakers, the backbone of the former ruling political party, who are among the losers in the new South Africa. For example, the South African Quality of Life Trends Study found that white South Africans, in particularly Afrikaners, who were willing to subscribe to the collectivist myth of the rainbow nation, were more likely to experience national pride and to score higher on subjective well-being (Dickow & Møller, 2002).

Diener and Oishi (2000) argue that poor people may be better off in a wealthy than in a poorer nation due to shared community resources. By definition, a divided society has difficulty in sharing resources. So far South Africa has not introduced a wealth tax as such. However, measures to promote affirmative action and black economic empowerment opportunities as well as cross-subsidization of services in poorer areas are being put in place to bring the benefits from islands of wealth to the more dispersed poor. In her introduction to the study of income and life satisfaction in transitional Russia, Peggy Schyns (2001) makes reference to a guilt factor, which might mediate the satisfaction of the better-off. In the South African case, there appear to be no indications that the guilt factor has depressed the subjective well-being of economically more advantaged South Africans.

OUTLOOK

What then are the prospects for a less divided South Africa? There are encouraging signs that the fault lines between South Africa's divides may be softening.

A nationally representative survey conducted in 2001 in advance of the world conference on racism found that ordinary South Africans saw race discrimination as the least of their problems. Typical problems of transition, such as unemployment and crime, rather then race discrimination were perceived to be unresolved in the new South Africa (Schlemmer, 2001). A more recent survey by the Institute for Justice and Reconciliation in October 2002 found widespread willingness among South Africa's youth to coexist. Youth are optimistic about the country's chances of finding solutions to the problems their parents and grandparents created. Almost 80 % of young people surveyed are confident of a happy future for all races in the country (Sapa, 2003).

Returning to the income/satisfaction curve, the South African Quality of Life Trends Study, referred to above, shows that subjective well-being appears to be remarkably sensitive to changing living conditions. In South Africa higher incomes and improved living standards do appear to translate into increased happiness and life satisfaction. For example, in 1999, for the first time in the history of South African social indicators research, a sufficiently large number of black householders gained entry into the highest-ranking living levels group, which allowed for comparisons of black elites with their white counterparts. General levels of satisfaction among black and white high-income earners were identical and equally high (Møller & Dickow, 2002, p. 289).

At both city and national level, other survey evidence demonstrates that householders report higher levels of satisfaction with living conditions in line with increased access to services. Even black rural households below the poverty line register increased satisfaction if they have gained access to services such as electricity and a basic old-age pension[7] (Møller, 2000; Devey & Møller, 2002).

Thus, we might conclude that South Africa is slowly working towards the day when its country statistics will be a truer reflection of the quality of life of all of its citizens. South Africans have come a long way since their first democratically elected president, Nelson Mandela, began his long walk to freedom on his release from prison in February 1990. In terms of the income/satisfaction graph, South Africans still have a long way to go to reach the happiness set-level equal to those of other democracies. It will take time for South Africa's fledgling democracy to match the success of a once divided Switzerland whose happy citizens now "prosper under democracy" according to research by Bruno Frey and Alois Stutzer (2000).

Meanwhile, a sign of some blurring of the deep divides in South African society may be that South Africans have not lost their sense of humor in the transition period. In fact, they are learning to laugh at themselves in harmony. Since the coming of democracy, a new daily cartoon series, Madam and Eve, has captured daily life in a South African home against the background of unfolding national events. Now in its tenth year, the cartoon is so popular that the book on Madam and Eve is a best seller (Francis & Schachterl, 2002). The book has been translated into several European languages, and made into a television series. The ten-year retrospective of the cartoon series shows how far South African divides have softened in social discourse in everyday life. This should make it much easier for South Africans to adhere to a single cultural script to achieve happiness.

NOTES

1   Actually, two questions were posed. The first question was whether QOL research had ever actually improved anyone's life. One might suggest that the development of the millennium goals reported by Abbot Ferris (2002) in our own newsletter, *SINET*, might be regarded as a step in the right direction of defining quality-of-life targets in the global effort to fight poverty.

2   The other half made no country reference in title or abstract. No specific country reference would appear to be appropriate in the case of international, cross-cultural or cross-country studies. I also included the few cross-cultural studies that involved a specific developed and developing country in the 'no label of origin' category.

3   In the last 90 articles I trawled through in *Social Indicators Research*, I went to the additional trouble of checking out the social setting or identity of samples if there was no label of origin in title or abstract. I found a country label in title or abstract might have been appropriate in some 12 of the 90 articles or in only 13 % of cases. Similarly, I felt some 6 of 42 *Journal of Happiness Studies* papers or some 14 % could have made bolder mention of the study context.

Methodology papers and general discussions are obviously exempt from country labeling. Reports on small-scale laboratory studies, health studies or studies of older populations also tended to be devoid of social origin labels, possibly because authors assume that their subjects are representative of humankind. As exemplary, one might cite an article with the title: "Cross-cultural Variations in Predictors of Life Satisfaction: an Historical View of Differences among West European Countries". However, one might argue that origin labels tend to clutter titles and should be avoided to save space. In this respect, exemplary is an article with the punchy, eye-catching title "Does Choice of Poverty Index Matter?", which makes reference to use of US census data in the short abstract.

Among western authors, Canadians and Australians usually dutifully mention the locality of their studies in the paper's abstract with some allowances; say assuming that most quality-of-life researchers will know that the Victorian Panel Study is run by colleagues based in Melbourne, Australia. In contrast, I traced the origins of several unlabelled articles back to Norwegian samples and one to a large Swedish database. However, most of the 13 % of culprits who shy away from labels of origin understandable to the rest of the world appear to be US-based researchers. I assume this is oversight not arrogance. Typically, reference to sample characteristics are buried in the methods section. Databases may be referred to as "national" or the "current population survey" without a country reference. In labeled articles, minority and subpopulations are sometimes referred to in title or abstract by local labels such as "farm families" or "back-to-landers". Whereas a title specifying hyphenated African-Americans or Chinese-Americans would be clearly country-specific, one mentioning "black women" might also refer to half the population on the African continent rather than a minority group in the US.

4   As an exercise, take the major social divides in your own society. Are they deep enough to manifest significant differences in quality-of-life indicators? If they do, then they probably should not be routinely overlooked in our quality-of-life studies. Say if cultural identity explains more variance in subjective well-being than other demographics taken together such as sex, age, education, or possibly even income, it should be recognized and taken into consideration in the quality-of-life equation. As a rule of thumb, if within-nation differences are greater than the cross-national difference in international studies, then perhaps we should take notice.

5   South Africa's Gini co-efficient is close on .60, with 1 indicating the most extreme division of income in society (Cf. Devey & Møller, 2002).

6   South Africa's violent crime rates are among the highest in the world with a murder rate of 47.4 per 100 000 population in 2001/2002 (SAIRR, 2002: p. 4).

7   In an unpublished 2002 study of pensioner households in the rural Eastern Cape province, the state old-age pension was identified as one of the "good things" in life by the small group of householders who perceived an improvement in their financial situation in the past two years (Møller & Ferreira, 2003).

REFERENCES

Afrobarometer (2002): Afrobarometer Briefing Paper No. 1 (www.afrobarometer.org).
Cummins, R. A. (2000): Personal Income and Subjective Well-being: A Review. Journal of Happiness Studies 1, 133-58.

Devey, R. & V. Møller (2002): Closing the Gap between Rich and Poor in South Africa: Trends in Objective and Subjective Indicators of Quality of Life in the October Household Survey. W. Glatzer (ed.): Rich and Poor: Disparities, Perceptions, Concomitants, Dordrecht: Kluwer Academic Publishers, 105-22.

Dickow, H. & V. Møller (2002): South Africa's "Rainbow People", National Pride and Optimism: A Trend Study. Social Indicators Research 59 (2), 175-202.

Diener, E. & R. Biswas-Diener (2002): Will Money Increase Subjective Well-being? A Literature Review and Guide to Needed Research. Social Indicators Research 57, 119-69.

Diener, E. & C. Diener (1995): The Wealth of Nations Revisited. Social Indicators Research 36, 275-86.

Diener, E., E. Sandvik, L. Seidlitz, & M. Diener (1993): The Relationship between Income and Subjective Well-being: Relative or Absolute? Social Indicators Research 28, 195-223.

Diener, E. & S. Oishi (2000): Money and Happiness: Income and Subjective Well-being across Nations. E. Diener & E. M. Suh (eds.): Culture and Subjective Well-being, Cambridge, Mass.: MIT Press, 185-218.

Easterlin, R. A. (1974): Does Economic Growth Improve the Human Lot? P. A. David & M. W. Reder (eds.): Nations and Households in Economic Growth. Essays in Honor of Moses Abramovitz, New York: Academic Press, 89-125.

Easterlin, R. A. (1995): Will Raising the Incomes of All Increase the Happiness of All? Journal of Economic Behavior and Organization 27, 35-47.

Easterlin, R. A. (2002): The Income-Happiness Relationship. W. Glatzer (ed.): Rich and Poor: Disparities, Perceptions, Concomitants, Dordrecht: Kluwer Academic Publishers, 157-75.

Ferris, A. (2002): World Development Indicators 2002: Poverty is the Enemy. Social Indicators Network News (Sinet) 73, 6-7.

Fielding, R. (2003): Response to Editorial – QOLNL 28: The Value of Quality of Life Research – Two. MAPI Research Institute Quality of Life Newsletter 30, 22.

Francis, S. & R. Schachterl (2002): Madam and Eve: Ten Wonderful Years, Johannesburg: Rapid Phase.

Frey, B. S. & A. Stutzer (2000): Happiness Prospers in Democracy. Journal of Happiness Studies 1 (1), 79-102.

Glatzer, W. (ed.) (2002): Rich and Poor: Disparities, Perceptions, Concomitants, Dordrecht: Kluwer Academic Publishers.

Hanf, T. (1999): The Sacred Marker: Religion, Communalism, and Nationalism. Th. Hanf (ed.): Dealing with Difference. Religion, Ethnicity and Politics: Comparing Cases and Concepts, Baden-Baden: Nomos, 385-95.

Huntington, S. P. (1998): The Clash of Civilizations and the Remaking of World Order, New York: Touchstone Books.

Inglehart, R. & H.-D. Klingemann (2000): Genes, Culture, Democracy and Happiness. E. Diener & E. M. Suh (eds.): Culture and Subjective Well-being, Cambridge, Mass.: MIT Press, 165-183.

Johnson, P. (1996): Modern Times: A History of the World from the 1920s to the 1990s, London: Phoenix, Orion Books.

Joyce, D. (2002): The Value of Quality of Life Research – Two. MAPI Research Institute Quality of Life Newsletter 28, 1.

Kernig, C. D. (1999): Violence, Conscience and Elites: Fundamentalism and Feminism as Signs of Cultural Crisis. T. Hanf (ed.): Dealing with Difference. Religion, Ethnicity and Politics: Comparing Cases and Concepts, Baden-Baden: Nomos, 8-53.

Kitayama, S. & H. R. Markus (2000): The Pursuit of Happiness and the Realization of Sympathy: Cultural Patterns of Self, Social Relations, and Well-being. E. Diener & E. M. Suh (eds.): Culture and Subjective Well-being, Cambridge, Mass.: MIT Press, 113-61.

Knox, P. L. (1974): Social Well-being: A Spatial Perspective, London: Oxford University Press.

Michalos, A. C. (1985): Multiple Discrepancies Theory (MTD). Social Indicators Research 16, 347-413.

Michalos, A. C. (1991): Global Report on Student Well-being. Volume 1: Life Satisfaction and Happiness, New York: Springer.

Møller, V. (1993): Quality of Life in Unemployment, Pretoria: Human Sciences Research Council Publishers.

Møller, V. (ed.) (1997): Quality of Life in South Africa, Dordrecht: Kluwer Academic Publishers.

Møller, V. (1998): Quality of Life in South Africa: Post-apartheid Trends. Social Indicators Research 43, 27-68.

Møller, V. (1999a): Happiness and the Ethnic Marker: The South African Case. T. Hanf (ed.): Dealing with Difference. Religion, Ethnicity and Politics: Comparing Cases and Concepts, Baden-Baden: Nomos, 283-303.

Møller, V. (1999b): South African Quality of Life Trends in the Late 1990s: Major Divides in Perceptions. Society in Transition 30 (2), 93-105.

Møller, V. (2000): Monitoring Quality of Life in Durban, South Africa. F. T. Seik, L. L. Yuan & G. W. K. Mie (eds.): Planning for a Better Quality of Life in Cities, Singapore: School of Building and Real Estate, National University of Singapore, 313-29.

Møller, V. (2001): Happiness Trends under Democracy: Where Will the New South African Set-level Come to Rest? Journal of Happiness Studies 2, 33-53.

Møller, V. & H. Dickow (2002): The Role of Quality of Life Surveys in Managing Change in Democratic Transitions: The South African Case. Social Indicators Research 58 (1-3), 267-92.

Møller, V. & M. Ferreira (2003): Just Getting By, Cape Town: Walter and Albertina Sisulu Institute for Ageing in Africa, University of Cape Town.

Møller, V. & L. Schlemmer (1983): Quality of Life in South Africa: Towards an Instrument for the Assessment of Quality of Life and Basic Needs. Social Indicators Research 12, 279-91.

Saris, W. E. & A. Andreenkova (eds.) (2001): Happiness in Russia. Journal of Happiness Studies 2 (2), 95-109.

SAPA (2003): Youth Confident in SA Future. Daily Dispatch, East London, June 12, 1.

Schlemmer, L. (2001): Race Relations and Racism in Everyday Life. South African Institute of Race Relations Fast Facts, Johannesburg, 9, 2-12.

Schyns, P. (2001): Income and Satisfaction in Russia. Journal of Happiness Research 2 (2), 173-204.

Sen, A. K. (1999): Development as Freedom, Oxford: Clarendon Press.

Shisana, O. & L. Simbayi (2002): Nelson Mandela/HSRC Study of HIV/AIDS 2002: South African National HIV Prevalence, Behavioural Risks and Mass Media, Household Survey 2002, Cape Town: Human Sciences Research Council Publishers.

South African Institute of Race Relations (SAIRR) (2002): Crime Watch, Fast Facts No. 10, October.

South African Institute of Race Relations (SAIRR) (2003): Fast Facts No. 7, July.

Triandis, H. C. (2000): Cultural Syndromes and Subjective Well-being. E. Diener & E. M. Suh (eds.): Culture and Subjective Well-being, Cambridge, Mass: MIT Press, 13-36.

United Nations Development Programme (1994): Human Development Report 1994, New York: Oxford University Press.

Veenhoven, R. (2002): Why Social Policy Needs Subjective Indicators. M. R. Hagerty, J. Vogel & V. Møller (eds.): Assessing Quality of Life and Living Conditions to Guide National Policy: The State of the Art, Dordrecht: Kluwer Academic Publishers, 33-45.

Vogel, J. (1997): The Future Direction of Social Indicators Research. Social Indicators Research 42, 103-16.

19. SATISFACTION WITH HEALTH CARE SYSTEMS

A Comparison of EU Countries

Jürgen Kohl and Claus Wendt

University of Heidelberg and University of Bremen, Germany

ABSTRACT

Apart from the market and the family, welfare state institutions undoubtedly have a major impact on the living conditions of individuals and social groups. As a matter of fact, welfare state institutions can be differently organized and geared towards different goals (e.g. supplementing vs. replacing markets, equality vs. security, minimum standards vs. optimal standards), and hence are likely to have different consequences. The focus of this article, however, is not directly on measuring the impact of welfare state programs on living conditions, but rather on the subjective perception of social security as well as on the acceptance of welfare state institutions.

"Quality of life" has been conceptualized by Zapf (1984) as the combination of objective living conditions and subjective well-being, thereby distinguishing various welfare constellations. In a similar vein, we regard subjective social security as an element of the quality of life, and ask for the degree of correspondence between particular institutional arrangements of providing social security and citizens' satisfaction with the performance of these institutions. The area of health care policy is taken as an example, but the general methodology could be applied to other fields of social policy as well.

Based on objective health system indicators from OECD sources and Eurobarometer survey data, patterns of satisfaction with health care systems are explored cross-nationally. Welfare state regime types, level of health expenditure and "real" level of health services are taken into account as potential determinants. The findings basically point to the importance of institutional characteristics, almost regardless of the level of health expenditure. Since the analysis allows to evaluate the "success" of national health care systems to find popular satisfaction and approval, it may yield important clues for social policy reform.

INTRODUCTION[1]

"Quality of life" has been conceptualized by Zapf (1984) as the combination of objective living conditions and subjective well-being. By dichotomizing the two dimensions and cross-tabulating them, four types of welfare constellations can be distinguished (table 1).

Wolfgang Glatzer, Susanne von Below, Matthias Stoffregen (eds.), Challenges for Quality of Life in the Contemporary World, 311-331.
© *2004 Kluwer Academic Publishers. Printed in the Netherlands.*

Table 1: Individual Welfare Positions

Objective Living Conditions	Subjective Well-being	
	Good	Bad
Good	Well-being	Dissonance
Bad	Adaption	Deprivation

Source: Adapted from Zapf (1984, p. 25).

It is the merit of this conceptualization that it draws our attention to the fact that subjective well-being does not simply "reflect" objective living conditions, but that seemingly inconsistent constellations of high satisfaction despite bad living conditions and dissatisfaction despite good living conditions are also possible.

It is then a matter of empirical analysis to explore how often these paradoxical constellations occur and by which intervening factors they can be explained.

Likewise, when exploring "contributions of the welfare state to the quality of life", one may ask either for the contribution of the welfare state to the improvement of objective living conditions, for instance, by means of income redistribution or by granting access to social services, *or* for the contribution of the welfare state to the subjective well-being of the citizens. Mostly, only questions of the first type are asked and investigated. We do believe, however, that questions of the second type should not be neglected. If we take the goal of "social security" seriously, it denotes not only a state of objective social welfare, but comprises subjective feelings of social security as well. Moreover, it can even be argued that attaining the goal of social security crucially and ultimately requires that social security arrangements and provisions are experienced and evaluated by the citizens as contributing to their subjective well-being (Veenhoven, 2001).

Furthermore, the evaluation and appreciation of existing welfare state arrangements is of crucial importance in a policy context. A certain degree of satisfaction with their performance seems to be a prerequisite that citizens put their trust into the institutions. If it cannot be demonstrated that certain institutions are working fairly well, they will probably not be accepted by the citizens and voters in the long run which, in turn, will give rise to demands for change. Likewise, public acceptance and support seem to be a precondition for the political feasibility of reform proposals.

The issue of legitimation of the welfare state is closely related to the issue of trust in welfare state institutions. Trust in institutions can be generated in two ways: by a normative belief in the guiding principles *("Leitideen")* of an institution, or by the experience of successful performance of existing institutions (table 2).

Table 2: Sources of Trust in Institutions

Trust in the Performance of Institutions	Belief in the Guiding Values *("Leitideen")* of an Institution	
	High	Low
High	A	C
Low	B	D

Source: Adapted from Wendt (2003, p. 65).

With regard to the health care system, such basic principles may be found in the idea that the system provides universal and equal access to medical services in the case of need, and that the costs of the system are collectively and equitably shared, taking into account the individual's ability to pay. The actual performance of the system is experienced and continuously evaluated by the citizens. These experiences may conform and reinforce their beliefs in the principles of the system, or they may jeopardize them.

Trust will be highest and the legitimacy of the institution most stable when both conditions are met simultaneously (A); conversely, there will be a lack of trust when neither condition is met (D), with the likely consequence of institutional destabilization. But one source of trust can also be substituted for the other, to some extent at least. Even if there is initially not much trust in the principles of the system, trust can be built up by the continued experience of well functioning institutions, i.e. when they produce benefits for the citizens (C). On the other hand, even when an institution is not functioning well, e.g. when it faces organizational or financial problems, trust in the institution may still be sustained as long as there is a basic belief in its values and virtues (B).

In our analysis, we try to apply the basic idea of different constellations of objective conditions and subjective perceptions to a comparison of welfare state arrangements in EU countries at the aggregate level.[2] We are asking (and trying to answer) questions like these:

- How are "objective" welfare state arrangements related to subjective satisfaction with these arrangements?
- Are high outlays for health care really a good indicator for a high level of benefits and services?
- Do increased welfare efforts and improved benefits and services really result in higher satisfaction?
- Which specific institutional arrangements are likely to lead to a high level of satisfaction on the part of the citizens?

The analysis of such issues can be understood as a sort of "macro-evaluation" of welfare state arrangements, in this case in terms of citizens' satisfaction with these arrangements.[3] Drawing inferences from the findings of micro-level quality-of-life studies, we are prepared to find also in international comparisons examples of consistent and inconsistent combinations.

Table 3: Objective and Subjective Components of Welfare State Arrangements

Objective Welfare State Arrangements	Level of Subjective Satisfaction	
	High	Low
High	A	C
Low	B	D

Source: Own adaptation.

Such findings may provide important clues for social policy reform. As a null hypothesis, we would expect a positive association between objective levels of welfare effort and subjective satisfaction (type A and D in table 3). But if we find, for example, low degrees of satisfaction despite strong efforts and performance (type C), this may raise doubts about the rationality of the underlying arrangements. If, on the other hand, we find high satisfaction scores despite low levels of expenditure (type B), this may be interpreted as a high degree of cost efficiency in producing welfare or social security.

"Welfare state arrangements" can be operationalized in different ways:

a) in *qualitative* terms as "regime types" guided by certain principles and goals, e.g. the distinction between the Bismarckian and the Beveridgean approach in social protection, or the well-known distinction of "three worlds of welfare capitalism" suggested by Esping-Andersen (1990, 1999). Because most welfare states nowadays represent a mix of programs following different organizational principles, we believe it makes sense to break down such general typologies by policy area in order to reach more specific conclusions. In the field of health policy, for example, one can distinguish between a *social insurance* approach and a *national health service* approach; or in the field of pension policy, between a *basic security* approach (with flat-rate benefits) and an *income security* approach (with earnings-related benefits).[4]

b) in *quantitative* terms as resources allotted to a certain social policy area, e.g. share of health expenditures in GDP. As a rule, one would expect improving objective conditions when (absolute and relative) expenditures are rising. But strictly speaking, such expenditures are only monetary inputs which have to be transformed into *real* outputs in order to make a contribution to citizens' welfare. And it was just because of the inadequacy of monetary indicators to measure "welfare" that, 40 years or so ago, social indicators have been developed, designed to measure "welfare" more directly.

c) Thirdly, one may attempt to measure the "quality" of social policy arrangements in terms of performance indicators such as "doctors per 1,000 inhabitants" or "hospital beds per 1,000 inhabitants". In a second step, it has then to be examined whether quantitative differences in the provision of such services are really perceived and reflected in the subjective satisfaction on the part of the citizens.

In this paper, we will confine ourselves to exploring these issues with regard to health policies although the general methodology could be applied to other fields of social policy as well.

As *objective* indicators of welfare effort and performance, we make use of data collected by OECD (OECD Health Data 2002). At present, OECD data are considered to be the best available data base for comparisons of health care systems (Schieber & Poullier, 1990; Saltman, 1997; NOMESCO, 2001). As *subjective* indicators, we use question items from the Eurobarometer survey 44.3, 1996, on "Health Care Issues and Public Security"[5] (cf. also Mossialos, 1997). Our main dependent variable, subjective satisfaction with the health care system, is aptly captured by question Q.123: "In general, would you say you are very satisfied, fairly satisfied, neither satisfied nor dissatisfied, fairly dissatisfied or very dissatisfied with the way the health care runs in (our country)?". With regard to the two sources of trust in institutions (cf. figure 2), this item relates to the instrumental aspect of the actual performance of institutions, while the normative aspect of belief in the guiding values is better captured by a question asking for the public commitment in the field of health care (see below).[6]

SATISFACTION WITH HEALTH CARE IN DIFFERENT WELFARE STATE REGIME TYPES

In comparative welfare state research, Western welfare states are often clustered into "regime types" according to their ideological stance and broad visions of society. In the probably most influential typology developed by Esping-Andersen, it is assumed, moreover, that the political-ideological tendencies are reflected in the existing institutional arrangements so that different regime types can be identified by certain institutional characteristics.

Table 4: Satisfaction with Health Care Systems by Welfare State Regime Type (1995/96)

Social Democratic		Conservative		Liberal		Rudimentary	
Denmark	90.0						
Finland	86.9						
Netherlands	72.8						
		Luxembourg	71.0				
		Belgium	70.7				
Sweden	67.8						
		Germany	66.0				
		France	65.9				
		Austria	63.3				
				Ireland	48.8		
				UK	47.8		
						Spain	35.7
						Portugal	20.8
						Greece	18.4
						Italy	16.3
Average	79.4	Average	67.4	Average	48.3	Average	22.8

Source: Own calculation based on Eurobarometer 44.3, 1996. The level of satisfaction is defined as the percentage of the population that is very or fairly satisfied with the health care system.

Esping-Andersen (1990, 1999) distinguished "three worlds of welfare capitalism", the liberal, the conservative-corporatist and the social democratic regime type. Since his analysis did not include the Southern European countries (except Italy) and since these countries show some distinct features from the "three worlds", a fourth regime type has been suggested by Leibfried (1992) and called the "rudimentary welfare state" (cf. also Ferrera, 1998).

Classifying EU member states by these four regime types[7] and ranking them by the level of subjective satisfaction with the health care system yields a surprisingly clear pattern (cf. table 4): At the top, we find three social-democratic welfare states with levels of satisfaction of more than 70 %, followed by the countries of the con-servative regime type which all show levels of satisfaction of more than 60 %. The United Kingdom and Ireland, the closest approximations to the liberal welfare state type in Western Europe, follow suit with a level of satisfaction of about 50 %, while the rudimentary welfare states of Southern Europe are trailing with levels of satisfaction as low as 20 %. There is an almost perfect fit in the sense that no country of the conservative type exceeds the average level of satisfaction in the social-democratic type, no liberal country exceeds the average level of the conservative type, and no rudimentary welfare state exceeds the average level of the liberal type. While there can be no doubt about the empirical validity of this finding, one should not jump to precipitate conclusions, for the causal mechanism remains unclear: Do the countries of the social-democratic regime type rank so high because they organize health care services in a specific way, or because they give a special emphasis on health care and spend more, or simply because they are among the wealthiest and most affluent countries in Western Europe?

SATISFACTION BY TYPE OF HEALTH CARE SYSTEM

In order to explore these various possibilities, as a next step we classified the EU member countries according to the organizational type of their health care systems. In principle, we can distinguish between a national health service approach and a social insurance approach. In a national health service approach, as exemplified by the British NHS, health care services are provided free of charge to all citizens, and the bulk of health care expenditure is financed out of general revenues.

Table 5: Satisfaction with Health Care System by Type of System (1995/96)

National Health Service		Social Insurance	
Denmark	90.0		
Finland	86.9		
		Netherlands	72.8
		Luxembourg	71.0
		Belgium	70.7
Sweden	67.8		
		Germany	66.0
		France	65.9
		Austria	63.3
Ireland	48.8		
U.K.	47.8		
Spain	35.7		
Portugal	20.8		
Greece	18.4		
Italy	16.3		
Average	48.1	Average	68.3

Source: Own calculation based on Eurobarometer 44.3, 1996. The level of satisfaction is defined as the percentage of the population that is very or fairly satisfied with the health care system.

In contrast, according to the social insurance approach, the provision of health care benefits is restricted to insured people only, typically the employed labor force who pay their contributions as a percentage of their earnings (family members may be included under this approach, by virtue of "derived entitlements"). The bulk of health care expenditure is, hence, financed by earmarked social security contributions.

A major difference between the two types of organization lies in the fact that in the national health service scheme, the state (government) is directly involved in the provision and delivery of health care services, whereas under a social insurance regime, health care is collectively financed, but mostly delivered by private providers.

When classified according to these types of organization, no systematic advantage is apparent for either type with regard to subjective satisfaction (cf. table 5). At the top, we find two countries with a national health service, followed by a number of "social insurance" type countries with also fairly high levels of subjective satisfaction. But it has to be noted that those six countries which rank lowest in terms of subjective satisfaction are also characterized by some sort of national health service. While the "social insurance" type countries form a fairly homogeneous cluster in terms of satisfaction, the countries with national health services fall apart into two sharply different clusters at the top and at the bottom.

This should caution us against making any generalizing statement about the merits and shortcomings of the national health service approach as such. The level of satisfaction which can be achieved under this form of organization seems to depend largely on additional variables.

When comparing the classification of countries in tables 4 and 5, it becomes evident that the organizational form of a national health service is used by social-democratic, liberal and rudimentary welfare states alike (while the social insurance approach is typical of the conservative welfare states). Therefore, it seems likely that, due to their different ideological stance, the role of the state and the level and quality of services a public health system should provide, will be differently defined within each regime type. For example, the social-democratic welfare states may aim at an extended range of services for all citizens, while the liberal welfare states may want to provide only basic services for all citizens and leave supplementary services to private provision. Likewise, in the liberal welfare states, with their attempt to limit social expenditures, the state-controlled health system will tend to be underfunded, while the "redistributive" social-democratic welfare states will put a higher priority to health services which may result in more generous funding. This consideration may help explain why there is practically no correlation between "type of system" and satisfaction, although there is a strong association with "welfare state regime type".

Satisfaction with the health care system then depends on whether the institutionalized priorities of the existing system are in line with the preferences of the citizens, or not. If they are, i.e. if the citizens by and large get what they want – be it a health care system with basic services only or with extended services – satisfaction will result. But if there is a conflict between the demands of the citizens and the scope and character of the existing system, dissatisfaction will probably emerge.

In order to examine this hypothesis, we used the following question item: "The government should only provide everyone with essential services such as care for serious diseases and encourage people to provide for themselves in other respects (agree strongly, agree slightly, neither agree nor disagree, disagree slightly, disagree strongly)" and recoded disagreement with this statement as support for an extended role of the state with regard to health care. We then correlated these scores with the share of public financing of (total) health expenditures (as an indicator of the state's institutionalized influence in the health sector) (cf. figure 1).

Figure 1: Share of Public Health Expenditure and Support for Public Commitment in the Field of Health Care (1995/96)

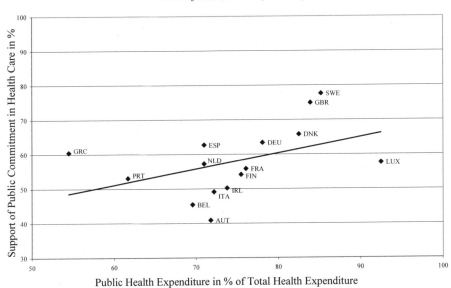

Source: Own calculation based on OECD Health Data 2002 and Eurobarometer 44.3, 1996.
Correlation: r=+0.43.

One can see quite clearly that the general tendency is a correspondence between *public support* for an extended role of the state in providing health care and the *actual degree of state involvement* in the health system. In countries with a high share of public health expenditure, the population also supports a high public commitment in the field of health care. From this perspective, the strong support for state commitment in Sweden, Great Britain, Denmark, and Germany, but also in Spain and Greece, can be interpreted as a high level of trust in the government's ability to guarantee security and equality (Flora, Alber & Kohl, 1977) by providing comprehensive health care services. This is the case despite the fact that in Great Britain, Spain and Greece (and some more countries) people's satisfaction with their *currently existing* health care systems is rather low.[8] On the other hand, especially in Austria, but as well in Belgium or Luxembourg, the government would receive popular support when *reducing* state involvement and increasing private expenditure for health care.

SATISFACTION BY LEVEL OF EXPENDITURE

When it comes to analyzing the impact of health care expenditures on satisfaction with health care systems, one should distinguish between absolute and relative expenditure levels.

Table 6: Indicators of Health Expenditure (1995/96)

	Total Health Expenditure in % of GDP	Total Health Expenditure in US$ per capita	Public in % of Total Health Expenditure	Support for the Increase of Health Care Costs in %
Austria	8.6	1,831	70.5	16.4
Belgium	8.7	1,896	88.8	39.6
Denmark	8.2	1,882	82.4	34.8
Finland	7.5	1,415	75.9	32.3
France	9.6	1,980	76.3	30.9
Germany	10.2	2,184	78.3	25.7
Greece	8.9	1,131	58.7	86.8
Ireland	7.2	1,300	72.5	71.6
Italy	7.4	1,486	67.8	52.0
Luxembourg	6.4	2,122	92.8	34.3
Netherlands	8.4	1,787	67.7	49.6
Portugal	8.3	1,146	66.7	79.2
Spain	7.7	1,184	78.5	53.9
Sweden	8.1	1,622	84.8	57.5
United Kingdom	7.0	1,315	83.7	81.9
EU Average	8.1	1,619	76.4	49.8

Sources: OECD Health Data 2002; Eurobarometer 44.3, 1996. Total health expenditure comprises public *and* private health expenditure.

Relative expenditure levels, measured as a percentage of GDP, are an indicator of the relative priority a society is willing to attach to health care on the current level of economic development and wealth, i.e. *under given resource constraints. Absolute* expenditure levels have to be converted into a common currency, using purchasing power parities (PPP) as exchange rates. They reflect both, the general economic wealth of a country *and* the social-political priority given to health care (table 6).

In terms of *relative* expenditures, we find no correlation between the level of health expenditure and subjective satisfaction with the health care system (cf. figure 2). Very diverse country profiles stand out: Portugal and Greece spend "above average" shares of GDP for health care, but citizens' satisfaction with their health care systems remains at very low levels of about 20 %. Italy and Spain do hardly any better. By contrast, the systems of Denmark and Finland are able to generate very high levels of satisfaction (of about 90 %) with similar shares of GDP. Likewise, the Danish and the Finnish system attain also higher levels of satisfaction than the French and the German system which are much more expensive. The German health system is undoubtedly the most expensive one in terms of relative as well as absolute expenditures; the level of satisfaction it generates is certainly above the EU average, but falls short of what one would expect on the basis of its expenditure level. We hypothesize that such striking differences as between Denmark and

Finland on the one side and France and Germany on the other (which are on a similar level of economic development) can only be explained by taking into account the different organizational forms of providing health care. We will come back to this point at a later stage of our argumentation.

Figure 2: Total Health Expenditure (in % of GDP) and Satisfaction with Health Care Systems (1995/96)

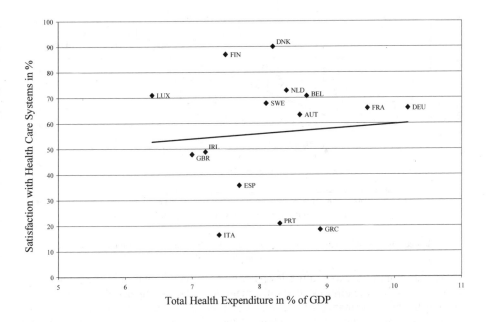

Source: Own calculation based on OECD Health Data 2002 and Eurobarometer 44.3, 1996.
Correlation: r=+0.08.

In contrast to *relative* expenditures, *absolute* health expenditures, measured in US$ per capita, show a correlation of r=+0.68 with subjective satisfaction (cf. figure 3). It seems that in welfare states allocating high absolute amounts of resources to health care, citizens are, on average, more satisfied with the performance of these systems. It also becomes evident that the rudimentary welfare states of Southern Europe, despite the fact that they spend 7-9 % of their GDP on health care, are only able to raise limited absolute amounts of resources, due to their lower level of economic development. These rudimentary welfare states with their low-cost health care systems, consequently, meet with a rather low approval, whereas the above average expenditure levels in the conservative welfare states result in higher levels of satisfaction of about 70 %. The conservative welfare states are all among the "big spenders", but exhibit lower levels of satisfaction than one would expect taking the regression line as a reference line. But especially noteworthy are the scores of about 90 % in Denmark and Finland, although their health expenditure in US$ per capita is lower than the average of the conservative welfare states – in Finland even below the EU average. This can be interpreted as a high degree of cost efficiency in the provision of health care in both countries.

Figure 3: Total Health Expenditure (in US$ per capita) and Satisfaction with Health Care Systems (1995/96)

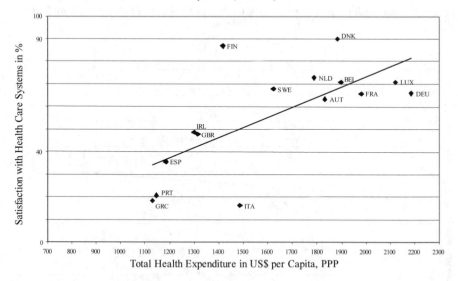

Source: Own calculation based on OECD Health Data 2002 and Eurobarometer 44.3, 1996.
Correlation: r=+0.68.

Thus, with regard to expenditure levels, we can conclude that absolute input of re-sources (health expenditures) certainly matters in improving people's satisfaction, but the better performance of the social-democratic welfare states and the poorer performance of the rudimentary welfare states still hold – even if we control for the absolute level of expenditures.

When focusing on "trust in health care institutions", the assessment of future de-velopments is of paramount importance. A suitable indicator for trust in the future viability of a system seems to be whether people are willing to accept or even sup-port future increases in health expenditures. This is captured by the question: "Do you think that the (national) government should spend more, the same amount as today or less on health care?" Figure 4 shows that support for expenditure increases the lower the higher health care costs (in US$ per capita) already are.

The strong negative correlation has an important political implication: While higher absolute expenditures, by and large, are associated with higher levels of satis-faction (cf. figure 4), a strategy of further increasing expenditures in order to im-prove satisfaction is blocked by strong tax resistance on the part of the citizens, at least in the high-spending countries. In these countries, the only feasible option seems to be to increase efficiency by improved organization of services, without further expenditure increases. When taking into account that, due to demographic ageing, there will be a need for further increases in health expenditure in all EU countries, the low support for such a development in Austria and Germany indicates the potential for future conflicts about this issue in both countries.

Figure 4: Absolute Level of Health Expenditure and Support for the Increase of Health Care Costs (1995/96)

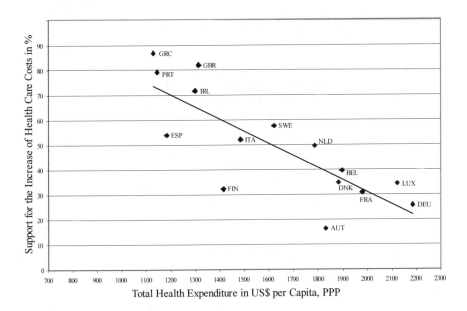

Source: Own calculation based on OECD Health Data 2002 and Eurobarometer 44.3, 1996.
Correlation: r=-0.80.

At the other end of the scale, we find relatively high support (of more than 70 %) for such a strategy in the low-cost health care systems of Greece and Portugal. Here, higher investments in the field of health care are accepted as necessary in order to overcome the perceived deficits of the existing health systems. Not only in these rudimentary systems, but in the early institutionalized national health systems of Great Britain and Ireland as well, there seems to be an awareness among citizens that these health systems are currently underfunded. Higher expenditure, because of demographic changes as well as for health service improvements, would therefore be supported. On the other hand, in Austria, Germany, France, and presumably Luxembourg and Denmark the limits for raising expenditures have already been reached. The consequence of further expenditure increases without improvements of service quality here would probably be a loss of trust followed by institutional destabilization.

SATISFACTION BY LEVEL OF HEALTH SERVICES

While in most countries cost containment of health *expenditure* is the main focus of reforms, the production side of health *services* is often neglected in the health policy debate – probably due to the difficulties of measuring the level and/or quality of health services. Jens Alber (1988), for example, used as indicators for the "quality of health care" the density of medical doctors and hospital beds in OECD countries.

Compared with these input indicators, the "quality of health service index", developed by Olli Kangas (1994), is more complex and takes into account the earnings replacement ratio of sickness benefits, the coverage rates of health care systems, the number of waiting days, and the length of the contribution period required for the access to benefits. For a comparison of the *level* of health care services, however, further or, more precisely, different health care indicators have to be included.

We selected two indicators from the in-patient health care sector (total hospital employment and hospital beds), two indicators from the out-patient health care sector (total out-patient health employment and general practitioners), one indicator from the dental health care sector (dentists) and one indicator from the pharmaceutical health care sector (pharmacists).

Table 7: Indicators of Health Care Services (per 1000 Population) (1995)

	In-Patient Care		Out-Patient Care		Dental Health Care	Pharm. Health Care	Index of Health Care Services
	Total Hospital Employm.	In-Patient Beds	Total Out-Patient Employm.	General Practitioners	Dentists	Pharmacists	% of EU-Average
AUT	15.4	6.6	14.4	1.2	0.5	0.5	117.0
BEL	11.5	4.7	9.6	1.5	0.7	1.4	127.3
DNK	15.9	3.6	7.3	0.6	0.9	0.5	92.5
FIN	13.0	4.0	25.6	1.4	0.9	1.4	158.4
FRA	17.8	4.6	8.6	1.5	0.7	1.0	123.9
DEU	12.1	6.9	16.4	1.1	0.7	0.5	121.2
GRC	8.9	4.0	5.2	0.8	1.0	0.8	94.5
IRL	12.4	3.1	6.0	0.5	0.4	0.7	73.3
ITA	11.2	5.5	7.7	0.9	0.5	1.0	101.1
LUX	11.1	5.7	1.2	0.8	0.5	0.7	81.6
NLD	15.4	3.8	8.4	0.4	0.5	0.2	73.6
PRT	9.1	3.3	2.9	0.6	0.3	0.7	63.8
ESP	9.4	3.0	4.5	0.8	0.4	0.6	69.5
SWE	24.4	3.0	14.6	0.5	1.0	0.7	118.6
GBR	21.1	2.5	7.5	0.6	0.4	0.6	83.7
EU	14.0	4.3	9.3	0.9	0.6	0.8	100.0

Source: Own calculation based on OECD Health Data 2002.

While indicators of health care provision like the ones we used are sometimes considered as objective indicators of health care quality, we would like to insist upon the difference between "real input" and "real output". In our view, the number of doctors and other medical personnel and the number of medical facilities are only the "production factors" which may be combined in various ways to produce services which meet the needs and demands of the citizens (table 7).

We aggregated these indicators into an index of health care services in the following way:

First, the raw values for the various indicators, expressed per 1,000 of population, were standardized and recalculated as percentages of the EU average. Our index of health care services was then calculated as the average value for all six health service indicators (where all indicators were weighted equally, thus approximating the relative importance of the various health care sectors).

For Great Britain, for example, the number of total hospital employment is above EU average, but all the other indicators are below EU average. The total index of health care services is 83.7 and therefore below EU average. Finally, we correlated this index with the level of satisfaction, as explained before (cf. figure 5).

Not surprisingly, the higher the index of health care services, the higher is the level of satisfaction with the health care system. The correlation is r=+0.50. However, it is somewhat surprising that this correlation is lower than the one between absolute expenditure levels and level of satisfaction (r=+0.68) because one would expect that the availability of health care facilities is closer to the average citizen's experience and, therefore, has a more direct impact on his evaluation of the health care system.

Figure 5: Index of Health Care Services and Satisfaction with Health Care Systems (1995/96)

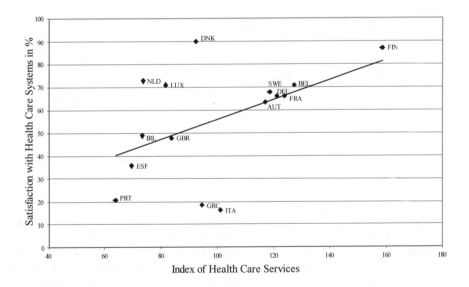

Source: Own calculation based on OECD Health Data 2002 and Eurobarometer 44.3, 1996.
Correlation: r=+0.50.

Finland can be taken as an outstanding example that it is possible to provide a high level of services that contributes to the subjective well-being of the citizens with below-average health expenditure. Most health insurance systems provide above-average health services as well – but at much higher (relative and absolute) costs. The Danish system, on the other hand, provides health care services that are at EU average – but enjoys the highest support of its population. As mentioned before, further organizational information about the respective health care systems is necessary to better understand which specific welfare arrangements result in a high level of subjective well-being. In the case of Denmark, for example, we would argue that the close cooperation between the health care sector and the social service sector relieves the health care system in financial terms and provides flexible services according to the needs and individual preferences of patients (for example home care instead of hospital care). The close cooperation is strengthened by the organizational structure of the Danish health care system, where health services are mainly financed and delivered at the local level with direct access of citizens and patients, respectively, to health care providers as well as to politicians to be held responsible for health care reforms. Transparency of the organizational structure and decision-making process and participation chances are likely to increase the citizens' support of the health care system (cf. Wendt, 2003, p. 277ff.). Likewise, further information on the institutional structure would be necessary to explain the departure from the general trend, for example in Italy or Greece.

DISCUSSION

Finally, we return to the issues raised at the beginning. The production process of health services can be schematically outlined in the following way (figure 6):

Figure 6: The "Production Process" of Health Care Services

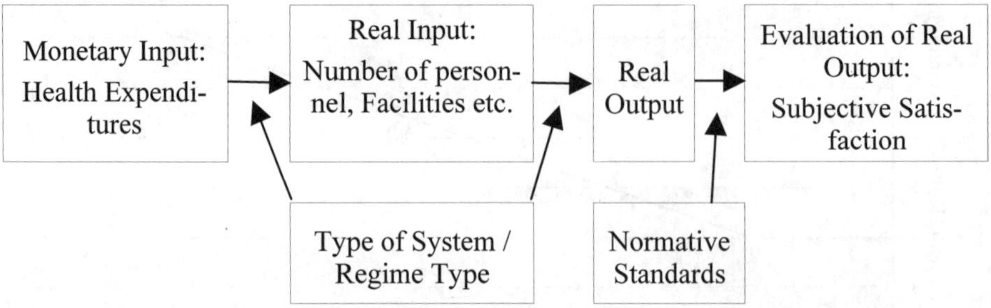

Source: Own Adaptation.

Health expenditures can be considered the *monetary input* into the system. These expenditures are used to establish a specific organizational structure with doctors, hospitals, and other medical personnel and facilities. This constitutes the *real input* to the system. The real inputs of resources are then used to produce and deliver a range of health-related services which constitute the *real outputs* of the system.

Unfortunately, our database did not provide good indicators to measure the quality of services directly (real outputs). Instead, we have focused on the subjective dimension of social security, on citizens' satisfaction with the health care system which can be considered as the *subjective evaluation of real outputs*.

Hence, we assumed that, as a rule, good quality of services should lead to high levels of satisfaction. Low satisfaction despite high expenditures, on the other hand, would then indicate either that the input resources have not been efficiently converted into health services or that the services provided do not match the needs of the citizens.

Although it seems reasonable to assume that, in general, health expenditures, the provision of health care services and subjective satisfaction with the health care system are positively correlated with each other, we also take into account that this correlation is far from perfect and that different constellations of objective and subjective measures of health care may emerge.

This assumption is based on the following reasoning: The transformation of monetary into real inputs as well as the transformation of real inputs into real outputs is *mediated by the prevailing institutional structures*. These comprise the political-institutional structure which provides a framework for political decision-making about the priorities of goals and the adequacy of instruments to achieve these goals, as well as the institutional arrangements of organizing and delivering health services. In the end, political and administrative decision-making processes may lead to a more or less efficient use of resources.

The second intervening variable are the normative expectations of citizens of what constitutes a good or optimal health care system. For the degree of satisfaction which people express derives from a subjective evaluation of the health care system, in which the actual performance of the system is compared with some pre-conceived notion of how it *should* be organized which reflects the value preferences of the citizens. These may or may not be in accordance with the institutionalized priorities of the system.

We have found that there is an almost perfect fit between welfare state regime types and citizens' satisfaction with the performance of health care systems, but that there is no systematic difference with regard to the organizational form of how health care is provided: whether it is organized as a national health service or as a (branch of a) social insurance system.

In further explorations, we found that the level of citizens' satisfaction is practically unrelated to the *relative* level of health expenditure, as measured by the share of GDP spent on health care. But there is a fairly strong correlation with the *absolute* level of health expenditure, as measured in US$ per head of population ($r=+0.68$). This leads us to conclude that the general wealth of a country is a more important factor than the specific efforts a country undertakes when it raises the share of GDP spent on health care, and that the impact of the relative level of expenditures (welfare effort) is crucially mediated by the welfare state regime type.

The economically more advanced countries of the European Union are able to spend more on health in absolute terms, and this leads to better satisfaction with the performance of the health care system. However, there is a counterbalancing factor which sets limits to a strategy of generous spending for health care in order to increase popular satisfaction: people in "big spender" countries are much less willing to agree to further increases in health care costs than people in those countries with a low absolute level of spending ($r=-0.80$). There is also a moderately strong correlation between the index of health care services (which is intended to measure the "real input") and the level of subjective satisfaction ($r=+0.50$).

In addition to the general tendencies expressed in regression lines and correlation coefficients, a closer inspection by countries yields additional insights. Making use of the various constellations of objective health care arrangements and subjective satisfaction with the health system, referred to in the beginning (cf. table 3), we are able to identify countries which conform to the general tendencies described above (as expressed in the regression lines) and those countries which deviate from the general pattern in a positive or negative sense.

For this purpose, we have cross-classified countries in two dimensions according to whether they fall above or below the EU average in the respective dimensions (table 8).

We are arguing that countries in box B realize *superior* welfare constellations because they are able to combine "above average" satisfaction scores with "below average" health expenditures (monetary inputs) or "below average" health care provision indicators (real inputs), respectively. Conversely, countries in box C represent *inferior* welfare constellations because they reach "below average" satisfaction scores despite "above average" monetary or real inputs of resources.

Table 8: Relative Level of Health Expenditures and Subjective Satisfaction with Health Care System (1995/96)

Relative Level of Health Expenditures	Subjective Satisfaction with Health Care System			
	Above Average (>56 %)		Below Average (<56 %)	
Above Average (>8.2 %)	Germany	10.2	66.0	Greece	8.9	18.4
	France	9.6	65.9	Portugal	8.3	20.8
	Belgium	8.7	70.7			
	Austria	8.6	63.3			
	Netherlands	8.4	72.8			
Below Average (<8.2 %)	Denmark	8.2	90.0	Spain	7.7	35.7
	Sweden	8.1	67.8	Italy	7.4	16.3
	Finland	7.5	86.9	Ireland	7.2	48.8
	Luxembourg	6.4	71.0	United Kingdom	7.0	47.8

Source: Own calculation based on Eurobarometer 44.3, 1996, and on OECD Health Data 2002.

In terms of the relative expenditure level, i.e. the welfare efforts countries undertake according to their economic position, Greece and Portugal fall into this "inefficient" pattern, but Spain and Italy hardly do any better. Subjective satisfaction with the health system is lowest in these countries although they spend about the same share of GDP for health care as do the countries in box B: Denmark, Sweden, Finland, and Luxembourg.

With regard to the index of health care services, a similar picture emerges (cf. table 9). 11 out of 15 countries conform to the general tendency. There is only one country in the "inefficiency" box (C), namely Italy which has the lowest satisfaction score although the index for health service provision is very close to the European average. Greece is also very similar with regard to the dissatisfaction of the citizens, but its index score for health service provision is slightly below the EU average so it has to be classified in the "consistency" box (D).

But three countries excel with "above average" satisfaction despite the fact that their index score for health service provision is "below average": Denmark, Luxembourg and the Netherlands. We suppose that these countries are able to organize their health systems in an efficient way so that they produce good quality care with limited real resource input, and that this is reflected in high popular satisfaction.

Two of these countries, Denmark and Luxembourg, have also been in the "efficiency" box (B) in table 8. The remaining two countries in that box in table 8, Sweden and Finland, are good examples that it is possible to provide "above average" health care service structures with relatively limited monetary resource inputs, and that this performance is finally honored by high citizens' satisfaction.

Table 9: Index of Health Care Services and Subjective Satisfaction with Health Care System (1995/96)

Index of Health Care Services	Subjective Satisfaction with Health Care System			
	Above Average (>56 %)		Below Average (<56 %)	
Above Average (>100)	Finland	158	86.9	Italy	101	16.3
	Belgium	127	70.7			
	France	123	65.9			
	Germany	121	66.0			
	Sweden	118	67.8			
	Austria	117	63.3			
Below Average (<100)	Denmark	92	90.0	Greece	94	18.4
	Luxembourg	81	71.0	United Kingdom	83	47.8
	Netherlands	73	72.8	Ireland	73	48.8
				Spain	69	35.7
				Portugal	63	20.8

Source: Own calculation based on Eurobarometer 44.3, 1996, and on OECD Health Data 2002 (cf. table 7).

The logic of the inquiry suggests that when it comes to emulate models for reform, one should have a closer look at those countries which show a superior performance with regard to the goals to be achieved *("best practices")*. When the goal is "high satisfaction of the citizens with their health care systems", our analysis has identified the following countries which should be scrutinized in greater detail: Denmark, Finland, the Netherlands, Sweden, and Luxembourg.

Since four of these five countries fall into the social-democratic welfare state regime type, our first impression from the beginning (cf. table 4) appears to be corroborated: The fact that these countries are at the top with regard to citizens' satisfaction with their health care systems cannot simply be attributed to "disruptive factors" (like level of economic development), but appears to be rooted in institutional characteristics specific to this regime type.

NOTES

1   The authors gratefully acknowledge the critical and helpful comments by Roland Eisen and Andreas Hoff.
2   A similar macro-level analysis of the constellations of objective living conditions and subjective well-being in EU member countries has been undertaken by Noll (1997).
3   For such a macro-evaluation of welfare state regime types with regard to objective performance indicators, cf. Kohl (1999).
4   Note, however, that any such type of scheme may be institutionalized providing more or less generous benefits and resulting in higher or lower aggregate expenditures. Empirical analysis then has to clarify whether subjective satisfaction with welfare arrangements is more affected by the type of schemes and services or by the level of benefits and services.
5   Data for the Eurobarometer data set 44.3 were collected from February to April 1996. The survey includes about 1,000 persons above the age of 14 in each country.
6   Following a different conceptualization developed by Roller (1992), the first item relates to the output dimension (intended consequences), the second one to the goal dimension (extent of public responsibility) of policies.
7   In our classification, we largely follow the clustering of welfare states suggested by Esping-Andersen (1990, Tables 2.2 and 3.3, pp. 52 and 74).
8   This can be taken as evidence that the two sources of trust in institutions depicted in table 2 may not always coincide.

REFERENCES

Alber, J. (1988): Die Gesundheitssysteme der OECD-Länder im Vergleich. M. G. Schmidt (ed.): Staatstätigkeit. International und historisch vergleichende Analysen. PVS, Sonderheft 19/1988, Opladen: Westdeutscher Verlag, 116-50.
Esping-Andersen, G. (1990): The Three Worlds of Welfare Capitalism, Cambridge: Polity Press.
Esping-Andersen, G. (1999): Social Foundations of Postindustrial Economies, Oxford: Oxford University Press.
Eurobarometer (1996): 44.3: Health Care Issues and Public Security. February – April 1996, Cologne: Central Archive for Empirical Social Research.
Ferrera, M. (1998): The Four 'Social Europes': Between Universalism and Selectivity. M. Rhodes & Y. Mény (eds.): The Future of European Welfare: A New Social Contract?, London: Macmillan, 79-96.
Flora, P., J. Alber & J. Kohl (1977): Zur Entwicklung der westeuropäischen Wohlfahrtsstaaten. Politische Vierteljahresschrift 18, 707-72.
Kangas, O. (1994): The Politics of Social Security: On Regressions, Qualitative Comparisons, and Cluster Analysis. T. Janoski & A. M. Hicks (eds.): The Comparative Political Economy of the Welfare State, Cambridge: Cambridge University Press, 346-64.
Kohl, J. (1999): Leistungsprofile wohlfahrtsstaatlicher Regimetypen. P. Flora & H.-H. Noll (eds.): Sozialberichterstattung und Sozialstaatsbeobachtung, Frankfurt/Main: Campus, 111-39.
Leibfried, S. (1992): Towards a European Welfare State? On Integrating Poverty Regimes Into the European Community. Z. Ferge & J. E. Kolberg (eds.): Social Policy in a Changing Europe, Frankfurt/Main: Campus, 245-78.
Mossialos, E. (1997): Citizens' Views on Health Care Systems in the 15 Member States of the European Union. Health Economics 6, 109-16.
Noll, H.-H. (1997): Wohlstand, Lebensqualität und Wohlbefinden in den Ländern der Europäischen Union. S. Hradil & S. Immerfall (eds.): Die westeuropäischen Gesellschaften im Vergleich, Opladen: Leske & Budrich, 431-73.
NOMESCO (2001): Health Statistics in the Nordic Countries, Copenhagen: NOMESCO.
OECD (2002): OECD Health Data 2002. Comparative Analysis of 29 Countries, Paris: OECD.
Roller, E. (1992): Einstellungen der Bürger zum Wohlfahrtsstaat der Bundesrepublik Deutschland, Opladen: Westdeutscher Verlag.
Saltman, R. B. (1997): The Context of Health Reform in the United Kingdom, Sweden, Germany, and the United States. Health Policy 41, 9-26.
Schieber, G. J. & J.-P. Poullier (1990): Overview of International Comparisons of Health Care Expenditure. OECD: Health Care Systems in Transition. The Search for Efficiency. OECD Social Policy Studies No. 7, Paris: OECD, 9-15.

Veenhoven, R. (2001): Why Social Policy Needs Subjective Social Indicators. WZB Working Papers FS III 01 – 404, Berlin: WZB.
Wendt, C. (2003): Krankenversicherung oder Gesundheitsversorgung? Gesundheitssysteme im Vergleich, Wiesbaden: Westdeutscher Verlag.
Zapf, W. (1984): Individuelle Wohlfahrt: Lebensbedingungen und wahrgenommene Lebensqualität. W. Glatzer & W. Zapf (eds.): Lebensqualität in der Bundesrepublik, Frankfurt/Main: Campus, 13-26.

20. THE QUALITY OF DEATH AS A COMPONENT OF QUALITY OF LIFE

María-Angeles Durán

Consejo Superior de Investigaciones Científicas, Madrid, Spain

ABSTRACT

According to the most recent data available from Eurostat, in the EU-15, there are 3.7 million deaths per year. Death is one of the very few experiences that we can be sure that will happen to us. But it is a rare circumstance: It only happens to 9.9 out of one thousand persons every year, and it happens mostly among very aged people, over 80 years old, who have little chances to fight for organizing themselves to improve their conditions. The main causes of death are circulatory diseases, cancer, respiratory diseases, and other causes, including accidents and suicides: but causes vary significantly by age, sex, and life style. Not surprisingly, in 1995 the standard death rates per 100.000 were, in the EU-15, for men, 896.2, while women only reached 529.9, a third less than men.

During the twentieth century, some great technological and social improvements permitted the modification of natural borders of life: birth and death. Concerning birth, the major improvements resulted in new ways of defining "quality of birth" in all developed countries, which nowadays includes four aspects: free decision, low risk for child and mother, absence of pain, comfort, and economic and social coverage for both child and parents. About the second life border, death, fewer changes have taken place. The only really big one is its delay, the general increase of life expectancy. But public opinion is changing, and probably the twenty-first century will see similar changes in attitudes about death, as already happened in the past century towards birth.

This paper analyses the conditions of the "ideal model of death" as it has been studied in several samples of population in Spain by Jesús de Miguel and Marga Mari-Klose, as well as half a dozen surveys done in Spain about the frequency of thoughts about death, worries about it, and attitudes towards intervention in the case of terminal patients who ask to die. The results are analyzed in the context of a society that is getting more and more non-confessional, and that recognizes a rising respect for the personal autonomy of subjects during all their life. The associations of patients and their relatives can play an important role as modifiers of conditions of death; especially the people involved in sicknesses like cancer in which death can be anticipated long in advance, when the patients and their families are still in a socially active age. Quality of death (pre-death, death itself, and post-death periods) is increasingly becoming part of the aspirations and expectancies for a good quality of life.

FROM QUANTITY TO QUALITY OF DEATH

According to the most recent data available from Eurostat, in the EU-15 there are 3.7 million deaths every year. Death is one of the very few experiences that we can be sure that will happen to us. But it is a rare circumstance: It only happens to 9.9 out of one thousand people every year, and it happens mostly among very aged people, over 80 years old, who have little chances to fight for organizing themselves to improve their conditions. The main causes of death are circulatory diseases, cancer, respiratory diseases and other causes, including accidents and suicides: But causes

Wolfgang Glatzer, Susanne von Below, Matthias Stoffregen (eds.), Challenges for Quality of Life in the Contemporary World, 333-345.
© 2004 Kluwer Academic Publishers. Printed in the Netherlands.

vary significantly by age, sex, and life style. Not surprisingly, in 1995 the standard death rates per 100,000 were in the EU-15, for men, 896.2, while women only reached 529.9, a third less than men.

During the twentieth century, some major technological and social improvements permitted the modification of the natural borders of life: birth and death. Concerning birth, the major improvements resulted in new ways of defining *"quality of birth"* in all developed countries, which nowadays include four aspects: free decision, low risk for child and mother, comfort, and absence of pain as well as economic and social coverage for both child and parents.

Concerning the second life border, namely death, fewer changes have taken place. The only really big one is its delay, the general increase of life expectancy. But public opinion is changing, and probably the twenty-first century will see similar changes in attitudes about death, as has already happened in the past century towards birth.

This paper analyzes the conditions of the "ideal model of death" as it has been studied in several samples of population in Spain by Jesús de Miguel and Marga Mari-Klose, as well as half a dozen of surveys conducted in Spain about the frequency of thoughts about death, worries about it, and attitudes towards intervention in the case of terminal patients who ask to die. The results are analyzed in the context of a society that is becoming more and more non-confessional, and that recognizes a rising respect for the personal autonomy of subjects during all their life. The associations of patients and patients' relatives can play an important role as modifiers of conditions of death; especially the people involved in sicknesses like cancer in which death can be anticipated long in advance when the patients and their families are still in a socially active age. *Quality of death* (pre-death, death itself and post-death periods) is increasingly becoming part of the aspirations and expectancies for a *good quality of life*.

THE PRESENCE OF DEATH IN DAILY LIFE

The frequency of thinking about death is an index of the degree of presence of this topic in daily life. Data presented in table 1 were obtained in a national survey conducted in Spain in 2002 on several topics of public opinion, with a sample of 2,500 personal interviews, interviewees being over the age of eighteen..

The first conclusion could be that death is not a frequent motive of thought. Only 14.1 % of the population devotes frequent thoughts to it, and 18.6 % never think about it. However, the addition of the answers "frequently" and "sometimes" covers 55.8 %, the majority of the population.

Age is a variable associated with the frequency of thoughts about death. In the youngest group of the sample (18-24 years old), only 9.2 % think about it frequently, and 23.9 % never do so. In contrast, in the group aged 65 years old and over, the percentage of people who think frequently about death is almost three times higher than among the youth. The synthetic index gives a result of 2.32 points for the general population, but 2.06 for the youth and 2.73 for the elder.

The accumulation of experiences related to death (death of own parents, relatives, and friends) as well as approaching the age that marks the end of life expectancy, and the passage through other vital thresholds as retirement, own sickness, etc., favors the reflection on death. In the group over 65 years old, more than two thirds of the interviewees declare to think about it frequently.

Table 1: Frequency of Thoughts about Death, by Age

		Total	18-24 Years	65 Years and Over
4	Very Frequent	14.1	9.2	24.7
3	Sometimes	41.7	36.2	42.1
2	Almost Never	25.2	30.4	15.9
1	Never	18.6	23.9	16.3
-	No Answer	0.5	0.3	1.9
	Average	2.32	2.06	2.73

Source: Centro de Investigaciones Sociológicas, Spain, 2002. National Survey, 2,500 personal interviews, population aged 18 years and over.

Women live longer than men, and just this difference in age would explain that they think more about death (table 2). However, the difference is too high to be explained by the personal experience of death. It reveals a cultural and structural pattern of relationship to death, personal as well as others, which is different for male and female. Women are more affected by death because they have to face their own death, but also the death of their relatives and closest friends, caring for them during illness, inability, old age and final moments. Besides, the post-death processes of mourning, burying, and symbolic maintenance relies on them. The task of facing other's death is not easy: All of us can remember with closed eyes the pathetic image of the *"Pietá"*, of Maria receiving the dead body of Jesus. Or the Greek myth of Antigone, going to death at her spring age because she has to solve the conflict between loyalty to her brother (burying and honoring him) and loyalty to the political rules of the city. Even from the economic and social perspective, women are more affected by the passing of her family males. Women depend more on the earnings of men (breadwinners), and because they are usually younger than their partners, their probability of experiencing the spouse's death is high.

The definition of pre-death not only comes from medical considerations, but also from faith and the cultural atmosphere. For some philosophies, the pre-death period is as long as life, because for interpreting life, the focal point is its end or the period of over-natural life that starts when natural life comes to its final point.

For other philosophies or vital positions, death is seen from the opposite perspective, just the end of what really matters, that should be mastered to control it and to adapt it to the same values (for instance, freedom, reason, absence of pain, even joy) that should preside over any other period of life.

Other socio-demographic variables such as education level or socioeconomic status do not present such clear associations with the frequency of thoughts about death. Our available data are not good enough to filter the effect of them disaggregated from age. In very raw data, the high and high-middle classes manifest a slightly higher frequency of thought about death (15.3 % and 14.2 %, respectively).

Manual workers get the highest percentage of answers saying they "never" think about death (22.8 % the qualified ones, 19.1 % the non qualified ones).

Table 2: Frequency of Thoughts about Death, by Gender

		Total	Male	Female
4	Very Frequent	14.1	10.4	17.5
3	Sometimes	41.7	38.3	44.9
2	Almost Never	25.2	27.4	23.0
1	Never	18.6	23.4	14.0
-	No Answer	0.5	0.4	0.5
	Average	2.32	2.12	2.51

Source: Centro de Investigaciones Sociológicas, Spain, 2002. National Survey, 2,500 personal interviews, population aged 18 years and over.

Thinking about death does not necessarily mean a preoccupation with or special fear about it. Even among the elder, who think about death much more than youngsters, death is not one of their main worries. Two surveys of Centro de Investigaciones Sociológicas, one on the general population and the other on the population older than 65 years, underline that this topic is not central among the worries of the elder.

In the survey among the general population (2,500 interviews, national scope, to 18 years old and over), people were asked about "the three main worries of old people".

Table 3: The Three Main Worries for the Elder

	Total	Age		Gender	
		18-24 Years	65 Years and Over	Male	Female
Inactivity	16.6	14.9	13.3	19.7	13.8
Loss of Memory	27.6	23.9	38.4	23.8	31.0
Loneliness	76.9	78.8	71.0	75.5	78.3
Dependency	33.9	34.5	27.1	32.4	35.5
The Feeling of Being Useless	32.8	41.0	21.7	33.8	31.9
Pain	13.3	11.7	20.2	12.7	13.9
Physical Deterioration	26.3	26.9	24.6	28.7	24.1
Sickness	38.1	34.2	45.0	37.1	39.0
Death	13.3	17.1	12.0	14.6	12.2

Source: Centro de Investigaciones Sociológicas, 1997, survey number 2244, April 1997, 2,500 personal interviews, general population, up to three answers.

Table 3 shows the image projected by the general population and an extract of two segments of the population, the youngest and the oldest. No matter having three possible answers, death was mentioned by only 13.3 % of the interviewees as one of the main worries of the elder. The youth projected an image of the elder as being more worried about it (17.1 %) than the elder themselves (12.0 %). Instead of death, loneliness received a very high number of mentions in all age groups (76.9 %), a little more among youngsters than among the elder. Sickness is the second motive for worry and is mentioned more frequently by the elder than by the youngsters. The loss of memory is the third cause mentioned by the elder, but it is not so much mentioned by the younger. There are two other causes which are more often underlined by the youngsters: dependency from other persons and the feeling of being useless. Perhaps both segments of the population perceive the intergenerational relationship in a different way; or, perhaps, simply the elder perceive it in the same way but give a different value to it, that is, they assume it as an "acquired right" which they do not bother to claim.

By contrast, the mentioning of pain as a motive for worrying is mentioned twice as often by the elder than by the youngsters.

Gender does not mark a difference in mentioned worries, at least not as much as age. Males mention slightly more inactivity and physical deterioration while women mention slightly more the loss of memory. If we already noted that women said more frequently than men that they thought about death, we should underline now that, however, women interviewed in such general population surveys attribute to the elder slightly less worry about death than is attributed by the male in the same survey.

Table 4: Main Worries of the Elder

	1997		1998
	General Popula- tion	Aged 65 and over	Aged 65 and over
Loss of Memory	27.6	38.4	32.9
Loneliness	76.9	71.0	22.4
Dependency	33.9	27.1	17.1
The Feeling of Being Useless	32.8	21.7	13.0
Pain	13.3	20.2	14.1
Sickness	38.1	45.0	47.1
Inactivity	16.6	13.3	-
Physical Deterioration	26.3	24.6	-
Death	13.3	12.00	-
Loss of Friends	-	-	5.5
Loss of Spouse or Partner	-	-	0.5
Other Causes	-	-	2.5

Source: Centro de Investigaciones Sociológicas (1997/98): Survey Number 2244, Madrid.

Another survey of 1998 enriches the just quoted survey. Results are shown in table 4. In this survey there were also multiple answer choices, although only two answers. The formerly mentioned survey questionnaire was maintained, but the explicit mention of death was suppressed, as well as physical deterioration and inactivity. Instead, it was added the possible answers: "loss of friends", "loss of spouse or partner" and "other causes".

It is remarkable that, in both surveys, there is no mentioning of economic problems or lack of safety, although this last point could be partly included in loneliness. What is good from the comparison between the 1997 and 1998 surveys is the methodological reflection on the extent to which we rely on the way we ask. Within a single year it is unlikely that the attitudes of the general population about such topics vary greatly. As in the second survey only two answers were possible, in case the answers were distributed similarly, all the percentage of mentions should have decreased 33 %. However, after the explicit mention to death as cause of worry disappeared, nobody seems to feel the lack of such response, and "other causes" only get 2.5 % of the total answers.

Not mentioned, forgotten. Or just not explicitly mentioned? In Spain, especially in some regions, the term death is still a taboo, there are many words and circumlocutions to avoid its mention. The same happens in many other cultures, in the developed as well as in the non-developed world, where ancient, almost magic beliefs attribute to words the power of causing what they mean. And words have, consequently, to be handled with extreme care and caution.

In the 1998 survey that we are commenting, the percentage of references to sickness increased, probably because they received some of what could be in the former one of 1997 expressed as physical deterioration. The mention to loneliness strongly decreased, revealing that it is more a "third level cause" than a real "first level cause" of worry. Finally, we cannot avoid underlining that the mention of "loss of friends" is eleven times higher than the "loss of spouse". Why? Perhaps because what has already happened can not be feared, or because the circle of friends and relatives includes such a large number of persons, that the risk of losing some of them within a short term is almost a certainty. In any case, this is a surprising result that invites to reflection about the boundaries of identity and about the role that spouse and friends play in the definition of the self and the quality of life.

THE "HIGH QUALITY" MODEL OF DEATH

At present, and according to Jesús de Miguel, a third of the Spanish population dies in hospitals, very often connected to machines, tubed, isolated and with no possibility of talking to their relatives. Some famous "bad deaths" under extreme medical attention and care, especially Franco's death in 1975, after ruling the country for forty years, impacted public opinion as something to be avoided for oneself. In some, not infrequent cases, life is prolonged under painful and very costly conditions, and covered economic interests (both in favor of maintaining the high medical business and the opposite) make it complicated to take a decision in behalf of the different parts involved in the affair: the patient, the hospitals or health professionals, the relatives, the tax-payers, the ideologists and the insurance companies, whose interests are legitimate but not always coincident.

Jesús de Miguel and Marga Mari-Klose (2000) have done one of the few empirical studies in Spain about the "*canon of death*" or ideal way of dying. They conducted interviews in several samples of the population although they did not use a traditional random survey. The main features of the ideal death, or "high quality death" are the following: a) painless; b) unconscious, sleeping; c) fast, although not by accident; d) accompanied by relatives and close friends; e) at an old age; f) at home. It is not easy to combine in the same case points b), c), and d), although this last one can be interpreted as a rejection of the "social death" that so often precedes the physical death, and that causes abandonment and loneliness.

Table 5: Opinions about Death

	Yes	No	Don't Know	No Answ.
"Do you think that, no matter his/her age, the life of a sick person should be artificially prolonged when there are no possibilities of curing?"	24	64	11	1
"Should the doctors give medicines to alleviate the pain of an incurable sick, even if it shortens the patient's life?"	78	13	8	1
"Does an incurable sick suffering great pains have the right to get from doctors some product that ends his/her life without pain?"	59	28	12	1
"In such cases, should the laws allow doctors to end his/her life and pain, if the patient asks for it?"	66	22	11	1
"In case the patient cannot ask himself and the relatives do it for him, should the law permit it?"	49	33	17	1

Source: Centro de Investigaciones Sociológicas, survey number 1996, 2,492 interviews, March 1992, general population over 18 years old.

THE BOUNDARIES OF WILL: ASPIRATIONS AND IMPOSED LIMITS

The main social debate about death is nowadays about the limits of will, the degree of intervention allowed to ourselves and to the health system in the pre-death, imminent death period. A survey from the Center for Sociological Research (1992), the most recent available including several questions about this topic, obtained the results displayed in tables 5 and 6.

The answers are above 50 % in the sense of favoring quality of death, administering medicines against pain even if it shortens life, and absence of punishment to the doctors who help patients to die when asked to do it.

The few exceptions to the majority come from people with a very low level of education, a high level of religious practice and of extreme right ideology. But even within such segments of the population the answers are not frequent, and they are not more numerous than the answers in favour of applying medical technology at the service of a death more rapid and less painful.

Table 6: Personal Behavior in Some Cases of Terminal Sickness

"In case a member of your family would suffered an incurable and very painful sickness, and would ask you repeatedly to help him/her to die: Which of the following decisions would you be ready to take and which ones not?"	Yes	No	Don't Know	No Answer
A) "I would ask doctors to give him enough analgesics to calm pain, even if it advances the end of his life."	74	13	12	1
B) "I would ask the doctor to intervene and put an end to his/her life."	44	36	18	2
C) "If necessary, I personally would contribute to advance the end of his/her life."	24	54	20	2
D) "I would oppose to any medicine or treatment that could shorten his/her life."	24	54	20	3

Source: Centro de Investigaciones Sociológicas, survey number 1996, 2,492 interviews, March 1992, general population over 18 years old.

Another research institution, the Center for Studies on Social Reality (CIRES), conducted a survey in 1992 on "Social Ethic" and a survey on "Health" in 1994, where some related questions were asked. Results are shown in Table 8. Opinions in favor of euthanasia are in a majority throughout all social segments, both in absolute and relative terms. The contrary is only slightly more frequent, in relative terms, among persons of low social positions and over fifty years old.

Table 7: Opinion about Euthanasia, by Socio-economic Characteristics, November 1992

	Total	"It should be permitted to help to die persons asking for it."	"Only in certain circumstances should it permitted."	"It should never be permitted."	"Don't know."/ No Answer
Total	1,200	33 %	43 %	18 %	5 %
Age					
18-29 Years	311	41 %	47 %	9 %	3 %
30-49 Years	421	35 %	47 %	13 %	5 %
50-64 Years	272	30 %	39 %	26 %	6 %
65 and over	196	20 %	38 %	32 %	10 %
Social Position					
Low	465	30 %	39 %	24 %	8 %
Middle	537	34 %	45 %	17 %	4 %
High	198	38 %	49 %	10 %	3 %
Ideology					
Left	370	39 %	47 %	11 %	3 %
Center	144	27 %	45 %	24 %	4 %
Right	126	28 %	44 %	24 %	5 %
Religiosity					
High	344	21 %	37 %	32 %	9 %
Middle	243	27 %	48 %	19 %	6 %
Low	550	40 %	46 %	11 %	3 %

Source: CIRES, November 1992, Survey on Social Ethic. 1,200 interviews to population over 18 years old.

Table 8: Attitude that the Health Professionals Should Take about Passive and Active Eutha-nasia, by Socio-economic Condition, February 1994

	Total	"Health professionals should respect the will of the patients who do not want to continue living under extreme circumstances."	"The duty of all health professionals is to maintain human life, no matter under what circumstances."	None	Don't Know/ No Answer
Total	1,200	63 %	27 %	2 %	7 %
Sex					
Male	576	64 %	27 %	2 %	7 %
Female	624	63 %	28 %	2 %	7 %
Age					
18-29 Years	311	69 %	23 %	2 %	5 %
30-49 Years	421	69 %	24 %	2 %	5 %
50-64 Years	272	55 %	34 %	2 %	9 %
65 and over	196	55 %	33 %	2 %	10 %
Level of Education					
Low	726	59 %	31 %	2 %	9 %
Middle	340	73 %	22 %	2 %	2 %
High	128	67 %	24 %	4 %	5 %
Social Position					
Low	507	59 %	30 %	2 %	9 %
Middle	525	65 %	28 %	2 %	6 %
High	168	72 %	19 %	4 %	5 %

Source: CIRES, February 1994, Survey on Health, 1,200 interviews to population over 18 years old.

Another opinion poll from 2001, conducted among people 15-29 years old, showed results clearly in favor of the intervention for ending life under certain circumstances. These results are in contrast to the negative opinions about suicide (only 10.4 % in favor, 82.0 % against, 6.2 % don't know, 1.5 % without an answer).

Table 9: Independently of What You Would Do Personally, Are You in Favor or against of Helping to Die to an Incurable Sick that Asks for it?

Against	In Favor	Don't Know	No Answer
17.8	72.2	8.4	1.6

Source: Centro de Investigaciones Sociológicas, 2001. Survey number 2440/0, question number 12. Sample of 2,500 personal interviews to population 15-29 years old.

ANTICIPATED WILLS: APPROACHING PERSPECTIVES FROM DIFFERENT IDEOLOGICAL POSITIONS

The explicit manifestation of wishes about one's deaths is not frequent. The traditional "testament" is a document of last wills, but its content is almost only economic, about the distribution of patrimony. The civil law has regulated this field and it is much more frequent among high classes and the well-off population than among the low-middle or lower classes. However, in Spain 84 % of the families own their apartments or place of lodging and the existence of a will could help to make clear the sharing of the inheritance. According to a survey from the CIS (the only one that asks about this topic), only 18.7 % of the population over 18 years old have prepared their will and a similar percentage expects to do it. But the majority of population (61.0 %) has not thought about doing it. Of those who expect to do it, one third expects to do it when ageing and 5 % when they will feel sick. Of course, many people make economic decisions oriented towards distributing their patrimony among relatives while they are still in good physical and mental condition, thereby avoiding the need for a formal document of will. They do it, mostly "against" the Ministry of Economies, in other words to avoid taxes on income, patrimony and inheritance.

A signal of new coming times is the "vital will", a document in which people state their wishes about the way they want to be treated during the last period of sickness. What reveals the change of times is the explicit solicitude of "not prolonging life" under certain conditions, i.e. strong pain or reasonable lack of expectancies of cure. This new attitude requires a full revolution in the medical system, the abandonment of the agonic insistence of "fight against death" at any price, at any pain, at any time. What brings hope – at least in Spain – to patients suffering from terminal diseases and not finding any sense in the prolongation of their situation is that, for the first time in history, two associations of such different ideological roots as the "*Conference of Bishops*" (Conferencia Episcopal) and the "*Association for the Right of Dying with Dignity*" have agreed on the essentials in their respective documents (a form to be signed) of *vital testament*. The reasons and founding are very different, religious on the one hand and secular on the other, but the essence is the same; the recognition that quality of death is a human right which nobody should steal, and that death should be as human, and as good as life should be for all of us.

REFERENCES

Miguel, J. de & M. Mari-Klose (2000): El Canon de la Muerte. Revista Politica y Sociedad, 35.
Centro de Investigaciones Sociológicas (1992): Survey Number 1996, Madrid.
Centro de Investigaciones Sociológicas (1997): Survey Number 2244, Madrid.
Centro de Investigaciones Sociológicas (2001): Survey Number 2440/0; Madrid.
Centro de Investigaciones Sociológicas (2002): National Survey, Madrid.
CIRES (1992): Survey on Social Ethic, Madrid.
CIRES (1994): Survey on Health, Madrid.

21. LIFE SATISFACTION: CAN WE PRODUCE IT?

Richard A. Easterlin

University of Southern California, Los Angeles CA, USA

ABSTRACT

What do social survey data tell us about the determinants of life satisfaction? First, that the psychologists' setpoint model is questionable. Life events in the nonpecuniary domain, such as marriage, divorce, and serious disability, have a lasting effect on life satisfaction, and do not simply deflect the average person temporarily above or below a setpoint given by genetics and personality. Second, the assumption by economists that in the pecuniary domain "more is better", is problematic. An increase in income, and thus in the goods at one's disposal, does not bring with it a lasting increase in life satisfaction because of the negative effects of adaptation and social comparison on feelings of well-being.

Because individuals fail to anticipate the extent to which adaptation and social comparison undermine expected life satisfaction in the pecuniary domain, they allocate an excessive amount of time to monetary goals, and shortchange nonpecuniary ends such as family life and health, reducing their life satisfaction. Most people could increase their life satisfaction by devoting more time to family life and health, and less, to making money.

INTRODUCTION[1]

Most of us, I think it is safe to say, would like to be happier, and to hold the "keys to happiness." For centuries this subject was the exclusive preserve of philosophers and theologians, who speculated and offered prescriptions on "the good life." Only fairly recently has it come into the domain of social science, first in psychiatry (where the inverse of happiness, depression, was the object of concern), and then, since around 1950, in the mainstream social sciences. The impetus for social science research in the last half century has been the development of population surveys inquiring into people's feelings of well-being. A very simple survey question, for example, might ask a respondent "How satisfied are you with your life as a whole – very, somewhat, so-so, not very, or not at all?" Another question might be, "In general, how happy would you say you are – very happy, pretty happy, or not so happy?" Each of us, I imagine, could readily respond to such queries on our overall feelings of well-being, as do survey respondents generally.

Over the years a substantial methodological literature has developed evaluating the answers to such questions. The professional consensus is that the responses, though not without their problems, are meaningful and reasonably comparable among groups of individuals (Diener, 1984; Frey & Stutzer, 2002a; Frey & Stutzer, 2000b; Veenhoven, 1993). Although there are subtle differences between life satis-

Wolfgang Glatzer, Susanne von Below, Matthias Stoffregen (eds.), Challenges for Quality of Life in the Contemporary World, 347-357.

faction and happiness, I will treat them for the present purpose as interchangeable measures of overall feelings of well-being, that is, of *subjective* well-being. My focus will be on what we are learning from the survey data on the causes of subjective well-being, and, based on this, what we might do to improve it.

As I go along I shall discuss two prominent and contrasting theories of well-being, one in psychology, one in economics. In psychology, "set-point theory" has gained increasing attention in the last decade or so (Costa et al., 1987; Cummins et al., 2003; Lykken & Tellegen, 1996; Myers, 1992; for a recent overview, see Lucas et al., 2002). Each individual is thought to have a fixed setpoint of happiness or life satisfaction determined by genetics and personality. Life events such as marriage or divorce, loss of a job, and serious injury or disease may temporarily deflect a person above or below this setpoint, but in time each individual will adjust to the new circumstances, and return to the given setpoint. Psychologists call this adjustment process "hedonic adaptation." One setpoint theory writer states flatly that life circumstances have a negligible role to play in a theory of happiness (Kammann, 1983, p. 18). If this is correct, then there is little that you or I can do to improve our well-being, and public policies aimed at making people better off by improving their social and economic conditions are largely fruitless (cf. Diener & Lucas, 1999, p. 227).

In contrast, economics places particular stress on the importance of life circumstances to well-being, particularly one's income and employment situation. The view that money makes you happier finds ringing endorsement in economic theory (see, e.g., the discussion of "revealed preferences" in Easterlin & Schaeffer, 1999; Samuelson, 1947; Varian, 1987). The implication is that one can improve one's happiness by getting more money, and that public policy measures aimed at increasing the income of society as a whole will increase well-being.

I shall argue here that the accumulating survey evidence indicates that neither of these theories is correct. Contrary to setpoint theory, life events such as marriage, divorce, and serious disability or disease do have lasting effects on life satisfaction. Contrary to what economics says, more money does not make people happier. Then I will discuss what this implies for what we might do as individuals to produce more life satisfaction for ourselves.

SOURCES OF LIFE SATISFACTION

My discussion is guided by what people themselves say about what makes them happy. In the early 1960s, social psychologist Hadley Cantril carried out an intensive survey in fourteen countries worldwide, rich and poor, capitalist and communist, asking open-ended questions about what people want out of life – what they would need for their lives to be completely happy (Cantril, 1965). I would like to stress the open-ended nature of Cantril's survey. There have been many surveys of people's values and goals, but almost all present the respondent with a list predetermined by the interviewer. Cantril, in contrast, lets each respondent speak for him- or herself.

Despite enormous socio-economic and cultural disparities among the countries, what people said was strikingly similar. In every country, material circumstances, especially level of living, are mentioned most often. Next in importance are family concerns, such as a happy family life. This is followed by concerns about one's personal or family health. After this, and about equal in importance, are matters relating to one's work (an interesting job) and to personal character (emotional stability, personal worth, self-discipline, etc.). Concerns about broad international or domestic issues, such as war, political or civil liberty, and social equality, are rarely mentioned. Abrupt changes in these circumstances do affect people's sense of well-being at the time they occur, but ordinarily they are taken as a given. Instead, it is the things that occupy most people's everyday life, and are somewhat within their control, that are typically in the forefront of personal concerns – especially making a living, marriage and family, and health. The universality of these concerns helps explain why comparisons of life satisfaction among groups of individuals are meaningful. Although the survey questions leave it open for each individual to define life satisfaction or happiness for him or herself, most people are basing their judgments of well-being on essentially the same considerations.

In what follows I shall discuss the evidence on the relation to life satisfaction of the three circumstances most often named by people as their sources of well-being – material living level, family circumstances, and health. I will focus throughout on average relationships. Needless to say, what is true on average is not necessarily true for each individual, but it is important to be clear on what is typical.

Usually, I will be looking at survey data – some, but not all, from my own research – that show how life events affect well-being as people progress through the adult life cycle, from early adulthood through middle age to their retirement years. Most of the generalizations in the social science literature on subjective well-being are based, not on life cycle, but point-of-time studies. As shall be seen below in regard to money and happiness, point-of-time relationships are not always replicated over the life course. Even in those studies that do try to follow the same individuals over time, the period covered is rarely more than a year or two; hardly ever are data representative of the national population as a whole available for as long as five to ten years. The life cycle approach that I use here employs the demographers' technique of birth cohort analysis. Annual surveys are used to track the experience as they become older of a group of individuals born in a particular year or decade, a "birth cohort." Although the same individuals are not interviewed in each successive year, we do have a nationally representative random sample of the same group of individuals. The special advantage of this approach is that we can follow birth cohorts over a substantial segment of the life cycle – in American data on happiness for almost three decades.

HEALTH AND LIFE SATISFACTION

Let me start with health. The critical issue is whether significant changes in health have a lasting effect on life satisfaction. One might suppose, on the one hand, that a serious accident or major disease would permanently reduce one's life satisfaction. On the other, people may bounce back from such occurrences, especially if helped by medications and health devices such as wheelchairs, and by a support network of friends and relatives.

Indeed, the psychologists' setpoint theory sees people as adapting fully, and re-turning to the level of life satisfaction they had before the adverse turn in health. The seminal article, repeatedly cited in the psychological literature as evidence of this is a study of 29 paraplegics and quadriplegics (Brickman, Coates & Janoff-Bulman, 1978). The principal conclusion of this study is that the accident victims, when compared with 22 others comparable in all respects except that they had not experi-enced serious disability, "did not appear nearly as unhappy as might have been ex-pected" (ibid., p. 121).

It is a puzzle to me why this study is seen as supporting the setpoint model. The statement I have just quoted simply asserts that the accident victims were not as unhappy "as might have been expected," and what the latter phrase means is never spelled out. Elsewhere, it is clearly stated that relative to the comparison group, accident victims "rated themselves significantly *less* happy" (ibid., p. 924, emphasis added).

In any event, there have been a number of studies since, some supporting the conclusion of complete adaptation – as the 1978 study is claimed to show – others, contradicting it. To my knowledge the most comprehensive investigation is an American study that examines the life satisfaction of large national samples of dis-abled and nondisabled persons (Mehnert et al., 1990). The conclusion is the same as the actual finding of the 1978 study, namely, that the life satisfaction of disabled persons is, on average, significantly *less* than those who report no disabilities. Of even more importance is the finding that when persons with disabilities are classi-fied in several different ways – according to the severity of the disability, whether the respondent suffers from one or multiple conditions, to what extent the respon-dent is limited in daily activities, and whether close others are thought to perceive the respondent as disabled – life satisfaction is less for those with more serious prob-lems on every single one of these dimensions.

It is extremely unlikely that these systematic differences in life satisfaction arise because those with more serious disabilities simply have not had enough time to adjust to their health problems. Rather, the plausible interpretation is that, on aver-age, an adverse change in health permanently reduces life satisfaction, and the worse the change in health, the greater the reduction in life satisfaction. The results do not mean that no adaptation to disability occurs. But the evidence does suggest that even with adaptation, there is, on average, a lasting negative effect on life satisfaction of an adverse change in health.

Let me turn from point-of-time to life cycle evidence (Easterlin, 2004). As we all know, among adults real health problems increase as people age. But what do people *say* about their health? If people adapted completely to adverse changes in health, as setpoint theory asserts, then there should be no change in self-reported health over the life course, because people would continuously adjust to worsening health. Is it true that self-reported health does not change?

The answer is no, self-reported health declines throughout the life cycle. If one follows Americans born in the decade of the 1950s over the 28-year segment of the life span for which data are available, one finds a clear and statistically significant downtrend in their average self-reported health. This downtrend in self-reported health as people get older is also true of people born in earlier decades as far back as 1911-1920.

This finding, of course, assesses adaptation in terms of self-reported health, not life satisfaction, as in the disability analysis. Perhaps health might get worse, but people do not feel unhappy about it. However, this is not the case – people who report poorer health also say that they are less satisfied with their health, and that they are less happy generally. At a point in time among adults of all ages reported happiness is always less, on average, the poorer the state of self-reported health. The negative impact of poorer health on life satisfaction is due in part to loss of income, but also importantly to nonpecuniary effects such as the unhappiness caused by limits on one's usual activities. It seems clear from comprehensive survey evidence that, contrary to the psychologists' setpoint theory, adverse health changes have a lasting and negative effect on life satisfaction, and that there is less than complete adaptation to deteriorating health.

MARRIAGE AND LIFE SATISFACTION

Let me turn to the effect on life satisfaction of marriage and marital dissolution. One might suppose that establishing close and intimate relationships of the sort represented by marriage would make the partners in such a relationship happier and more satisfied with life in general. Correspondingly, the loss of a partner and consequent dissolution of such relationships, through widowhood, separation, or divorce, would affect life satisfaction negatively. Some of the initial pleasure of a new union might be expected to wear off in time; similarly, persons who have lost a partner might adjust somewhat to single status. But, on average, the close relationships embodied in marriage would be expected to have a lasting positive effect on one's life satisfaction, and the loss of such relationships, a permanently negative effect. – I am using marriage here as a proxy for the formation of unions. These days marriage is often preceded by a period of cohabitation, and the real "union" consequently takes place some time prior to marriage.

The psychologists' setpoint theory would argue, however, that adaptation to marriage and marital dissolution is complete. Indeed, there is a recent study of the German population claiming to support this conclusion (Lucas et al., 2002) Around the time of marriage, life satisfaction reportedly increases briefly during what might be called a "honeymoon period," but after one year of marriage it returns to the level that prevailed more than one year before marriage. Widowhood takes a somewhat longer time for complete adaptation to occur, eight years (separation and divorce are not included in the study.).

American life cycle data, however, contradict the results of the German study, and suggest enduring effects of the formation and dissolution of unions. As young Americans increasingly shift from unmarried to married status from ages 18 through 29, the average happiness of those who are married is consistently higher than the unmarried, and quite constant (Easterlin, 2004).

This result is counter to that which finds for the German population only a "honeymoon period" elevation of life satisfaction. If Americans were simply experiencing a temporary increase in well-being when they married, then the life satisfaction of *married* persons should start out at its highest value at ages 18 to 19 when virtually all of those married are in the honeymoon period. Then, the life satisfaction of married persons should progressively decline after age 19 as the honeymoon happiness of those newly marrying is increasingly offset by the return to their setpoint level of those who were married first.

The American results also contradict another argument, namely that the higher life satisfaction of the married group stems from a "selection effect," that is, that those getting married had greater life satisfaction to start with. If those who marry were happier to start with, then the life satisfaction of the *combined* group of married and unmarried persons would not increase as more and more persons marry. But contrary to the selection effect argument, life satisfaction of the group as a whole, married and unmarried, does increase as the proportion married rises from ages 18 to 29.

Beyond the early adult years the survey evidence continues to suggest lasting effects on life satisfaction associated with marital status. The happiness of married persons remains significantly greater than that of the unmarried throughout the life cycle. Persons who *re*marry are just as happy as those still in their first marriage, and even after 35 years of marriage, the happiness of those still in their first marriage continues to be significantly greater than their unmarried counterparts.

Results consistent with these are reported by American sociologist Linda Waite and her collaborators (2002) in a study that follows 5,000 married Americans over a five year period. At the end of the period, the happiness of those who remained married is virtually unchanged, while the happiness of those who separated, or divorced and did not remarry is significantly below that of those who remained married. The happiness of those who divorced and *re*married is not significantly different from the happiness of those who stayed married. The lesson is clear: On average, marriage brings greater happiness, marital dissolution, less.

Another variant of the selection effect argument is sometimes invoked to explain these results, in this case, that those who divorced were, on average, always less happy – before, during, and after marriage. But this claim is countered by the life satisfaction of widowed persons. At a given age, there is no significant difference between their happiness and that of the divorced. Because of the involuntary nature of widowhood, the widowed are unlikely to be an especially selected group, and the fact that their happiness and that of the divorced is the same suggests that the divorced also are not specially selected.

Evidence of people's desires for a "happy marriage" is also inconsistent with the notion that people adapt completely to their marital circumstances (Easterlin, 2004). I think it is reasonable to say that women over 45 years old have quite low prospects for remarrying if they are widowed, divorced, or separated; hence one might expect them to be fully adjusted to their status as single women, and have largely dismissed marriage from their minds. Yet, when asked about their conception of the good life as far as they *personally* are concerned, six in ten cite a happy marriage. Even more remarkable are the responses of women over age 45 who have never been married. Among these women more than four in ten cite a happy marriage as part of the good life. Perhaps some have adapted, and doubtless some never wanted to marry in the first place, but a sizeable proportion of these women, *who have been single their entire lives*, have not fully adjusted to their unmarried status, and continue to wish they were married.

These are substantial reasons, I believe, for concluding that adaptation with regard to marital status is less than complete, and that the formation of unions has a lasting positive effect on happiness, while dissolution has a permanently negative effect. This does not mean that no adaptation occurs after unions are formed or dissolved, but the adaptation that does occur is less than complete. If the psychologists' setpoint model is correct that life circumstances are of negligible importance to long run happiness, then it is hard to see how one can reconcile it with the bulk of population survey evidence on either marriage or health.

Let me briefly mention, finally, two pieces of survey evidence other than those on health and marriage that are difficult to square with the setpoint model. Throughout the life cycle blacks in the United States are, on average, consistently less happy than whites (Easterlin, 2001). One would be hard put, I believe, to argue that this difference by race is due simply to different setpoints given by genetics and personality, and that differences in the life circumstances of the two races are of negligible importance. Second, beyond age 60 the life cycle excess of female over male happiness is reversed. Clearly, this cannot be explained by genetic and personality factors; rather an important life event – the much higher incidence of widowhood among females than males – is chiefly responsible (Easterlin, 2003a).

MONEY AND LIFE SATISFACTION

I would like to turn now to the source of life satisfaction that is mentioned most often by people – one's material living level, or standard of living. Does more money make people happier? To judge from survey responses, most people certainly think so, although there is a limit. When asked how much more money they would need to be completely happy, most people name a figure greater than their current income by about 20 %. Indeed, when life satisfaction and income are compared in any given year, those with more income are happier, on average, than those with less.

But what happens to happiness over the life cycle as income goes up – does happiness go up too? The answer is no; on average, there is no change. Consider, for example, Americans born in the 1940s. Between the years 1972 and 2000, as their average age increased from about 26 to 54 years, their average income per person – adjusted for the change in the price of goods and services – more than doubled, increasing by 116 %. Yet, their reported happiness in the year 2000 was not different from that 28 years earlier (Easterlin & Schaeffer, 1999; Easterlin, 2001). They had a lot more money and a considerably higher standard of living at the later date, but this did not make them feel any happier.

Consider, further, two subgroups of persons born in the 1940s, those with at least some college education, and those with only a secondary education or less. At any given age, the more-educated are more satisfied with life in general than the less-educated. This is consistent with the point-of-time relation between happiness and income I just mentioned, the more-educated being, on average, more affluent and happier.

But what happens over the life course for the two educational groups? As one might expect, the income of the more educated increases more than that of the less educated. If life satisfaction were moving in accordance with the income of each group, then the life satisfaction of both groups should increase, with that of the more-educated increasing more, and the difference between the two groups widening. In fact, life satisfaction remains constant over the life course for both educational groups, and the happiness differential, unchanged (Easterlin, 2001). Although those fortunate enough to start out with higher income and education remain, on average, happier than those of lower socio-economic status, there is no evidence for either group that happiness increases as income grows.

These results – both point-of-time and life cycle – hold for other birth cohorts as well, for persons born in the 1950s, 1930s, and 1920s (ibid.). Although the point-of-time result seemingly confirms the economists' assumption that more money produces more life satisfaction, the life cycle result contradicts it.

Why this paradoxical pattern? A simple thought experiment brings out the basic reason. Imagine your income increases substantially while everyone else's stays the same – would you feel better off? The answer most people give is yes. But now, let us turn the example around. Think about a situation in which your real income stays the same, but everyone else's increases substantially – how would you feel then? Most people say that they would feel less well off, even though their real level of living has not, in fact, changed at all.

Now what this thought experiment is demonstrating is that so far as material things are concerned one's satisfaction with life depends not simply on one's own *objective* condition, but on a comparison of one's objective situation with a *subjective* (or internalized) living level norm, and this internal norm is significantly affected by the average level of living of people generally. At any given time, the living conditions, or real incomes, of others are fixed, and happiness differences depend, therefore, on differences in people's own, actual, income. This is the point-of-time relationship. Over time, however, as everyone's income increases, so too do the internal norms by which we are making our judgments of life satisfaction. The increase in internal norms is greater for those with higher income, because as we go through the life cycle, we increasingly compare ourselves with those with whom we come in closest contact, and contacts tend increasingly to be confined to those of similar income. The increase over time in one's internal norm undercuts the effect on well-being of the growth of one's own, actual, income, and, as a result, life satisfaction remains unchanged (for evidence of the rise in norms, see Easterlin, 2001).

The subversive effect of rising internal norms also explains why people think that over the life course more money will make them happier, when, in fact, it does not. When people think about the effect of higher income in the future, they conclude they will be happier, because they assume that their own income increases while everyone else's stays the same. What actually happens, of course, is that when their own income increases, so too does that of everyone else. This means the internal norms used to evaluate life satisfaction also increase. In thinking about the effect of future higher incomes on well-being, people fail to factor this prospective increase in their internal norms into their judgments of how well-being will be affected, and hence mistakenly conclude that more money will make them happier.

But it does not – happiness stays the same as income goes up. Here, at last, we seemingly have a validation of the psychologists' model – in the material domain there does appear to be complete hedonic adaptation.

IMPLICATIONS

Let me try to pull together now these several strands of analysis to see what they suggest for producing more life satisfaction. The survey evidence indicates that typically family and health circumstances have lasting effects on life satisfaction, but more money does not.

Each of us has only a fixed amount of time available for family life, health activities, and work. Do we distribute our time in the way that maximizes our satisfaction? The answer, I believe, is no, for a reason that has already been suggested. We decide how to use our time based on a "money illusion," the belief that more money will make us happier, failing to anticipate that in regard to material conditions the internal norm on which our judgments of well-being are based will rise, not only as our own income grows, but that of others does as well. Because of the money illusion, we allocate an excessive amount of time to monetary goals, and shortchange nonpecuniary ends such as family life and health.

As evidence of this money illusion, let me cite another survey in which Americans were asked about the likelihood of their taking a more highly rewarding job that would take away family time, because it would require more work hours and take one away from one's family more often (Glenn, 1996, p. 28). Out of four response options, not one of the 1,200 respondents said it was "very unlikely" he or she would take the job, and only about one in three said it was "somewhat unlikely". The large majority of respondents said it was either "very likely" or "somewhat likely" that they would take the job, each of those categories accounting for about one-third of the respondents. Most Americans, it would seem, would readily sacrifice family life for what they think will be greater rewards from their working life, not knowing that these rewards are likely to be illusory.

Although I have been critical here of two prominent theories of happiness in psychology and economics, I want to make clear that there is much valuable work in both disciplines, without which this article would not have been possible. Some may feel that I have given too little attention to genetic and personality determinants of happiness. This is so, but there is a reason for this. There is nothing one can do, at least at present, about one's genes, and very little that can be done about one's personality (except, perhaps, consult at considerable cost a psychologist). But everyone has the potential for managing his or her life more efficiently to produce greater life satisfaction.

In my discussion of life circumstances, I have focused on the three – money, family, and health – that people cite most often as important for their happiness. There are, of course, other nonpecuniary domains that have enduring effects on life satisfaction. Take friendships, for example. Is it not true that for many of us, there are certain people whom, when we see them, continue to evoke in us, year after year, special feelings of pleasure? And yet, how often do "work" commitments interfere with the enjoyment of such friendships? Each of us, I am sure, could name similar sources of satisfaction that we have sacrificed to the money illusion.

This article started with the question, can we produce more life satisfaction? The tentative answer, based on the survey evidence at hand, seems clear. Most people could increase their life satisfaction by devoting less time to making money, and more to nonpecuniary goals such as family life and health.

NOTE

1   Public lecture, Johann Wolfgang Goethe – University Frankfurt/Main, Germany, July 21, 2003. This is an expanded version of "What Makes People Happy?" Daedalus, 2004, forthcoming.

REFERENCES

Brickman, P., D. Coates & R. Janoff-Bulman (1978): Lottery Winners and Accident Victims: Is Happiness Relative? Journal of Personality and Social Psychology 36 (8), 917-27.

Cantril, H. (1965): The Pattern of Human Concerns. New Brunswick, N.J.: Rutgers University Press.

Costa, P. T. Jr., A. B. Zonderman, R. R. McCrae, J. Cornoni-Huntley, B. Z. Locke & H. E. Barbano (1987): Longitudinal Analyses of Psychological Well-Being in a National Sample: Stability of Mean Levels. Journal of Gerontology 42 (1), 50-5.

Cummins, R. A., R. Eckersley, J. Pallant, J. van Vugt & R. A. Misajon (2003): Developing a National Index of Subjective Well-Being: The Australian Unity Well-Being Index. Social Indicators Research 64 (2), 159-90.

Diener, E. (1984): Subjective Well-Being. Psychological Bulletin 95 (3), 542-75.

Diener, E. & R. E. Lucas (1999): Personality and Subjective Well-Being. D. Kahneman, E. Diener & N. Schwarz (eds.): Well-Being: The Foundations of Hedonic Psychology, New York: Russell Sage Foundation, 213-229.

Easterlin, R. A. (2001a): Income and Happiness: Towards a Unified Theory. The Economic Journal 111 (473), 465-484.

Easterlin, R. A. (2001b): Life Cycle Welfare: Trends and Differences. Journal of Happiness Studies 2, 1-12.

Easterlin, R. A. (2003a): Happiness of Women and Men in Later Life: Nature, Determinants, and Prospects. M. Joseph Sirgy & J. Samli (eds.): Advances in Quality of Life Research: Dordrecht: Kluwer Academic Publishers, pp. 13-26.

Easterlin, R. A. (2004): Explaining Happiness. Proceedings of the National Academy of Sciences, forthcoming.

Easterlin, R. A. & C. M. Schaeffer (1999): Income and Subjective Well-Being over the Life Cycle. C. D. Ryff & V. W. Marshall (eds.): The Self and Society in Aging Processes. New York: Springer, 279-302.

Frey, B. S. & A. Stutzer (2002a): Happiness and Economics: How the Economy and Institutions Affect Well-Being. Princeton: Princeton University Press.

Frey, B. S. & A. Stutzer (2002b): What Can Economists Learn from Happiness Research? Journal of Economic Literature 40 (2), 402-35.

Glenn, N. (1996): Values, Attitudes, and the State of American Marriage. D. Popenoe, J. Bethke Elshtain & D. Blankenhorn (eds.): Promises to Keep: Decline and Renewal of Marriage in America: Rowman and Littlefield, 15-33.

Kammann, R. (1983): Objective Circumstances, Life Satisfactions, and Sense of Well-Being: Circumstances Across Time and Place. New Zealand Journal of Psychology 12, 14-22.

Lucas, R. E., A. E. Clark, Y. Georgellis & E. Diener (2002): Re-Examining Adaptation and the Setpoint Model of Happiness: Reactions to Changes in Marital Status. Journal of Personality and Social Psychology 84, 527-39.

Lykken, D. & A. Tellegen (1996): Happiness Is a Stochastic Phenomenon. Psychological Science 7 (3), 180-9.

Mehnert, T., H. H. Kraus, R. Nadler & M. Boyd (1990): Correlates of Life Satisfaction in those with Disabling Conditions. Rehabilitation Psychology 35 (1), 3-17.

Myers, D. G. (1992): The Pursuit of Happiness. New York: Avon.

Samuelson, P. A. (1947): Foundations of Economic Analysis. Cambridge, MA: Harvard University Press.

Varian, H. R. (1987): Intermediate Economics: A Modern Approach. New York: Norton.

Veenhoven, R. (1993): Happiness in Nations, Subjective Appreciation of Life in 56 Nations 1946-1992, Rotterdam: Erasmus University.

Waite, L. J., D. Browning, W. J. Doherty, M. Gallagher, Y. Luo & S. M. Stanley (2002): Does Divorce Make People Happy? Findings from a Study of Unhappy Marriages. New York: Institute for American Values.

ABOUT THE AUTHORS AND EDITORS

SUSANNE VON BELOW, 38, Assistant Professor of Sociology at the Johann Wolfgang Goethe University Frankfurt am Main. She studied at the Leibniz Kolleg in Tübingen, earned her Diplom in Sociology at the University of Munich, and received her PhD in Sociology at the University of Frankfurt. Her research interests are social stratification, education, regional disparities, institutions, and the integration of migrants. Recent publications include "Bildungssysteme und soziale Ungleichheit" [Educational Systems and Social Inequality] (2002), "Schulische Bildung, berufliche Ausbildung und Erwerbstätigkeit junger Migranten" [Education, Training, and Employment of Young Migrants] (2003), "Can The North American Model Of Ethnicity Be Applied To Europe? The German Example" (with M. Bös, L. W. Roberts), in "The Tocqueville Review/La Revue Tocqueville" (2004), among others.

JEROEN BOELHOUWER, 34, is political scientist. He works at the Social and Cultural Planning Office in the Netherlands. There, he is engaged in research on living conditions and quality of life. He is one of the co-ordinators of a report called "Social State of the Netherlands". In this report, he also writes a chapter about the composite SCP living conditions index. Other publications include "Quality of Life and Living Conditions in the Netherlands", published in "Social Indicators Research" (2002); "The State of the City Amsterdam Monitor: Measuring Quality of Life in Amsterdam" (with P. Schyns), in "Community Quality-of-Life Indicators" (2004).

LAURA CAMFIELD, 30, current institutional affiliation: Wellbeing in Developing Countries (WeD) ESRC Research Group, University of Bath, UK (www.welldev.org.uk). Scientific Education: MA Anthropology of Development (School of Oriental and African Studies, London). PhD in Anthropology entitled "Measuring Quality of Life in Dystonia: An Ethnography of Contested Representations" (2002). Main topics of research: Quality of life approaches, narrative and discourse. Chronic illness, disability and HIV/AIDS. Qualitative and quantitative methodologies (especially creation and use of measures and participatory research).

FERRAN CASAS, 53, Professor in the Psychology Department and the Director of the Research Institute on Quality of Life Studies (IRQV), University of Girona, Spain. PhD in psychology. Main topics of research are quality of life, well-being, childhood, adolescence, social needs, youth, and media. His main publications include: "El bienestar psicológico de los adolescentes" [Adolescents' Psychological Well-being] (with M. Rosich, C. Alsinet), "Anuario de Psicología" (2000); "Subjective Well-Being and Socially Risky Behaviours of Youth" (with G. Coenders, S. Pascual),

359

in Casas/Saurina (eds.): "Proceedings of the Third Conference of the International Society for Quality of Life Studies" (2001).

GERMÀ COENDERS, 36, *Associate Professor in the Economics Department, University of Girona, and researcher of the IRQV. PhD in Business Administration. Main topics of research are survey methodology, structural equation models, multivariate analysis. His main publications include: "Alternative Approaches to Structural Modeling of Ordinal Data. A Monte Carlo Study" (with A. Satorra, W. E. Saris), in "Structural Equation Modeling" (1997); "Testing Nested Additive, Multiplicative and General Multitrait-Multimethod Models" (with W. E. Saris), in "Structural Equation Modeling" (2000); "Estimating Reliability and Validity of Personal Support Measures: Full Information ML Estimation with Planned Incomplete Data" (with T. Kogovšek, A. Ferligoj, W. E. Saris), in "Social Networks" (2002).*

JAAP DRONKERS, 58, *Professor for Social Stratification and Inequality at the European University Institute in San Domenico di Fiesole (FI) in Italy. He studied sociology at the Free University of Amsterdam. He published mostly research articles on the causes and consequences of unequal educational and occupational attainment; several issues in stratification and mobility research; changes in educational opportunities; effect-differences between public and religious schools; education of Dutch elites; relations between school and labor; the effect of parental divorce on their children. Recent example: "Family Policies and Children's School Achievement in Single- Versus Two-Parent Families" (with S.-L. Pong, G. Hampden-Thompson), "Journal of Marriage and Family" (2003).*

MARÍA ANGELES DURÁN *is Professor of sociology and research Professor at the Council for Research of Spanish (Department of Economy, Madrid). She has been president (1998-2001) of the Federación Española de Sociología, and since 2002 is a member of the Executive Committee of the International Sociological Association (ISA). In 2002, she received one of the main scientific prizes in Spain, the National Award for Research in Social Sciences. She has published more than a hundred studies on social structure, sociology of health, work, family, and gender. Her more recent books are: "The contribution of unpaid work to Spanish economy" (2000) and "The invisible cost of sickness" (2003). She has published (2003) an autobiographic book entitled "Diario de Batalla" [Diary of a Battle], which reflects her own experiences with cancer. She is married and has three children.*

RICHARD A. EASTERLIN *is currently University Professor and Professor of Economics, University of Southern California. He is a member of the National Academy of Sciences, past president of the Population Association of America and the Economic History Association, a former Guggenheim Fellow, and a Fellow of the American Academy of Arts and Sciences. He is editor of "Happiness in Economics" (2002) and author of "Growth Triumphant: The 21st Century in Historical Perspective" (1996). His recent articles on happiness and life satisfaction include "Explaining Happiness" (Proceedings of the National Academy of Sciences, 2003),*

"The Income-Happiness Relationship" in Glatzer (ed.):, "Rich and Poor" (2002), and "Will Raising the Incomes of All Increase the Happiness of All?", in "Journal of Economic Behavior and Organization" (1995).

PATRICK A. EDEWOR, 44, Department of Sociology, Olabisi Onabanjo University, Ago-Iwoye, Ogun State, Nigeria. PhD in Sociology. His main topics of research are fertility, the value of children, and reproductive health. His publications include "Social Life and Problems of Liberian Refugees in Nigeria", in "African Population Studies" (1999).

ANDREW EGGERS, 26, is Senior Research Analyst in the Governance Studies Program at the Brookings Institution. He has a BA from Harvard University, where he studied Japanese history, and an MA in economics from Tufts University. His current research includes a study of the link between unemployment and well-being in Russia and a project on the political economy of corporate financial disclosure. He is also completing publications on IMF board governance and the stabilization of US output growth.

CRISTINA FIGUER, 27, Assistant Professor in the Psychology Department and researcher of the Research Institute on Quality of Life Studies (IRQV), University of Girona, Spain. MA in psychology; now doctoral student in the Psychology Department program. Her main topics of research are quality of life, well-being, childhood, adolescence, social needs, youth, and media. Her publications include "Estrategias de búsqueda de información y bienestar psicológico en la adolescencia" (with F. Casas, C. Figuer, C. Alsinet), in "Proceedings of the VIII National Congress on Social Psychology" (2003); "Los valores y su influencia en la satisfacción vital de los adolescentes entre los 12 y los 16 años: Estudio de algunos correlatos" (with F. Casas et al.) (2004).

WOLFGANG GLATZER, 59, Professor of Sociology at the Johann Wolfgang Goethe University at Frankfurt am Main. Doctorate from the University of Mannheim. His main topics of research are on social structural change, quality of life, household production and technology, especially in comparative perspective. Latest books "Sozialer Wandel und gesellschaftliche Dauerbeobachtung" [Social Change and Social Monitoring] (co-ed. 2002); "Rich and Poor: Disparities, Perceptions, Concomitants" (ed., 2002); President of the International Society for Quality of Life Studies (ISQOLS); founding member of the international research group "Comparative Charting of Social Change" (CCSC).

MÒNICA GONZÁLEZ, 29, Researcher of the Research Institute on Quality of Life Studies (IRQV), University of Girona, Spain. MA in psychology. Doctoral student in the Psychology Department program. Her main topics of research are quality of life, well-being, childhood, adolescence, social needs, youth, and media. Her publications include "Indicadores Sociales y Psicosociales de la Calidad de Vida de las

Personas Mayores en un Municipio" [Social and Psychosocial Quality of Life Indicators of Older Persons in a Municipality] (with F. Casas et al.), in "Intervención Psicosocial" (2001); "Life-Satisfaction, Values, and Goal Achievement: The Case of Planned Versus by Chance Searches on the Internet" (with F. Casas, C. Figuer, G. Coenders), in "Social Indicators Research" (2004).

CAROL GRAHAM, 41, is Vice President, Director of the Governance Studies Program, and Senior Fellow in Economic Studies at the Brookings Institution. She has an AB from Princeton University, an MA in international economics from the Johns Hopkins University School of Advanced International Studies, and a DPhil in Political Economy from Oxford University. Her research focuses on poverty, inequality, social welfare policy, and well-being in developing and transition economies. Her publications include "Private Markets for Public Goods: Raising the Stakes in Economic Reform" (1998); and "Happiness and Hardship: Opportunity and Insecurity in New Market Economies" (2001) (with Stefano Pettinato), as well as articlesamong others in "The Journal of Happiness Studies".

MARKUS HADLER, 31, is a social researcher at the department of sociology (University of Graz). His main areas of research are international comparisons, methods of empirical research, and political sociology. He is also a member of the International Social Survey Programme (ISSP) and has published various articles about inequality, mobility, and modernization processes, most of them in a comparative perspective?

MAX HALLER, 57, Professor and Head of the Department of Sociology at the University of Graz (Austria), and (part-time) Professor at the Facoltà di Sociologa, Università degli Studi, Trento (Italy). Doctorate from the University of Vienna, Habilitation at the University of Mannheim. Main areas of research and teaching: international comparative research, social stratification, sociological theory; author and editor of 24 books; recent publications include "The Making of the European Union. Contributions of the Social Sciences" (ed., 2001), and "Soziologische Theorie im systematisch-kritischen Vergleich" [Sociological Theory in Systematic Critical Comparison] (2003, 2nd ed.).

HEINZ HERRMANN, 54, Head of Economic Research Centre, Deutsche Bundesbank. Doctorate from Saarland University; his main topics of research are macroeconomics and monetary economics in particular; editor of several books including "Aging, Financial Markets and Monetary Policy" (2002) and "Foreign Direct Investment in the Real and Financial Sector of Industrial Countries" (2003).

MICHAELA HUDLER-SEITZBERGER, 35, Psychologist at the Paul Lazarsfeld Institute for Social Research, Vienna. Her main topics of research are social indicators, quality of life, labor migration, and data quality in survey research. Her publications in the field of quality-of-life studies include: "Quality of the Current Politi-

cal System and Politics in East Central Europe after Transition", in "Proceedings of the Third Conference of the International Society for Quality of Life Studies" (2001); "Theoretical and Methodological Concepts for Future Research and Documentation on Social Reporting in Cross-sectional Surveys", EuReporting Working Paper 18 (2001) (with R. Richter); "Cross-national Comparison of the Quality of Life in Europe: Inventory of Surveys and Methods" (with R. Richter), in "Social Indicators Research" (2002).

LYDIA ILLGE, 34, MS ,Research associate at the German Institute for Economic Research (DIW Berlin) in the department of Energy, Transportation, Environment since 2001. From 1990 to 1994, she studied Business Management and Environmental Economics at Rostock University, Germany. From 1997 to 1999, she studied Ecological Economics at the Rensselaer Polytechnic Institute in Troy, NY, USA. E-Mail: lillge@diw.de

YOO-SUN KIM, 47, Deputy Director of the Korea Labour & Society Institute. He received his PhD in the economics department, Korea University. Main topics of his research are on the transformation of labor market structure and working conditions of non-regular employees. His recent publications are "The Change of Workers' Conditions After Exchange Crisis" (2002), "Determinants of Firm's Use of Nonstandard Workforce" (2003), "The Size and Working Conditions of Nonstandard Workforce – Analysis of EAPS" (2003).

JÜRGEN KOHL, 57, is Professor of Sociology at Heidelberg University since 1995. He received his PhD at Mannheim University in 1979 and his habilitation at Bielefeld University in 1994. His main teaching and research interests are in the areas of comparative social policy (especially on poverty and on old-age pension systems), political sociology, social structure and social indicators research. His publications include "The European Community – Diverse Images of Poverty", in Øyen/Miller/Samad (eds.): "Poverty: A Global Review. Handbook on International Poverty Research" (1996); "Wohlfahrtsstaatliche Regimetypen im Vergleich" [Welfare Regime Types in Comparison], in Glatzer/Ostner (eds.): "Deutschland im Wandel" (1999); "Einstellungen der Bürger zur sozialen Sicherung: Ein Überblick über die Forschungslage" [Citizens' Attitudes towards Social Security: An Overview over Research Results], in "Deutsche Rentenversicherung" (2002).

MARIA KONTOS is researcher at the Institute for Social Research and lecturer for sociology at the Johann Wolfgang Goethe University at Frankfurt am Main. She studied sociology, social psychology, and ethnology at the Universities of Göttingen and Frankfurt am Main. Her main topics of research are migration, gender, biography, self-employment, and quality of life. She is currently in charge of the coordination of the EU-project "The Chances of the Second Generation in Families of Ethnic Entrepreneurs: Intergenerational and Gender Aspects of Quality of Life Processes". She has published several articles on self-employment policies, ethnic entrepreneurship, women in ethnic business, and on the biographical method. Together with

Ursula Apitzsch, she is editor of the special issue of the "International Review of Sociology" on "Self-employment, Gender and Migration" (2003).

KENNETH C. LAND *is John Franklin Crowell Professor of Sociology at Duke University, where he also is Director of the Center for Demographic Studies and Senior Fellow in the Center for the Study of Aging and Human Development. He is the author of over 100 journal articles and other research publications on these topics. In the field of social indicators and quality-of-life studies, he has developed models for the construction, analysis, and forecasting of social indicators and the quality of life. He has been elected a Fellow of the American Statistical Association, the American Association for the Advancement of Science, the Sociological Research Association, and the International Society for Quality-of-Life Studies. In 1997, he received the Paul F. Lazarsfeld Award for distinguished contributions to the field of sociological methodology from the Methodology Section of the American Sociological Association.*

BYOUNG-HOON LEE, *45, Associate Professor at the Sociology department, Chung-Ang University. He received a PhD from the Industrial and Labor Relations School, Cornell University. His recent research focuses on the impact of globalization and information technology on employment relations and the quality of working life in Korea. His main publications are "A Study on the Conceptualization and Categorization of Non-regular Labor" (2001), "Employment and Industrial Relations in Korea" (2003), and "Globalization and Industrial Relations in Korea" (2003).*

URIEL LEVIATAN, *63, Professor, Department of Sociology and Anthropology, and senior researcher (and former director), The Institute for Social Research of the Kibbutz, University of Haifa, Israel. PhD in Organizational Psychology (1970), University of Michigan. His main research interests are social phenomena of Kibbutz society, organizational commitment, organizational leadership, social gerontology, health as resulting from organization structures and climate. Recent publications include "Contribution of Social Arrangements to the Attainment of Successful Aging – the Experience of the Israeli Kibbutz", in "Journal of Gerontology" (2000); "Leadership, P-E Fit, and Organizational Commitment – a Causal Flow: The Case of Israeli Kibbutzim", in Eckardstein/Ridder (eds.): "Personalmanagement in Non-Profit Organisationen" (2003). Leviatan is a Kibbutz member.*

ANNA LONT, *22, is a doctoral student of pedagogy at the University of Amsterdam. She wrote her contribution to this volume in the context of the course "Research Experience" given by Jaap Dronkers, who was then Professor of empirical sociology at the same university. In 2003, she followed a traineeship in an education service in which diagnostic skills and psychological testing were the main topics. For her thesis about the relationship between young children and their teachers, she tested the validity and reliability of a new Dutch interview for teachers. The subject of this interview are the feelings and emotions teachers have about their relationships with individual pupils.*

LAURENT J. G. VAN DER MAESEN, 63, director at the European Foundation on Social Quality in Amsterdam, holds an MA in political science and in economic science, as well as PhD for "Transformation Health Sector (Public Health)". In cooperation (see Alan Walker), he published two books about the theory of social quality and papers. His recent main topics of research concern the development of the theory of social quality and its application. His publications include "Continuing the Debate on the Philosophy of Modern Public Health: Social Quality as a Point of Reference" (with H. G. J. Nijhuis), in "Journal of Epidemiology and Community Health" (2000); "Social Quality, Social Services and Indicators: a New European Perspective?", Speech for the Conference on Indicators and Quality of Social Services in a European context, at the German Observatory for the Development of Social Services in Europe (2002) (website: www. socialquality.org).

VALERIE MØLLER, 58, born of British/Swiss parents, raised in the southern United States and Switzerland, came to Africa with her architect husband in a Volkswagen minibus in 1972. She has lived and worked in South and Southern Africa ever since, spending only the year of 1976 in Europe while writing her dissertation to earn a PhD in sociology from the University of Zürich. She is currently based in South Africa as Professor and Director of the Institute of Social and Economic Research, whose mission it is to undertake research to enhance the quality of life of people in the region and in South Africa generally. Together with colleagues she developed the first survey instruments in the 1980s to measure perceptions of personal well-being among South Africans – the study is regularly updated. To mark the transition to democracy in 1994, she compiled a reader on "Quality of life in South Africa" (1997).

BENJAMIN NÖLTING, 38, works at the Centre for Technology and Society at the Technical University Berlin. In 2002, he finished his dissertation in political sciences about local environmental groups. From 1988 to 1995, he studied history, political science, and economics. His research fields are sustainable development, agricultural and environmental policy, regional development, organic farming, and institutions.

THEO ROES, 61, studied sociology at the Radboud University, Nijmegen. He was journalist for several years. In 1975, he joined the Social and Cultural Planning Office of the Netherlands. He did research on a variety of subjects of social policies. Since 1991 he is deputy-director of the SCP and editor of "The social state in the Netherlands", a biannial publication.

MARTINA SCHÄFER, 40, is Professor for sustainability science at the department of Sociology at the Technical University Berlin and the head of the research project

"Reconsidering regional wealth" at the Centre for Technology and Society (ZTG) at the TU Berlin. In 1998, she received her PhD in sociology, in 1994 her PhD in biology at the TU Berlin. Her research topics are sustainability science, organic farming and the food sector, and gender.

MATTHIAS STOFFREGEN, *30, Research Assistant at the Department of Social Sciences at the Johann Wolfgang Goethe University Frankfurt am Main. He studied Political Science, History, and Philosophy in Hannover and received his PhD in Frankfurt. His research interests include political and sociological theory, constitutional law, party systems, welfare systems, and quality-of-life studies. In 2003 he was conference manager of the Fifth Conference of the International Society for Quality-of-Life Studies "Challenges for Quality of Life in Contemporary Societies".*

SANDIP SUKHTANKAR, *26, is Senior Research Assistant in the Governance Studies Program at the Brookings Institution and Research Assistant at the Center for Global Development. He has a BA from Swarthmore College. His research focuses on poverty, health, and well-being in developing countries. His publications include (with C. Graham) "Does Economic Crisis Reduce Support for Markets and Democracy in Latin America?", in the "Journal of Latin American Studies" (2004), and articles in the "Milken Institute Review" and the "Brookings Review".*

RUUT VEENHOVEN, *61, studied sociology. He is also accredited in social psychology and social-sexology. Veenhoven was Professor of humanism at Utrecht University in the Netherlands. Currently he is Professor of social conditions for human happiness at Erasmus University Rotterdam. Veenhoven's research is on subjective quality of life. He is director of the "World Database of Happiness". His major publications are "Conditions of Happiness" (1984), "Happy Life-expectancy" (1997), and "The Four Qualities of Life" (2000). Veenhoven also published on love, marriage, and parenthood. Veenhoven is editor of the "Journal of Happiness Studies".*

ALAN WALKER, *54, is Professor of Social Policy at the University of Sheffield, UK and co-founder and Chair of the European Foundation for Social Quality, Amsterdam. He attended the University of Essex (BA, DLitt in Sociology). His research focuses on social policy and social gerontology, particularly with reference to the European Union. He is Director of the ESRC Growing Older Programme on Extending Quality of Life (http://www.shef.ac.uk/uni/projects/gop/) and the UK National Collaboration on Ageing Research (http://www.shef.ac.uk/ukncar/). He has published more than 20 books, 200 reports and research monographs, and 300 scientific papers. Recent publications include: "Social Quality: A Vision for Europe" (ed. with Beck, van der Maesen, Thomèse) (2001); "Growing Older: Quality of Life in Old Age" (ed. with Hennessy) (2004).*

CLAUS WENDT, 35, earned his PhD at the Department of Sociology at Heidelberg University in 2003 and is now Research Fellow in the Collaborative Research Center 597 "Transformation of the State" at Bremen University. His main topics of research are political sociology, comparison of welfare states, and health system research. He is the author of "Krankenversicherung oder Gesundheitsversorgung? Gesundheitssysteme im Vergleich" [Health Insurance or Health Care? Health Care Systems in Comparison] (2003); "Vertrauen in Gesundheitssysteme" [Trust in Health Care Systems], in "Berliner Journal für Soziologie" (2003); "The Need for Social Austerity versus Structural Reform in European Health Systems", in "International Journal of Health Services" (forthcoming).